TECHNISCHE UNIVERSITÄT MÜNCHEN
Lehrstuhl für Betriebswirtschaftslehre
– Marketing und Konsumforschung
Univ.-Prof. Jutta Roosen, Ph.D.

An investigation of women's and men's perceptions and meanings associated with food risks

Andrea A. Bieberstein

Vollständiger Abdruck der von der Fakultät für Wirtschaftswissenschaften der Technischen Universität München zur Erlangung des akademischen Grades eines Doktors der Wirtschaftswissenschaften (Dr. rer. pol.) genehmigten Dissertation.

Vorsitzende:	Univ.-Prof. Dr. Isabell M. Welpe
Prüferinnen der Dissertation:	1. Univ.-Prof. Jutta Roosen, Ph.D.
	2. Univ.-Prof. Dr. Susanne Ihsen

Die Dissertation wurde am 11.07.2012 bei der Technischen Universität München eingereicht und durch die Fakultät für Wirtschaftswissenschaften am 15.11.2012 angenommen.

An Investigation of Women's and Men's Perceptions and Meanings Associated with Food Risks

Andrea Bieberstein

An Investigation of Women's and Men's Perceptions and Meanings Associated with Food Risks

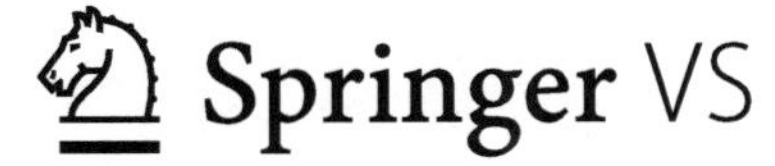

Andrea Bieberstein
München, Germany

Dissertation TUM (Technische Universität München) Munich, Germany, 2012

ISBN 978-3-658-03274-6 ISBN 978-3-658-03275-3 (eBook)
DOI 10.1007/978-3-658-03275-3

The Deutsche Nationalbibliothek lists this publication in the Deutsche Nationalbibliografie; detailed bibliographic data are available in the Internet at http://dnb.d-nb.de.

Library of Congress Control Number: 2013944912

Springer VS

Printed on acid-free paper

Springer VS is a brand of Springer DE.
Springer DE is part of Springer Science+Business Media.
www.springer-vs.de

Acknowledgment

Eine Dissertation ist laut Definition eine eigenständige wissenschaftliche Arbeit. Aber ohne die Unterstützung vieler Menschen wäre sie nicht möglich gewesen. Bei diesen Menschen möchte ich mich an dieser Stelle ganz herzlich bedanken.

Vor allem möchte ich mich bei meiner Doktormutter Prof. Jutta Roosen, Ph.D. bedanken. Ohne Ihre Vorlesungen im zweiten Semester hätte ich mich niemals für die Wirtschaftswissenschaften begeistern können. Danke für die große Offenheit meinen Ideen gegenüber, das Zutrauen in meine Fähigkeiten und Ihre große Unterstützung dabei, beides weiterzuentwickeln. Ich konnte viel von Ihnen lernen!

Weitherhin danke ich Prof. Dr. Susanne Ihsen für die Übernahme des Zweitgutachtens und der Deutschen Forschungsgemeinschaft für die gewährte finanzielle Unterstüzung.

Meinen KollegInnen und WegbegleiterInnen in Kiel und in Freising danke ich für unzählige Türrahmengespräche, Kaffees, Kickerturniere und die unschätzbare Zuarbeit unserer ‚Hiwis'!!

Ganz besonders danke ich meiner Familie in Bayern für ihr Interesse an mir und ihr Zutrauen, dass schon alles ‚passt'.

Ein großer Dank an die Vimy-WG, meiner Wahlfamilie im Norden, den BrüggerholzerInnen, meinen Herzensfreundinnen und meiner Liebsten: Für all das, was wirklich zählt!

Andrea Bieberstein

Table of Contents

List of Tables

List of Figures

List of Abbreviations

AIDS	acquired immunodeficiency sydrome
BSE	bovine spongiform encephalopathy
CES	Consumption Emotion Scale
DNA	deoxyribonucleic acid
e.g. *lat.*	exempli gratia (for example)
EHEC	enterohemorrhagic Escherichia coli
et al.	*lat.* et alii (and others)
HVM	hierarchical value map
i.e. *lat.*	id est (that is)
LTM	long-term memory
STM	short-term memory
MEC	means-end-chain
S&T	science and technology
US	United States
USTM	ultra short-term memory

1 Introduction

1.1 Statement of Problem

How people perceive and judge risks and what kind of risks motivate their behavior in which way, are crucial questions in consumer research (Mitchell, 1999). This is also the case in the food sector. People's perceptions of risks related to food products are important determinants of food choice, attitude towards technologies used in the food and agricultural sector, as well as behavior related to safety practices during the preparation of food (Frewer and Miles, 2001; Knox, 2000).

Risk and risk perception with regard to food is not a new phenomenon. Human beings are and have always been confronted with the choice between exploring new foods and avoiding foods that are unsafe in order to survive. This has become known as the omnivore paradox (Fischler, 1988; Rozin, 1976). Additionally, writings of the ancient Greeks show that concern about food safety is also historically an old phenomenon (Hohl and Gaskell, 2008; Zwart, 2000). However, for a long time, concern about food hygiene and availability of food was predominant (Knox, 2000) and these concerns were encountered with the development of local food customs that increased consumers' familiarity with and confidence in food (Buchler, Smith and Lawrence, 2010). This confidence in food seems to have eroded and concern about the safety of food is widespread (Hohl and Gaskell, 2008). Reasons for this development are diverse: Due to technological change the agricultural sector changes from small-scale labor intensive farming to large-scale industrialized farming. This development created distance between the production and consumption of food, bringing about a decrease in consumer knowledge about production processes and products and lack of control (Campbell and Fitzgerald, 2001; Gupta, Fischer and Frewer, 2011). Linked to that, complex technologies are increasingly applied in food production, confronting consumers with the possible risks from e.g. pesticides, irradiation, genetic modified foods or foods produced by means of nanotechnology. Moreover, several food scares such as bovine spongiform encephalopathy (BSE) in the United Kingdom in the mid-1990s and in several European countries in 2000/2001, the dioxin scandal in Belgian eggs in 1999 or entero-hemorrhagic Escherichia coli (EHEC) infections in Germany in 2011 increased consumer worries about the safety of food and undermined consumer confidence in the food industry and in public authorities responsible for the safety of food (Frewer and Miles, 2001; Knox, 2000). Furthermore, during the 1990s, the media and the academic world put food safety on their agenda (Buchler, Smith and Lawrence, 2010; Hohl and Gaskell, 2008).

Whereas concern about the safety of food seems to be a general phenomenon in many countries (Hohl and Gaskell, 2008), it has been found that people differ in their judgments about food risks. Since the 1960s, research in diverse scientific disciplines such as psychology and sociology has been conducted in trying to understand factors underlying risk perception, mainly concerning technological and environmental risks, and attempts have been made to explain differences of perceptions and judgments between different groups of people.

Scientists studying risk perception are not surprised when they find that women rate many risks higher than men. They can cite dozens of studies with similar findings to support their results. This is also the case in studies investigating food risk perception. However, the findings by Davidson and Freudenburg (1996) caution against accepting the gender[1] gap in risk perception as common sense. In their systematic literature review about gender and the perception of environmental and technological hazards, they found that in the majority of the studies women perceived risks as higher than men, but that the gender gap is very small in some cases. Moreover, their review shows that the gender gap is much more prevalent when the studies focused on risks that directly affect respondents' life or close environments in contrast to general national or global risks. Hence, the results of the systematic literature review by Davidson and Freudenburg (1996) show that a closer and more detailed look at the gender gap in risk perception is necessary in order to avoid generalizations. This concurs with general criticism by gender theorists. They criticize that commonsense knowledge and stereotypes about differences between men and women are also prevalent in the scientific community, which leads to exaggerated reporting of the gender gap (Lorber, 1991). In addition, systematic investigations that seek to understand the reasons and meaning behind the often reported gender gap in risk perception are sparse and based mainly on quantitative evidence (Gustafson, 1998). This is also the

---

1 'Gender' and 'sex' are used synonymously in this thesis. In general both terms refer to biological sex due to the thesis' focus on explaining differences in risk perception between women and men. For a detailed definition and further discussion of two terms see chapter 3.1.

case for food risks, where empirical evidence on the underlying reasons for the often cited gap in the perceptions of women and men is lacking.

1.2 Statement of Objectives

The overall objective of this thesis is to investigate differences or similarities in food risk perceptions between women and men in a systematic way by uncovering the meanings that women and men attach to various food hazards and by analyzing whether food hazards are differently constructed for women and men. But before investigating women's and men's food risk constructs, systematic knowledge of the gender gap is needed in terms of magnitude and direction as well as of variations with regard to different types of food hazards. This allows getting a deeper understanding of the character of gender differences or similarities in terms of their relevance and in terms of the big variety of food hazards. This understanding helps to avoid generalizations and taking gender differences for granted.

Literature analyzing consumer's perception of food hazards has found that a distinction can be made between natural (such as moulds), technological (such as pesticides) and lifestyle food hazards (such as a high fat diet) (Miles et al., 2004; Roosen, Thiele and Hansen, 2005; Siegrist, 2003). Previous research further reported gender differences in attitude towards science and technology and the acceptance of technology (Fox and Firebaugh, 1992), with women being more skeptical. Moreover, women and men are found to differ in their approach to food (Fagerli and Wandel, 1999). Due to this, it was concluded that different types of food risks are likely to be more or less gendered. Hence, the direction and magnitude of the gender gap in food risk perception is likely to differ for varying types of food hazards, such as technology-based versus natural versus lifestyle food risks.

Thus, the first main objective of this thesis is to find out if there exists a consistent gender gap in food risk perception and if a systematic pattern is prevalent with regard to type of food hazard. E.g., does the gender gap exist for all food hazards and/or is it especially small or large for some kinds of food hazards?

Following a psychological contextualist approach as proposed by Jackson, Allum and Gaskell (2006), the second aim of this thesis is to investigate whether women and men attach different meanings to food hazards.

A psychological approach is followed as it regards the perspective of individuals. In order to investigate gender differences in risk perception, it is important to understand first of all how individuals perceive risks. It is supposed that socialization processes and contexts influence people's self-concepts, identities, world views, preferences, values and expectations (Gustafson, 1998; Wharton, 2005). Thus possible gender differences in norms, values etc. are also expressed at the individual level through e.g. differences in risk perception. This thesis therefore focuses on risk perceptions and risk constructs from the perspective of individuals, which is related to approaches in cognitive psychology.

Getting a broad idea of risk constructs of individuals also demands a contextualist approach. Contextualist thinking in risk perception is derived from sociological approaches to risk perception, and especially recent socio-cultural approaches show that risk has different meanings to people depending on their social context (Zinn, 2006b). Regarding food risks as socially and culturally constructed, the aim is to investigate whether they are constructed differently for women and men.

Focusing on the meanings that women and men attach to different types of food hazards, a twofold approach was chosen:

First, women's and men's most salient concepts with regard to the hazards were investigated. Salient concepts are the first associations to be activated when a person is confronted with a stimulus, and from these concepts or images other cognitions in memory are activated (theory of spreading activation). These 'top of mind' cognitions are considered to be especially important in response-oriented studies (Wiedemann and Balderjahn, 1999), such as quantitative risk-perception studies, and might thus strongly influence consumer's risk evaluations. Furthermore, risk perception is found to be strongly influenced by affect (Loewenstein et al., 2001). The vividness or emotional intensity of the first images consumers have in mind when they are verbally confronted with a hazard is likely to influence people's cognitions and finally judgments about the stimulus (Jackson, Allum and Gaskell, 2006). It is therefore investigated whether there are gender differences in the vividness of the most salient associations.

Second, women's and men's motivational factors are the focus of this thesis. According to the means-end-chain (MEC) theory, knowledge is organized hierarchically in memory and the evaluation of an issue/object is based on how the issue/object is perceived to be related to principal life values (Olson and Reynolds, 1983). While a person's basic values are assumed to be relatively stable (Walker and Olson, 1991), different kinds of values and images are likely to be activated for different stimuli. This thesis analyzes whether women and men associate different kind of images to different food hazards and perceive threats to different kinds of values. Furthermore, the dominant cognitive paths in the minds of women and men are filtered. In addition to a meaning related to content in terms of individual images, associations, feelings, consequences and values linked to the food hazards, the structure of women's and men's cognitions is also investigated. More complex cognitive structures point to a higher level of involvement for the object or issue in question (Fotopoulos, Krystallis and Ness, 2003).

Finally, from a methodological point of view, this thesis applies a methodology called means-end-chain (MEC) theory and the related method called laddering to studying individuals' risk perceptions. MEC theory has been developed in the context of marketing and product innovation in order to understand why consumers choose products by uncovering the underlying motives of their consumption decisions. Only a few studies applied this methodology to research questions beyond marketing. Only Bredahl (1999), Wiedemann and Balderjahn (1999), Miles and Frewer (2001) and in a somewhat different way Barrena and Sánchez (2010) adopted it to investigate perceptions of risks. Based on these previous studies and problems encountered, this study adopted the laddering method developed for studying specific products to the study of more abstract issues such as food hazards.

The following research questions summarize the aims of this thesis:

- Do previous studies show a consistent gender gap and if so, how does the gender gap vary for different types of food risks?
- What are the differences and similarities of women's and men's most salient concepts and more underlying associations and values they attach to different food risks?
    - in terms of associations, consequences and values
    - in terms of emotional intensity
    - in terms of the complexity of cognitive structures
- How can the laddering method be adopted to the investigation of more abstract issues such as food hazards?

Overall, the investigation of food risk cognitions may contribute to a better understanding of people's risk perceptions in general. Getting to know people's food risk concepts is important for understanding people's risk evaluations and will contribute to research that is interested in explaining individual differences in risk perception. Moreover, people's risk constructs are interesting for risk communication strategies.

Most important, this thesis provides a comprehensive overview of previous work considering gender and risk perception. Based on this, the thesis further offers an approach to better understand women's and men's food risk constructs from a cognitive psychological point of view. According to the idea "that risk is culturally conditioned: what one defines as dangerous depends on where one stands" (Jackson, Allum and Gaskell, 2006: 11), similarities and more important differences in women's and men's risk constructs may further reflect gender relations in our society. What people or groups of people are concerned about and why they are concerned about it can throw light on their role and status in society.

1.3 Organization of the Thesis

In order to meet the objectives described above, this thesis is divided into eight chapters. Following this introduction, chapter 2 gives a comprehensive overview of theoretical approaches to risk perception and empirical work that has been conducted in the field of risk perception research. First of all, definitions and terminologies for risk and risk perception are introduced (2.1). Chapter 2.2 details the cognitive and affective factors and processes that have an impact on how individuals assess risks. The cognitive as well as affective processes are first introduced in the general context of consumer decision making (2.2.1), before the focus is put on their impact on risk perception more specifically (2.2.2). In chapter 2.3 different approaches to studying differences between individuals in risk perception are introduced starting with the psychometric paradigm (2.3.1), followed by the Cultural Theory approach to risk (2.3.2) and more recent approaches that have a more interdisciplinary approach (2.3.3). Chapter 2.4 presents in detail the factors that determine levels of risk perception. Empirical results with regard to the effect of socio-demographic factors such as gender and age, socio-structural factors such as education, socio-psychological factors such as world views and values as well as socio-political factors such as social trust or general scientific attitudes are presented.

Chapter 3 puts emphasis on gender and risk perception. After an introduction on the role gender plays in risk research in terms of how gender is considered and interpreted in chapter 3.1, chapter 3.2 presents results of previous studies on the impact of gender on levels of risk perception. Evidence on differences and similarities between women and men with regard to food risks are described.

Theoretical and empirical attempts to understand the underlying reasons for the often stated gender gap in risk perception are outlined in chapter 3.3.

Chapter 4 presents a systematic literature review of food risk perception studies with regard to the results for gender. Chapter 4.1 outlines its objectives, followed by the methodology (4.2) and results (4.3). Chapter 4.4 discusses the results of the systematic review.

Chapter 5 is devoted to the MEC theory. The MEC theory builds the methodological background of the empirical analysis in chapter 6. Among other theories, the MEC theory models how knowledge is organized in human memory as introduced in chapter 5.1. Chapter 5.1 also introduces network models of knowledge and explains similarities and differences between the two approaches. Before the widely accepted MEC models of Gutman and Reynolds (1979) and Olson and Reynolds (1983) are outlined (5.3), an overview of the historical development of the MEC theory is given (5.2). Chapter 5.3 relates the MEC theory to the theories of the self and involvement and the role that context or situation plays for the activation of self-relevant knowledge structures.

Chapter 6 presents the empirical investigation of women's and men's food risk constructs. After an introduction of the specific goals of the empirical analysis (6.1), chapter 6.2 describes and discusses in detail the design of the study in terms of sample selection (6.2.1), interview techniques (6.2.2 and 6.2.3) and data analysis (6.2.3.2). The results are presented in 6.3. Chapter 6.4 discusses the most important results against the background of general risk research and gender research. It also outlines the strength and limitations of the research and makes recommendations for future research.

Chapter 7 gives a summary of the thesis and its most important findings.

2 Background to Risk Perception

This chapter gives a theoretical and empirical account of risk perception research. Definitions of risk and an introduction to the concept of risk perception are presented in chapter 2.1, followed by an overview of the underlying cognitive and affective processes that affect human perception and decision making (2.2). The subsequent section 2.3 presents the theoretical approaches that have been developed in order to understand differences in risk perception between individuals and groups of individuals, and chapter 2.4 gives a detailed overview of the empirical evidence related to the factors that determine individual differences in the perception of risks.

2.1 The Concept of Risk and Risk Perception

Starting off with a brief introduction to the different conceptualizations of risk (2.1.1), the concept of risk perception and how it has evolved during the last few decades is presented in chapter 2.1.2.

2.1.1 The Concept of Risk

'Risk' is conceptualized in many different ways across research disciplines. However, most risk concepts are based on the distinction between 'reality' and 'possibility'. 'Reality' is related to adverse effects and its consequences and 'possibility' refers to the probability of adverse effects (Kogan and Wallach, 1964; Rayner and Cantor, 1987).

This probabilistic viewpoint dates back to Frank Knight (1921), who proposed a distinction between risk and uncertainty. Knight (1921) conceptualized risk as a measurable probability and uncertainty as a situation with lack of probabilistic information (LeRoy and Singell, 1987). According to Cunningham (1967), consumer decisions are in general decisions under uncertainty as they lack information about exact probabilities. Probabilistic thinking only gained importance when it was introduced in the debates around nuclear reactor safety in the sixties by Farmer (1967) and Starr (1969). Before, risk was mostly described in terms of (a) kind and (b) magnitude of damage following a deterministic approach to risk (Banse and Bechmann, 1998). Approaches solely based on this two-dimensional risk conceptualization are called formal-normative risk concepts that dominated early risk research and were introduced by the seminal work of Chauncey Starr (1969). Starr (1969) widened the approach to include technological risks.

The introduction of 'probability' led to a differentiation between 'risk' and 'hazards'. 'Hazard' is mostly described in terms of the source of an adverse effect and 'risk' refers to the possibility and probability of an adverse effect (Kaplan and Garrick, 1981). Whereas hazard is supposed to have an external cause, risk is internally produced by the acts and omissions of individuals (Ulbig, Hertel and Böl, 2010). In a similar way, the sociologist Niklas Luhmann differentiated between 'danger' and 'risk'. Whereas 'danger' is attributed to an external cause, 'risk' is produced inherently in the system itself (Luhmann, 1993). However, for Luhmann 'risk' is not necessarily related to the behavior of an individual, but the concept of risk entails a distinction between 'decision makers' (those who take risks) and those who are affected by the decisions of others (Japp and Kusche, 2008). Furthermore, the concept of 'probability' entails aspects of insecurity and uncertainty that are strongly linked to risk (Schütz et al., 2003). Taking 'uncertainty' into account, Rosa (2003: 56) defines risk as "a situation or event where something of human value (including humans themselves) is at stake and where the outcome is uncertain."

In addition to probabilistic approaches to risk, other conceptualizations of risk follow a contextualist approach (Thompson and Dean, 1996). The contextualist viewpoint treats probabilities as only one attribute among many others and focuses on the meaning of hazards for individuals and groups. For Mary Douglas (1990) risk, is, in addition to probability, determined by the meaning and value that is given to the outcome and consequences that depend on political, aesthetic and moral viewpoints. Accordingly, risk is associated with several risk characteristics such as familiarity or personal danger. Hence, the probability of occurrence is only one, albeit important, risk attribute among several others (Jackson, Allum and Gaskell, 2006; Thompson and Dean, 1996).

In addition to the probabilistic versus contextualist conceptualization of risk, a further helpful classification is built by Zinn (2008a). He classifies risk definitions and the related theoretical approaches on a continuum from whether risk is regarded as having an objective existence to being socially mediated/ constructed independent of its objective existence. Approaches that presuppose the objective existence of risks regard risk as real dangers. These objective dangers either exist independently of social factors or are subjectively perceived by individuals. Other approaches assume that real dangers are socially transformed into risks for the organization of society or that the subjective experience of a real danger is mediated by social factors. In addition, approaches that follow a constructivist view deny the existence of any objective risk and conceptualize it as a result of social processes.

Beck (1986; 1992) distinguishes three different kinds of risks according to time era: in pre-industrial societies, risks were conceptualized as hazards and regarded as coming from external forces such as gods or demons. In classical industrial society, the notion of hazards changed to the notion of risks that are taken voluntarily such as smoking and that can be calculated. Today, in what Beck (1986; 1992) calls 'risk society', risks are "man-made side effects of modernization". He characterizes these new risks as techno-scientifically produced risks that, compared to earlier risks, cannot be managed with the established scientific control strategies. New risks cannot be limited in time or place, questions of causality and liability are in general unanswerable, and thus compensation and insurance against these new risks is not possible (Banse and Bechmann, 1998; Beck, 1986; 1992; Zinn, 2008b). Thus, today's decisions are to an increasing extent decisions that have a probable but uncertain impact in the future (Banse and Bechmann, 1998). Linked to that, many decisions in our modern times are decisions under uncertainty as already claimed in the definition by Rosa (2003).

2.1.2 The Concept of Risk Perception[2]

Research into risk perception in the 1960s draws on the discussion around the evaluation and acceptance of man-made technical risks that are automatically linked to decision making processes (see above: Luhmann, 1993). Thus, cognitive processes that determine perception and evaluation of risks are central aspects of 'modern' risk research (Banse and Bechmann, 1998). Research into risk

2 Here, perception is used synonymously for assessment and evaluation. It does not refer to selection processes that play a role when human beings process information that they receive from the environment.

perception was inspired by the observation that experts and lay people often differ in their judgment about how risky hazards are. While experts were assumed to base their risk assessment on the analysis of probabilities, it has been found that lay people judge risks using manifold attributes. Findings in cognitive psychology by Tversky and Kahneman (1974) were critical for research into risk perception. They showed that people face cognitive limitations in dealing with probabilities and therefore deviate from the assumed rational behavior. They further found that people use a "limited number of heuristic principles which reduce the complex tasks of assessing probabilities and predicting values to simpler judgmental operations" (Tversky and Kahneman, 1974: 35).

Out of the assumed differences in risk assessment between experts and lay people arose the distinction between objective risks and subjective risks, with the idea that experts are the representatives of objectivity and lay people have to be supported for example with information to judge risks more realistically. Objective risk perception is the result of e.g. calculating probability distributions such as the probability of being killed in a plane crash, while subjective risk refers to the experiences and perceptions of individuals and thus the meaning of that risk for the individual person (Oltedal et al., 2004).

Whereas the distinction between subjective and objective risks is still made by researchers following a positivist philosophical belief, researchers following a relativist view deny the existence of any objective risks, arguing that risk is always a subjective and thus relative concept (Mitchell, 1999). For most sociologists, risk perception is a social and cultural construction process that reflects and is determined by values, symbols and ideology (Bøholm, 1998; Sjöberg, 2000b; Sjöberg, Moen and Rundmo, 2004). Independently of this philosophical orientation, research into risk perception is interested in people's subjective judgments and is trying to find out why people differ in their risk assessments (Slovic, 1987).

2.2 Cognitive and Affective Processes in Risk Perception

As the decision-making process itself is not observable, models of consumer behavior generally talk of a so-called Black Box where affect and cognition interact in influencing human behavior. Cognitions and affect also influence people's assessments of risks. Affects and cognitions are produced by the affective and cognitive system where each of them can react independently to stimuli of the environment, but the two systems are strongly interconnected and influence each other most of the time (Bänsch, 2002; Kroeber-Riel, Weinberg and

Gröppel-Klein, 2009). Organization and working of the cognitive and affective system is first introduced in 2.2.1, before the importance of cognitive and affective processes for consumers' perception of risk is outlined in 2.2.2.

2.2.1 Cognitions and Affect Influencing Decision Making

Dual-process theories of thinking distinguish two different modes by which information is processed (Chaiken, 1980; Chaiken and Trope, 1999; Epstein, 1994; Petty and Cacioppo, 1984; Sloman, 1996): a 'deliberative' and an 'experiential' style of reasoning. The 'deliberative', also called 'rule-based' processing (Sloman, 1996), is an analytical, formal and verbal style of thinking (see e.g. Epstein, 1994). It is a relatively controlled form of information processing and refers to the conscious, cognitive processing of information. The 'experiential' style of processing, also known as 'associative' processing (Sloman, 1996), is characterized as intuitive, automatic, natural, and nonverbal. In contrast to the 'deliberative' system of thinking that is based on conscious logic, the 'experiential' system is supposed to operate according to the principle of similarity and context and is thus quicker and more efficient (Sloman, 1996). According to the principle of similarity, the strength of activation from one concept to another depends on the similarity or strength of association between the concepts. Thus, the stronger the association between two concepts, the more activation is supposed to flow between the concepts. This activation is further dependent on situational context factors (Loewenstein et al., 2001). The 'experiential' system further encodes reality in the form of images, narratives and metaphors to which affect is attached. The 'deliberative' system results rather in cognitive processing, whereas the 'experiential' system results in an affective processing of information.

2.2.1.1 Cognitive Processes and Cognitive Structures

Peter and Olson (2010) define cognition as the thoughts and beliefs produced by the cognitive system (cognitive structures) and all mental processes (cognitive processes) performed by the cognitive system including understanding (interpretation of meanings of stimuli), evaluating (judging a stimuli as positive or negative), planning (developing solutions in order to reach a goal or solve problems), deciding (choice of the best solutions among alternatives) and thinking (cognitive activity necessary for the four processes).

According to approaches in cognitive psychology, human behavior is the result of an interaction between cognitive structures and cognitive processes (Grunert and Grunert, 1995; Peter and Olson, 2010). Consumers are exposed to information in their environment that is then processed by their cognitive system – the interacting cognitive structures and processes – and in turn influence consumers' decisions and behavior (Kroeber-Riel, Weinberg and Gröppel-Klein 2009; Peter and Olson, 2010). Cognitive structures or so-called knowledge structures define the already memorized knowledge that is the result of past experiences and past information. They are a representation of consumers' beliefs, values but also feelings (Grunert and Grunert, 1995, Kroeber-Riel, Weinberg and Gröppel-Klein, 2009; Olson and Reynolds, 1983). These knowledge structures are stored in long-term memory (LTM) and are called schemata. Schemata organize knowledge and canalize the perception and processing of information. They are linked with verbal and visual concepts in memory and can be applied to persons (schemata regarding another person or self-schemata), issues and events (Kroeber-Riel, Weinberg and Gröppel-Klein, 2009; Trommsdorff and Teichert, 2011). Cognitive structures strongly influence how people process new information (Olson and Reynolds, 1983). This processing of new information comprises processes through which information is perceived, processed and stored (Kuß and Tomczak, 2007). Cognitive processes change existing cognitive structures as a consequence of new information from the environment. Furthermore, cognitive processes retrieve information from cognitive structures in order to perceive and process new information (Grunert and Grunert, 1995). Thus, consumer decision-making behavior is the result of current, external information and of stored, internal information (memory) (Kuß and Tomczak, 2007).

Figure 1 details the functioning of cognitive processes and the role that cognitive structures play. It is based on the model of human memory by Atkinson and Shiffrin (1968) and describes the interaction between the key components of human's cognitive system and the processes within (Trommsdorff and Teichert, 2011): the ultra-short-term memory (USTM), the short-term memory (STM) and the long-term memory (LTM). The USTM receives external stimuli, e.g. visual and acoustic stimuli, and stores them for a very short time. By means of selection processes, also called perception, only a part of this information is transferred to the STM. This selection is part of the automatic cognitive processes that are unconscious and is influenced by the cognitive structures of the LTM (Kroeber-Riel, Weinberg and Gröppel-Klein, 2009; Trommsdorff and Teichert, 2011). The STM is the most active part of the cognitive system and works as its processor: it temporarily stores and processes current information (Keller, 1993).

The processes of the STM are part of the strategic cognitive processes and are conscious for humans. These processes refer to mental activities necessary for problem-solving tasks such as the interpretation of stimuli or combination of information in new ways in order to make evaluations and take decisions (Grunert and Grunert, 1995; Schneider and Shiffrin, 1977). By means of cognitive and behavioral processes, part of the processed information is transferred to the LTM, which is defined to be a subcomponent of human memory with an unlimited storage capacity (Dacin and Mitchell, 1986). The LTM is an active network that presents the knowledge structures (cognitive structures) (Kroeber-Riel, Weinberg and Gröppel-Klein, 2009) formed due to past experiences and past information.

Figure 1: Model of Consumer Information Processing

UNCONSCIOUS, AUTOMATIC PROCESSES

Ultra-short-term memory

Short-term memory

Long-term memory
Cognitive structures

Stimulation

Perception

Learning

Recall

External stimuli

Reaction

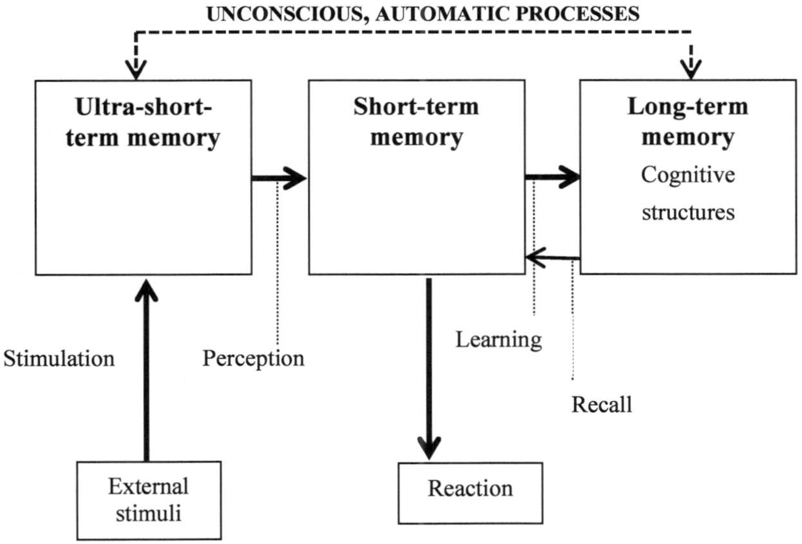

Source: Adapted from Trommsdorff and Teichert (2011)[3].

3 The model of consumer information processing is based on the human memory system by Atkinson and Shiffrin (1968).

Information from the LTM is retrieved (recall) and used to process new information (Marks and Olson, 1981) as it provides rules and heuristics that guide people's information processing in the STM and USTM (Grebitus, 2008; Wilkie and Farris, 1976). Also cognitive processes such as risk perception/evaluation are influenced by knowledge that is stored in the LTM (Slovic, 1987).

According to Kuß and Tomczak (2007), knowledge is defined as the information that is stored in memory and that can be retrieved. Two types of knowledge are usually distinguished: procedural and declarative knowledge (Squire, 1987; Trommsdorff and Teichert, 2011). Procedural knowledge contains scripts and skills, the knowledge how to do things, such as riding a bicycle or skiing (Anderson, 2007). This knowledge is unconscious and cannot be verbalized (Trommsdorff and Teichert, 2011). Declarative knowledge is formed by all kinds of stored information about the environment – facts, situations, objects, and causalities etc. It is thus factual and conscious knowledge and can be verbalized (Anderson, 2007). It comprises categories, concepts and associative networks (Brunsø, Scholderer and Grunert, 2004). Declarative knowledge is further subdivided into episodic and semantic knowledge. Episodic knowledge refers to a person's experiences and is mainly stored in the form of pictures. Semantic knowledge on the other hand is mainly stored in the form of words and refers to factual knowledge, meanings of words, rules of interpretation and analytical rules for solving problems (Kuß and Tomczak, 2007; Trommsdorff and Teichert, 2011). Semantic knowledge plays an important role in the formation of cognitive structures; due to its structured organization, it can be retrieved relatively fast (Anderson, 2007). Knowledge is assumed to be encoded and stored in LTM in the form of organized structures (knowledge structures) or semantic networks (Grebitus, 2008; Kroeber-Riel, Weinberg and Gröppel-Klein, 2009).

2.2.1.2 Affective Processes

Recent research into human decision making is increasingly interested in the impact of affect (Clore, Schwarz and Conway, 1994; Loewenstein et al., 2001; Zajonc, 1980). According to several authors, affect can be defined as a state of feeling that human beings experience such as 'sadness' or 'happiness' and is often also related to feelings of 'goodness' or 'badness' with regard to an external stimulus (Finucane et al., 2000a; Peters, Burraston and Mertz, 2004; Peter and Olson, 2010; Slovic and Peters, 2006). Affective responses are often linked to bodily reactions, e.g. increased heart rate or tears, and vary in terms of intensity. Peter and Olson (2010) distinguish four different types of affect that differ in terms of strength and physical reaction: emotions such as joy, fear or love are linked to intense bodily reactions and are very strong affective responses. Specific feelings such as disgust and sadness are linked to somewhat weaker physical reactions and are somewhat less intensive than emotions. Besides, moods such as boredom are rather diffuse affective responses that are not directed to a specific object or issue. Finally, evaluations such as liking and goodness are linked to the lowest level of bodily response and felt intensity (Kroeber-Riel, 1979; Peter and Olson, 2010)[4]. Moreover, in the empirical literature, the term affect is often used as a bipolar item contrasting positive and negative evaluation of an object or situation (Sjöberg, 2007).

Research into the influence of affective responses on judgment and decision making can be distinguished according to whether one is focusing on 'anticipatory' or 'anticipated' emotions (Loewenstein et al., 2001). Decision making research is interested in the effect of 'anticipated' or expected emotions. 'Anticipated' emotions are not experienced in the immediate situation, but it is assumed that during the process of decision-making, people anticipate how they would feel in different outcome situations, which constitutes an additional factor influencing decisions. With 'anticipated' emotions, the process of decision-making is still viewed as a mainly cognitive one (Loewenstein et al., 2001; Zinn, 2006a). Neuroscience and social psychology have mainly focused on the role of 'anticipatory' emotions by examining how immediate emotions (immediate visceral reaction in the decision-making situation) influence human decision-making. Lerner and Keltner (2000) further make a distinction between 'integral' and 'incidental' affect. Studies focusing on 'integral' affect analyze the impact of emotions that are related and relevant to the object of decision-making. 'Incidental' affect refers to emotions that are experienced during decision-making and that sometimes have an impact on judgment and choice even though these emotions are not linked to the object on which decisions are taken.

4 Damasio (1994) proposes a different classification. He distinguishes between (1) basic universal emotions such as happiness and anger, (2) subtle universal emotions such as jealousy and embarrassment and (3) background emotions such as wellbeing and fatigue. For Damasio (1994) 'feeling' is the experience of emotion.

2.2.1.3 The Interplay of Cognitive and Affective Processes

There exist several hypotheses about the interplay between cognitions and emotions, and their order and influence on judgment and choice. Those will be discussed in the following.

Stimulus→cognitions→affective responses→decision-making

Some researchers assume that people first cognitively evaluate a stimulus. This cognitive evaluation results in affective responses that directly influence human judgment and decision making. In other words, it is assumed that the effect of cognitions on decision making is mediated by affective reactions (Cottle and Klineberg, 1974; Damasio, 1994; Loewenstein et al., 2001). According to the 'somatic marker' hypothesis by Damasio (1994), emotions are the result of images related to the expected consequences or decision making outcomes. Due to past experiences these images are 'marked' by positive or negative feelings that are further linked to somatic states. Positive 'somatic markers' are likely to result in a positive evaluation of the outcome consequences, whereas negative 'somatic markers' are likely to lead to negative evaluations. These 'anticipatory' emotions linked to images of outcomes and consequences were found to guide people's judgment in an accurate and efficient way (Damasio, 1994) as they present a kind of summary of the likely consequences (Loewenstein et al., 2001). Studies supporting the 'affect-as-information' hypothesis found that affect can have a direct influence on decision-making outcome. When feelings during a decision-making process are perceived as relevant to the decision-making task by the person (referred to above as 'integral affect' according to Lerner and Keltner, 2000), then these feelings have an impact on the person's choice (Clore, Schwarz and Conway, 1994; Loewenstein et al., 2001).

Stimulus→affective responses→decision-making

In addition to the '*stimulus→cognitive→ affective*' path, affective reactions can also be a direct answer to a stimulus. Zajonc (1980) argues that people can emotionally react to a stimulus without being aware of the stimulus. For Zajonc affective responses are the first and automatic reactions to a stimulus that further guide cognitive processing of information and decision making. Neurological research approves this direct link to affective responses, as LeDoux (1996) found that there exists a direct neural projection from the sensory thalamus, which is responsible for the processing of signals to the amygdala, which in turn is important for the processing of affective reactions. Thus LeDoux (1996) proposed that emotional reactions are independent of (higher-order) cognitive processes.

Stimulus→peripheral cognitive processing→affective responses →cognitive processes→decision-making

More recent neurological research does not support the independence of emotional and cognitive processes. Storbeck, Robinson and McCourt (2006) found that prior to affective responses, a stimulus passes through a cognitive processing, called semantic analysis, within the visual cortex. Thus, a three-step processing is proposed with an initial peripheral cognitive processing that results in emotional responses that further guide more elaborate cognitive processes (Sjöberg, 2007; Storbeck, Robinson and McCourt, 2006). In this regard, the influence of affective reactions on cognitive processes is found to be stronger than the one from cognitive to affective reactions as in the human brain the connections from the affective system to the cognitive system are found to be stronger than vice versa (LeDoux, 1996).

2.2.2 Cognitive and Affective Factors in Risk Perception

Having reviewed the role of affect and cognition, the following section will apply these concepts to risk perception. Current psychological risk research considers not only cognitive processes but also the role of emotions and the interplay between affection and cognition.

2.2.2.1 Cognitive Factors Influencing Risk Perception

The majority of psychological studies investigating risk perception had a focus on the cognitive factors that influence risk perception and acceptance (Peters and Slovic, 1996; Slovic, Monahan and MacGregor, 2000).

Intuitive judgment of probability

Tversky and Kahneman's (1974) work on intuitive judgment of probability was a crucial milestone for research interested in how human beings assess risks. They tried to find out how people assess the probability of uncertain events or how people judge the value of an uncertain quantity. They found that there are several heuristic strategies used by humans in order to reduce the mental complexity of judging probabilities. This complexity reduction is often useful, but also leads to suboptimal outcomes. The deviation between optimal and actual outcome is defined as bias (Tversky and Kahneman, 1974).

The representative heuristic

In several empirical studies Tversky and Kahneman found that people use the representative heuristic as a cognitive shortcut. Tversky and Kahneman (1972: 430) defined representativeness as a heuristic "according to which subjective probability of an event, or a sample, is determined by the degree to which it (i) is similar in essential characteristics to its parent population; and (ii) reflects the salient features of the process by which it is generated." In other words, people compare a new or unknown event or sample with an event or sample they consider as comparable and judge the probability of the new event or sample as being similar to the known one. For instance, people judge the probability that a certain person is a farmer according to the similarity of that person with the stereotype of a farmer. And in applying this heuristic people tend to ignore base-rate frequencies such as the relative frequency of farmers in the sample or overall population (Kahneman and Tversky, 1973). In another study Tversky and Kahneman (1983) found that people rate the probability of a flood somewhere in the USA as lower than that of a flood that was caused by an earthquake in California, even though statistically the simultaneous occurrence of an earthquake and a flood is less probable than the occurrence of a flood. However, as earthquakes in California are known and highly probable events, people judged the simultaneous occurrence of flood and earthquake to be more likely. Besides, people expect a set of events that are generated by a random process to be a representative sequence even if this sequence is very small. Thus if a coin is tossed several times, people expect that sequences where the same side of the coin appeared subsequently to be less likely than sequences where coin sides alternated (Kahneman and Tversky, 1972; Tversky and Kahneman, 1974).

The results of a study by Visschers et al. (2007) point to the importance of the representativeness heuristic also for the assessment of risks. In their study they analyzed how people assess hazards that are unknown to them. They found that respondents related the unknown risks to risks they knew. This association was based on perceived similarities between qualitative characteristics of the two risks. In addition, judgments about risk similarity were very often based solely on semantic similarity between the unknown and known risk.

Availability heuristic

According to the availability heuristic, people's judgment about the probability of an event is affected by the ease with which knowledge concerning such an event can be retrieved (Tversky and Kahneman, 1974). If people can easily recall the occurrence of a certain event, people assess the probability of that event as high. Familiarity, salience and recency of an event play an important role. For instance, someone who lost a relative due to a heart attack can easily recall that experience and will assess the risk of heart attack as fairly high. As it was a relative that the person lost, the event of a heart attack is highly relevant and familiar. Furthermore, a person judges the probability of car accidents temporarily as higher after having seen an accident on the road, and sales of earthquake insurance increased considerably after a quake and then declined (Steinbrugge, McClure and Snow, 1969 as cited in Slovic, Fischhoff and Lichtenstein, 1982). Besides, risks that are often reported in the media are generally overestimated as a consequence of the availability heuristic. The availability heuristic has been regarded as especially relevant for understanding how people perceive risks (Tversky and Kahneman, 1973). Slovic, Fischhoff and Lichtenstein (1982) report that in the early years of recombinant DNA research, the communication of unlikely risks such as contamination with developed creatures led people to overestimate this risk. Moreover, in a study by Lichtenstein et al. (1978), they found a tendency of respondents to overestimate rare causes of death and underestimate common lethal risks. They further revealed that the hazards that were overestimated were often spectacular, while those that were underestimated were rather common and generally not fatal. Related to that, Combs and Slovic (1979) examined media coverage of causes of death and revealed that dramatic lethal risks were reported much more frequently in newspapers. Relating to the availability heuristic, Tversky and Kahneman (1974) further report bias due to differences in imaginability. When people are asked to assess the probability of a disaster, their assessment is highly influenced by the ease with which they can imagine reasons that would trigger such a disaster, but this evaluation is seldomly related to the statistical probability.

Adjustment and anchoring heuristic

The adjustment and anchoring heuristic is a mental short-cut in which a person estimates a probability or a frequency by using an initial value as a reference point called an anchor. From this starting point, people adjust new information in order to arrive at their final estimates. Tversky and Kahneman (1974) report on an experiment they conducted in which two groups of people were asked to estimate the percentage of African countries in the United Nations. Before respondents were asked about their precise estimates, one group was first asked if the percentage was higher or lower than 10, while the second group was asked if the percentage was higher or lower than 65. Average estimates in each group were closer to each group's reference point. The group with the reference point of 10% guessed on average 25%, while the group with the reference point of 65% guessed on average 45%. This anchoring effect is also prevalent in real life situations and often leads to biases in people's judgments (Tversky and Kahneman, 1974). This anchoring effect is also prevalent is real life-situations and often leads to biases in people's judgements (Tversky and Kahneman, 1974). This was also found in the above cited study by Lichtenstein et al. (1978), where respondents were asked to estimate the frequencies of 40 lethal incidents. Whereas one group was told that 50.000 people annually die in automobile accidents, another group was told that 1.000 people annually die from electrocution. They found that estimates of the first group were much higher for many hazards due to an anchoring effect.

Psychometric paradigm

The psychometric paradigm is the most influential approach in cognitive risk research that investigates factors determining risk perception. According to the psychometric paradigm, risk is an inherently subjective construct and risk perception is the subjectively defined severity of a risk and its characteristics. The paradigm aims at understanding and predicting the perception of different risks and seeks to classify hazards according to people's perceptions. In other words, researchers following the psychometric paradigm investigate why subjects judge some risks as being highly probable and less acceptable than other risks and why there are differences between risk judgments of lay individuals and experts (Slovic, 1987). The school of thought headed by Paul Slovic, Sarah Lichtenstein and Baruch Fischhoff focused on cognitive factors that influence people's judgments about risks. Using nine and later 18 bipolar psychological scales such as voluntary-involuntary or controllable-uncontrollable, subjects were asked to rate several kinds of hazards according to these possible risk properties. On the basis of overall mean ratings, it is possible to construct a cognitive map that shows how the rated hazards are perceived (Slovic, 1987). They found that laypersons' risk assessment is a function of general risk attributes such as the catastrophic potential of the risk, the extent to which a hazard is perceived as voluntary or controllable, inequitable and fatal. Further important characteristics determining the perceived riskiness of a hazard is the extent to which the hazard is perceived as familiar or new, chronic or entailing delayed effects (Fischoff et al. 1978; Slovic, Lichtenstein and Fischoff, 1979). More recent empirical studies added the dimensions 'unnatural' and 'immoral' (Sjöberg, 2000b). As it was further found that many qualitative risk attributes are correlated such as voluntariness and the extent to which the risk is seen as controllable, they condensed the specific characteristics by means of factor analysis to two main higher order factors, the 'dread risk' and the 'knowledge about risks': the 'dread risk' factor comprises the characteristics catastrophic, involuntary, the extent to which the hazard is dreaded and perceived as uncontrollable, inequitable (the judgment about the distribution of risks and benefits of a hazard), unobservable and fatal. The 'knowledge about risks' factor is characterized as degree of familiarity, the potential of chronic or delayed effects, and the risk's newness (Finucane and Holup, 2005; Slovic, 1987). In some psychometric studies a third factor referring to the 'number of people exposed' to a risk has been generated (Slovic, 1987). On the basis of the two main factors 'dread' and 'knowledge', a map of risks can be created with hazards being located along the four dimensions 'high dread, low knowledge', 'high dread, high knowledge', 'low dread, low knowledge' and 'low dread, high knowledge'. For example, nuclear power or DNA technology is mostly assessed as high in 'dread' and low in 'knowledge'. Furthermore, according to psychometric studies, 'dread' and 'knowledge' have been found to explain variances in people's assessments of different risks. In other words, hazards that are perceived as entailing 'high' dread and being unknown are assessed as more risky with a stronger impact of the 'dread' factor compared to the 'knowledge' factor (Schütz, Wiedemann and Gray, 2000).

2.2.2.2 Affective Factors Influencing Risk Perception

Alhakami and Slovic (1994) could show that risk and benefit are negatively correlated in people's minds and that this is related to the overall feelings about the object in question. Thus, when feelings about an object are positive, risks are perceived as low and benefits as high. Based on these findings, the 'affect heuristic' postulates that people evaluate risk and benefits of hazards or technologies also according to their feelings about it (Finucane et al., 2000a). Similar to the 'somatic marker' hypothesis by Damasio (1994), it is assumed that images referring to the hazard or technology in people's minds are marked with affect and that people refer to a pool of positive and negative feelings tagged to their associations in order to make judgments. The 'affect heuristic' proposes that if people's overall feelings about an object are positive, they judge risks to be low and benefits to be high and this overall 'summary' feeling serves as a mental shortcut in decision-making (Peters and Slovic, 1996). In their study Finucane et al. (2000a) tested the hypothesis for various technologies and found that giving people information stating that benefits are high results in positive affect, which further decreased perceived levels of risk. Similarly, in a study on the perception of flood risks, Keller, Siegrist and Gutscher (2006) found that the evocation of negative affect by means of photographs showing houses in the flood region resulted in higher perceptions of risk. According to Slovic et al. (2004), the affect heuristic is closely linked to the availability heuristic proposed by Tversky and Kahneman (1974) (see 2.2.1). They propose that the stronger the emotions tagged to images, the higher is the likelihood of these images to be remembered.

Based on the 'somatic marker' hypothesis (Damasio, 1994), on the 'affect-as-information' perspective (Clore, Schwarz and Conway, 1994) and on the 'affect heuristic' (Finucane et al., 2000a), Loewenstein et al. (2001) propose a 'risk-as-feelings' hypothesis that models how affective and cognitive processes influence people's responses to risky situations. The hypothesis postulates that feelings such as worry and fear, as well as people's cognitive assessments both have a direct impact on people's choices. Furthermore, cognitive evaluations affect people's feeling state, and emotional reactions have an influence on the cognitive evaluation. The 'risk-as-feelings' hypothesis further postulates that emotional responses often diverge from the cognitive assessments of a risk, since cognitive and affective responses have different determinants. Whereas cognitive assessments are based on subjective probabilities and desirability of outcomes, emotional reactions depend on factors such as vividness of mental images and sensitivity to probabilities (Loewenstein et al., 2001).

Sjöberg (2006: 104) describes the vividness of a mental image as an "underlying mental substrate, which drives the elicited beliefs and values connected to a concept or an object." The vividness with which outcomes or consequences are presented in memory has an impact on the emotional response and intensity (Damasio, 1994). The vividness and resonance of the image depends on the person's experience or contact with the risk in question (through own experience or someone's one knows, personal communication, the mass media) (Browne and Hoyt, 2000; Jackson, Allum and Gaskell., 2006), an individual's ability to form mental images (e.g. Carrol, Baker and Preston, 1979) and the way consequences of technologies or risks are described (Hendickx, Vlek and Oppewal, 1989). With regard to individual differences in mental imagery, several studies report that women are more capable of forming mental images than men (see Harshman and Paivio, 1987 for a review). In this context, the strength of emotions or emotional intensity that is linked to the vividness becomes important as it influences the mode of information processing: (a) a formal and numeric mode that is more linked to cognitive information processing, resulting in a more cognitive style of risk assessment; (b) a narrative, associative and intuitive mode applicable to affective information processing, leading to a more affective response to risk.

Whereas with low levels of emotional intensity, emotions were found to give good advice when people have to judge risks, high levels of emotional intensity seem to inhibit cognitive processes. In a study by Rottenstreich and Hsee (2001), people's behavior was hardly influenced by the probability of occurrence in the case of events linked to strong affections (such as a kiss from a favorite movie star or an electric shock), whereas probability judgments had an influence on decision with low levels of emotional intensity. Similarly, in risk judgment people reject any cognitive evaluation even when probabilities of occurrence are very small, when the possible negative consequences of a technology or hazards are perceived as catastrophic and too horrible (Loewenstein et al., 2001; Japp, 1997; Zinn, 2006a). In a study by Slovic, Monahan and MacGregor (2000), clinicians were asked to judge the risk that a hospitalized mental patient would become violent by presenting one group with statistics on that issue in the form of relative frequencies (20 of 100 patients), and the other group with the same statistics but in the form of probabilities (likelihood of 20% of committing a violent act). They found that the group of clinicians with relative-frequency condition judged the risk that the patient would relapse more highly than the other group. The relative-frequency condition is likely to activate images tagged with affect that lead to a higher perception of risk (Peters and Slovic, 1996). Furthermore, Slovic, Flynn and Layman (1991) elicited people's mental images and the affects tagged to them and found them to influence people's decision making with regard to nuclear waste disposal and people's likelihood judgments with regard to an accident on the disposal site.

Lerner and Keltner (2000) have criticized research into the impact of affective responses on decision making as it mainly differentiates between 'positive' or 'negative' emotions without taking into account the possible differing impact of different emotions with the same valence[5] (see e.g. Clore, Schwarz and Conway, 1994; Zajonc, 1980). Lerner and Keltner (2000) found that 'anger' and 'fear' resulted in opposite reactions on risk judgments. 'Fear' was related to pessimistic risk evaluations and risk-averse decisions, whereas 'anger' was related to optimistic risk judgments and rather risk-seeking decisions. They explain this by differing appraisal themes underlying each emotion according to cognitive appraisal theories of emotion. Smith and Ellsworth (1985) identified six major appraisal dimensions that underlie different emotions: certainty, pleasantness, attentional activity, control, anticipated effort and responsibility. These appraisal dimensions are assumed to be automatic and intuitive evaluations that are linked to the survival of human beings (Peters, Burraston and Mertz, 2004). Lerner and Keltner (2000) could show that 'fear' is defined by uncertainty, unpleasantness and situational control, whereas 'anger' is defined by certainty and individual control. Thus people reacting with fear might have different cognitive predispositions or recalled different memories in order to evaluate that risk and thus differ in their risk assessments.

In addition to cognitive factors such as subjective assessments of probabilities of negative consequences or the perceived ability to control, the evaluation of food hazards is likely to be also influenced by affective responses based on the vividness of mental images linked to possible consequences. Thus content and emotional intensity of mental images with regard to food hazards might provide interesting hints in understanding differences in risk evaluations between groups of people in general, and also between men and women. Furthermore, similar to the study by Lerner and Keltner (2000), affective reactions such as

5 Emotions of the same valence are different emotions that are all evaluated as positive or as negative. E.g. 'anger' and 'fear' are different emotions but both are generally judged as negative.

anger and fear might also in the case of food hazards be linked in opposite ways to their evaluations. Individual differences between these two emotions can reveal two different frameworks regarding specific food hazards due to differing appraisal dimensions linked to different mental images.

2.3 Approaches to Understanding Differences in Risk Perception among Individuals

Different disciplines like anthropology, geography, economics, psychology and sociology have contributed to risk perception research and proposed different theories why people perceive risks differently (Slovic, 1992; Bøholm, 1998). Hence, this section will summarize the findings of investigations that aimed at understanding individual differences in risk perception. Above (section 2.2.2), the general processes that are important in risk perception, as well as the impact of the hazards' characteristics were outlined. In the field of social science, one can distinguish two main largely independent strands: approaches footed in psychology and those mainly based on anthropological and sociological theories. Among the psychological approaches, the psychometric approach is the one most often considered. Its principal contributors are Paul Slovic, Sarah Lichtenstein, Baruch Fischhoff and their colleagues (Fischhoff et al. 1978; Slovic, Lichtenstein and Fischhoff, 1979). Moreover, socio-psychological approaches are often applied in empirical risk research that aims at understanding individual differences in risk perception. A further very influential approach is the Cultural Theory approach established by the anthropologist Mary Douglas and the political scientist Aaron Wildavsky (Douglas and Wildavsky, 1982) and further developed into the socio-cultural approach by Lupton (1999) and Tulloch and Lupton (2003). Additional sociological risk theories are the governmentality approach (Barry et al. 1996), approaches in system theory initiated by Luhmann (Japp, 1997; 2000) and reflexive modernization (Beck, 1992). Table 1 gives an overview over the main approaches that are relevant in empirical risk research.

Table 1: Main Approaches in Empirical Risk Perception Research

Core discipline	Perspective	Objective
Psychology	Psychometric approach (cognitive psychology)	Explaining why different risks are perceived differently; understanding the expert-lay gap
Anthropology	Cultural Theory approach	Explaining inter-group differences in risk perception
Current approaches		
Psychology	Socio-psychological approach (cognitive psychology)	Explaining individual differences in risk evaluation in social contexts
Sociology	Socio-cultural approach	Explaining individual risk perceptions in social contexts

Source: Own illustration.

In the following, the psychometric paradigm, the Cultural Theory approach and the two current approaches – the socio-psychological approach and the socio-cultural approach – are presented.

2.3.1 The Psychometric Paradigm

Apart from being able to give an explanation why some hazards are perceived as more risky than others, the psychometric paradigm also aimed at understanding differences in risk assessment between groups of individuals, in particular between lay persons and experts (Slovic, 1987). Research following the psychometric paradigm could show that people's risk perception is a complex phenomenon that depends on a variety of non-technical factors. For instance, lay people base their perception of risks on whether they perceive the risks as controllable, familiar or new (Finucane and Holup, 2005; Slovic, 1987). In contrast to experts, who are found to judge hazards on the basis of technical estimates and annual cases of death, lay people's risk assessment seems not to be based on the magnitude of a hazard and the probability of its occurrence (Schütz, Wiedemann and Gray, 2000). As such, psychometric approaches are able to show differences between individuals in terms on how risks assessments are made. They have, however, been criticized for neglecting social and cultural influences on risk perception and for thus not being able to explain differences between e.g. ethnic and social groups and the frequently reported differences between men and women (Flynn, Slovic and Mertz, 1994; Oltedal et al., 2004; Vaughan and Nordenstam, 1991). Another criticism refers to its inability to detect the cognitive, emotional and motivational processes linked to the evaluation of risks (Jackson, Allum and Gaskell, 2006; Johnson and Covello, 1987; Jungermann and Slovic, 1993). This criticism has been taken into account by anthropological and sociological approaches, which focus on social and cultural influences on risk perception.

2.3.2 The Cultural Theory of Risk

Anthropological and sociological approaches "rely (all more or less) on a weak constructivism as their normal epistemological approach to risk." (Zinn, 2006b: 8) Risk is conceived to be culturally and socially embedded and people relate each risk to its specific context. As Douglas (1990: 10) points out: "risk is not only the probability of an event but also the probable magnitude of its outcome and everything depends on the value that is set on the outcome. The evaluation is a political, aesthetic and moral matter." Hence individuals or groups may perceive risks differently as the hazard means different things to them: they might value differently, who or what is threatened, who or what is posing the threat or who is responsible for it. Thus relationships with who or what is threatened, possible responsibilities, trust in politics and risk management systems, institutions, perceived self-control and ability to protect self and others or what is eventually harmed are important for the judgment of a risk. Thus, according to Cultural Theory, risk perception is not governed by personal characteristics such as personality traits, needs, preferences, or by properties of the hazards. It is a socially, or culturally, constructed phenomenon. What is perceived as dangerous, and how much risk is acceptable, is a function of one's cultural adherence and social learning. Such adherences are described in Douglas' Cultural Theory (Douglas 1978; Douglas and Wildavsky, 1982; Thompson, Eillis and Wildavsky, 1990). Furthermore, risk perception is here a way of responding to dangers to the social order (Zinn, 2004).

Cultural Theory mostly focuses on the difference in risk perceptions between groups, and to a lesser extent between individuals. Human conceptions of what constitutes a risk may differ according to the organization of social relations in the society they live in. Douglas and Wildavsky (1982) developed four cultural types along a grid – group framework. The 'grid' dimension is a measure of constraint that is put on people by the social context. For example, in 'high grid' social environments, the individual has hardly any behavioral options, whereas in 'low grid' situations, individuals are free to select and negotiate their social relations (Oltedal et al., 2004). 'Group' stands for the degree of social interaction and the extent to which an individual's behavior depends on the group (Douglas and Wildavsky, 1982; Jackson, Allum and Gaskell, 2006). For example, variation in social participation is conceptualized as the interaction of these two dimensions (Tulloch, 2008). By combining the two dimensions, four kinds of social environments can be generated that are related with four different ways of life. The four ways of life are hierarchist ('high grid, high group'), egalitarian ('low grid, high group'), fatalist ('high grid, low group') and individualist ('low grid, low group') (see Figure 2):

Figure 2: The Grid-Group Classification of Douglas and Wildavsky

		Group	
		Low	High
Grid	High	Fatalist	Hierarchist
	Low	Individualist	Egalitarian

Source: Pidd (2005).

According to Cultural Theory, an individual's way of life and the linked worldviews are strongly tied to what the individual fears, since human beings are afraid of everything that endangers and questions their own way of life. As a consequence, depending on the organization of a social group, members of this group have also different concepts of risk.

People with a hierarchical worldview believe in a 'natural order' of society that has to be preserved, and fear is linked to everything that questions this order. Hierarchists further have great trust in the knowledge of experts. Egalitarian individuals fear inequality between people and everything that might engender inequality. They see nature as fragile and vulnerable and are opposed to activities and technologies that might cause irreversible damage to a large number of people or future generations (Tulloch, 2008). Fatalists hardly perceive themselves as an active part of a social group and tend to feel rather committed to others' decisions and behaviors. They believe that risks cannot be influenced and they thus try to ignore risks and not to worry about them. For members of the individualistic worldview, risk is an opportunity for gain. Individualists support market liberalism and fear everything that restricts their freedom. Moreover, they believe in the regeneration capacity of nature and they are not worried about damage to the environment. Sometimes a fifth way of life is mentioned, which refers to asocial individuals with no interaction with their environment.

According to Cultural Theory, every individual can be referred to one of these worldviews. Because some of the values and worldviews are shared in one culture and differ across cultures (Grunert and Juhl, 1995), risk concepts differ between groups of people and cultures.

To sum up the two main approaches in risk perception research, the psychometric paradigm has its roots in psychology and the Cultural Theory approach in anthropology. The first approach focuses on the characteristics of hazards that people take into account when making judgments about risks by applying approaches of cognitive psychology. However, it neglects the social context and cannot explain individual differences in risk perception. Cultural Theory focuses on the influence of culture and is able to explain inter-group differences, but it fails to take into account individual responses to risk (Jackson, Allum and Gaskell, 2006), and empirical applications usually have low explanatory power.

2.3.3 Current Approaches to Risk Perception Research

During recent years, both schools of thought have further developed and some researchers have attempted to combine the strengths of the two approaches. Jackson, Allum and Gaskell (2006) propose a contextualist psychological approach to risk and a sociological approach that also considers the individual perspective.

One dominant stream of research based on cognitive-psychological thinking is social-psychological research into risk perception. Socio-psychological approaches assume that individuals have a consistent system of attitudes and motives and that these general attitudes and also the more specific attitudes determine an individual's assessment of risks. It is proposed that the source of a risk with the related associations is central to people's evaluations. In addition, socio-psychological risk perception research is interested in the impact of social affiliation on people's attitudes towards risks and thus takes into account socio-economic and socio-demographic factors such as age, gender and income (Banse and Bechmann, 1998). Furthermore, socio-psychological risk research considers the role of attitudes towards and confidence in specific life domains such as science and technology and politics.

On the basis of the Cultural Theory approach, socio-cultural approaches (see Tulloch and Lupton, 2003) have been developed that overcome the very functionalist view on risk of the Cultural Theory approach. They suggest that worldviews are not stable but often dependent on the issue in question. For instance, a person might be an egalitarian in one sub-domain but a fatalist in another sub-domain (Knox, 2000; Rayner, 1992). Thus socio-cultural approaches focus on the individual's perception in cultural contexts. They "show that risk has different meanings to people depending on their social context and worldviews and take into account the role of identity-formation and –continuation, emotions, values and aesthetics, habituations and power-relations for people's perceptions and responses to risks." (Zinn, 2006b) Socio-cultural research into risk perception is mainly focused on an individual's perception of risks and how it is managed in cultural contexts. Empirical research based on socio-cultural approaches to risk that tries to understand individual differences in risk perception considers the role of personal values and worldviews, the role of religiosity or spiritual beliefs as important predictors in risk perception.

Work that follows socio-psychological and socio-cultural thinking in risk perception research is to a very large degree empirical and focuses on one or several of the above mentioned individual determinants of risk perception.

2.4 Literature Review on Factors Determining Risk Perception

Social, psychological, economic and political factors determine perceptions of risks in a complex and often interdependent way (Dosman, Adamowicz and Hrudey, 2001). Table 2 classifies and gives an overview of the different determinants of risk perception.

Table 2: Factors in Risk Perception[1]

Socio-demographic variables	**Socio-psychological variables**[2]
Gender/Sex	Worldviews[3]
Age	Personal values[3]
Ethnicity	Spiritual beliefs/religiosity
	Emotions
Socio-structural variables	**Socio-political variables**
Education	Attitude towards science and technology (S&T)
Income/Occupation	Political views
Knowledge	Social trust
Presence & age of children	

[1] The classification of the specific determinants of risk perception into the four groups might differ according to scientific disciplines. This table is based on the grouping of Slimak and Dietz (2006) since it provides the most comprehensive classification in the risk perception literature.

[2] Also called 'socio-cultural' factors according to other classifications.

[3] Sometimes classified as 'socio-political' factors.

Source: Adapted from Flynn, Slovic and Mertz (1994) and Slimak and Dietz (2006) with own extensions.

2.4.1 Socio-Demographic Factors

Many risk researchers were interested in understanding the relationship between socio-demographic factors such as gender, age and ethnicity and the evaluations and acceptance of risks and technologies (e.g. Adeola, 2007; Bord and O'Connor, 1997; Flynn, Slovic and Mertz, 1994; Krewski et al., 2006; Savage, 1993; Vaughan and Nordenstam, 1991).

2.4.1.1 Gender/Sex

The majority of studies that investigated the effect of sex on levels of risk perception found men rated many risks as lower, were less concerned, and showed higher acceptance of many technologies than women (see for instance: Dosman, Adamowicz and Hrudey, 2001; Dunlap and Beus, 1992; Krewski et al., 2006; Nayga, 1996; Ott and Maligaya, 1989; Pilisuk and Acredolo, 1988; Savage, 1993). However, in some studies no differences between women and men were found (see for instance: Slimak and Dietz, 2006). The effect of gender/sex is central to this work and is presented and discussed in detail in chapter 3.

2.4.1.2 Age

In contrast to gender, the direction of the effect of age on risk perception is not that evident, with some studies finding a positive relationship (Armaş, 2006; Cohn et al., 1995; Kirk et al., 2002; Krewski et al., 2006; Plapp, 2004; Renn and Zwick, 1997; Roosen, Thiele and Hansen, 2005), some a negative relationship (Freudenburg, 1993; Starr, Langley and Taylor, 2000; Viscusi, 1991), and in a few studies age had no effect on perceived risk (Hermand, Mullet and Rompteaux, 1999). For instance, in the study by Freudenburg (1993), older people perceived risks of a nuclear waste repository to be lower and another study found that older people rated risks due to smoking (Viscusi, 1991) to be lower compared to younger people. Similarly, a study performed in Australia by Starr, Langley and Taylor (2000) investigated people's assessment of health risks due to 28 different kinds of risks, such as pesticides contamination, cigarette smoking and AIDS, and found younger people to be more concerned than older respondents. However, studies investigating risk perception of natural catastrophes such as earthquake, flood and windstorm (Armaş, 2006; Plapp, 2004) could show that older people assessed higher levels of risks than younger people.

With regard to food risks, the causality shows a clearer pattern with mostly a positive relationship between age and risk perception. Younger respondents were less concerned about the risks of growth hormones, salmonella and residues in food (Kirk et al. 2002) and rated the risks of pesticides as lower (Dosman, Adamowicz and Hrudey, 2001; Ott and Maligaya, 1989). Furthermore, older people were found to be more concerned about natural food risks such as cholesterol in food and salmonella (Roosen, Thiele and Hansen, 2005), rated food safety issues as more important compared to younger people (Lin, 1995), and have a more pessimist attitude towards the safety of foods (De Jonge et al., 2007). In contrast, in the study by Nayga (1996) older respondents were more likely than younger respondents to perceive meat from animals that have been treated with antibiotics and food that was produced by using pesticides to be safe. Interestingly, Grobe, Douthitt and Zepeda (1999) in their study about consumers' assessments of recombinant bovine growth hormone found a non-linear relationship between age and risk perception: Consumers' concern increased with age up to a certain point and then decreased.

2.4.1.3 Ethnicity

Inspired by the Cultural Theory approaches of Douglas and Wildavsky (1982), who pointed to the importance of cultural background, several social scientists investigated the relationship between ethnicity and risk perception. Vaughan and Nordenstam (1991) reviewed the literature about environmental (such as natural hazards, water and air pollution) and technological (such as nuclear or toxic waste) risk perception with regard to their results in relation to ethnicity. They report that a consistent relationship between ethnicity and risk perception exists only for technological hazards such as nuclear power and nuclear waste, with ethnic minorities being more concerned and less willing to support nuclear technology. For other risks such as natural disasters or air and water pollution, results are mixed. In the study by Savage performed in the United States (1993) about the perception of four different kinds of hazards (aviation accidents, fires at home, automobile accidents, stomach cancer), African Americans dreaded all four hazards more strongly than Caucasians. More recently, Adeola (2004) found Caucasians to rate a wide range of different environmental and technological risks as posing a lower threat compared to African American respondents.

Some studies mostly conducted in U.S. found interesting interaction effects between gender and ethnicity. Flynn, Slovic and Mertz (1994), Finucane et al. (2000b) and Satterfield et al. (2004) found Caucasian men to be less concerned about several different hazards than Caucasian women, African American men and women. These results are often discussed in terms of status, power and control, and of who benefits from hazardous technologies (Adeola, 2004; Flynn, Slovic and Mertz, 1994; Slovic, 1999) that are relevant both in terms of gender and ethnicity. Following the idea of decision-making power and status, Adeola (2007) could further confirm the hypothesis that Native Americans would show lower levels of risk perception than immigrants.

Grobe, Douthitt and Zepeda (1999) found that African American, Asian, Native American and Hispanics were more likely than Caucasian Americans to be very concerned about the use of recombinant bovine growth hormone (r-BST) in rearing animals for milk production. Similarly, Pilisuk and Acredolo (1988) found that ethnic minorities in California were more concerned about food additives. Additionally, Nayga (1996) found that African American responsible for cooking are more likely than Caucasian meal planners to perceive meat from animals that were reared using antibiotics and hormones as unsafe. In the above-cited study by Finucane et al. (2000b), African American women showed the highest levels of worry with regard to risks due to hormones and antibiotics in meat products, whereas white men showed the lowest levels of concern compared to all other groups.

2.4.2 Socio-Structural Factors

The following presents studies that investigated the impact of the level of education and income as well as the presence of children in the household and consumers' level of technological knowledge or knowledge about risks and hazards.

2.4.2.1 Education and Income

Higher levels of education are often associated with lower levels of risk perception and a higher probability to accept certain technologies (Slovic et al., 1997). In the above-cited study by Savage (1993), people with low education dreaded the four investigated hazards more strongly than people with a higher education, and concern about technological risks was also negatively related with levels of education in the study by Pilisuk and Acredolo (1988). The inverse relationship between education and levels of concern about hazards has also been confirmed in two more recent studies (Krewski et al., 2006; Slimak and Dietz, 2006). In the investigation by Slimak and Dietz (2006), more highly educated respondents perceived environmental risks such as pesticides and global warming as well as global risks such as growth of human population to be lower than respondents with lower levels of education.

Considering perception of food hazards, Roosen, Thiele and Hansen (2005) also report a negative relation between education and concern about natural food hazards such as salmonella and moulds and, similarly, Dosman, Adamowicz and Hrudey (2001) found that with increasing levels of education, people were less concerned about bacteria in food. In the same way, levels of education determined also the likelihood of perceiving the technological food hazards antibiotics and hormones, irradiation and pesticides to be safe in the study by Nayga (1996).

Similar to education levels, income is often inversely related to levels of risk perception. The above-mentioned studies by Savage (1993) and Pilisuk and Acredolo (1988) found that poorer respondents indicated higher dread or concern about the investigated risks. Also, concern about pollution was especially strong among poor respondents even after controlling for levels of pollution of respondents' communities (Cutter, 1981). Social vulnerability due to unemployment and low incomes were further found to be related to overestimations of the probability of death due to various risks, while higher income and stable social status was rather related to underestimation (Bastide et al., 1989; Nyland, 1993; Sjöberg et al., 1996 as cited in Bøholm, 1998).

With regard to food hazards, this pattern is not that evident. Several studies confirmed the postulated negative relationship between income and risk perception for natural and technological food hazards (Dosman, Adamowicz and Hrudey, 2001; Nayga, 1996; Roosen, Thiele and Hansen, 2005; Siegrist, 2003). However, according to the German National Nutrition Survey II (Federal Research Centre for Nutrition and Food, 2008), consumers with lower socio-economic background were found to be more concerned about natural food hazards such as spoilt food, whereas wealthier consumers were more concerned about the technological food hazards of pesticides. Additionally, a positive relationship between income and concern about unhealthy diet was reported for the German population.

2.4.2.2 Knowledge

The 'familiarity hypothesis' approach, also known as the 'knowledge deficit' approach, suggests that knowledge about science and technology or about hazards relates to lower levels of risk assessment with regard to (technological) risks (Slovic, 1987). In other words, for a long time, lay people's inability to understand complex scientific information has been seen as a reason for the gap between expert and lay risks judgments (Bettman et al., 1987; Cross, 1998). Whereas several studies found support for the familiarity hypothesis (Cobb and Macoubrie, 2004; Vandermoere et al., 2010), the knowledge deficit model has been questioned by several social scientists (for a detailed discussion see: Hansen et al., 2003), and more complex relationships between scientific knowledge, attitudes towards technology and science, trust and risk perception have been proposed (Kahan et al., 2009b; Siegrist and Cvetkovich, 2000; Vandermoere et al., 2010). It is suggested that a positive attitude towards technology encourages people to learn more about these issues (Kahan et al., 2009b; Vandermoere et al., 2010) and scientific literacy is rather an expression of general attitudes such as attitudes towards science and technology. This is especially the case when subjective technological knowledge is elicited that is related to people's values and general attitudes (Costa-Font, Gil and Traill, 2008) or influenced by people's identities (Bieberstein et al., 2011).

The rather complex and inconsistent relationship between knowledge and risk perception is also prevalent in the case of food hazards. Vandermoere et al. (2010) found a positive relationship between knowledge about food hazards and nanotechnology and respondents' attitudes toward the application of nanotechnology in food packaging. Similarly, several studies indicated that increasing levels of knowledge about gene technology was related to respondents' higher level of acceptance of genetically modified food (Moerbeck and Casimir, 2005; Moon and Balasubramanian, 2004). However, the German study by Roosen, Thiele and Hansen (2005) found a positive relationship between people's knowledge and concern about natural food risks. Interestingly, according to a finding by the European Commission (1999), higher knowledge levels lead to polarized views about biotechnology and thus have differing effects on people's attitudes dependent on their prior beliefs. This was confirmed in the study by Christoph, Bruhn and Roosen (2008) about consumers' acceptance of genetic modification.

2.4.2.3 Presence of Children

The above-cited studies by Dosman, Adamowicz and Hrudey (2001) and Roosen, Thiele and Hansen (2005) found a positive relation between the presence of young children in the household and concern about natural food hazards and also about pesticides in the first study. According to Hamilton (1985) the age of the children also plays an important role and respondents with younger children are shown to be more worried about environmental risks. However, the presence of children did not have an effect on the perception of food irradiation, antibiotics and hormones in food and pesticides in the study by Nayga (1996).

2.4.3 Socio-Psychological Factors[6]

This chapter presents empirical evidence about the impact of general worldviews on risk perception as proposed by the Cultural Theory of risk, followed by studies that analyzed how risk perceptions varies according to consumers' personal values as proposed by socio-psychological classifications of human values such as the list of values by Kahle, Beatty and Homer (1986). Finally, results of studies that examined the relationship between more specific values such as environmental values and risk perception are presented.

2.4.3.1 Worldviews and Values

People's assessments of risks have been found to be related to their worldviews and values that are perceived to be advocated by or inhibited by related risks (Rohrmann and Renn, 2000; Slovic, 1999). Empirical work based on the Cultural Theory of risk has investigated the role of worldviews in people's assessment of risks. Worldviews are general cultural and political attitudes towards the world and how the world should be organized (Dake, 1991; Peters, Burraston and Mertz, 2004; Slovic, 1999). Thus, it is proposed that an individual's assessment of a risk depends on how this risk is managed by industry, government and science and how this management is judged in terms of the individual's view on the social organization of society (Peters and Slovic, 1996). Wildavsky and Dake (1990) and Dake (1990; 1991) were the first to try to empirically verify the Cultural Theory approach to risk perception and concern. They developed scales in order to measure the above-described social environments or world views and correlated them with concerns about social issues. Measuring bivariate correlations and using an American sample, they found that worldviews were significantly correlated with societal concerns such as poverty and unemployment. Later, studies added ratings of risk perception to investigate the impact of

6 The role of affect and emotions will not be detailed here as it was discussed in detail in 2.2.2.2.

worldviews on technological risk perception (Palmer, 1996; Peters and Slovic, 1996; Sjöberg, 1998). Also within a U.S. context, Palmer (1996) could show that people with a 'hierarchical' worldview consider possible dangers and benefits of technological risks, whereas 'egalitarians' only focus on the dangers of technological risks. Sjöberg (1998) found that similar to the study by Dake (1991), worldviews and societal concerns are considered to be significantly correlated, but correlations between worldviews and risk ratings were minor. Similarly, in a study by Peters and Slovic (1996) the correlations between risk ratings and worldviews were very low. The 'Dake worldview scales' were adapted for the European context and a British version of the scales was developed that became known as the 'scales of cultural biases' or 'World View Scales' (Marris, Langford and O'Riordan, 1998; Sjöberg, 1998). However, the explanatory power of the 'world view scales' is strongly questioned as in most of the studies using multiple regression analysis the worldviews accounted for only a maximum of 5% of variance in risk perception (Brenot, Bonnefous and Mays, 1996; Marris, Langford and O'Riordan, 1998; Sjöberg, 1997; Steg and Sievers, 2000). More recent research using a different way of measuring the worldviews according to Douglas (1990) has shown that when people have some information about technology (here nanotechnology), worldviews are important predictors for people's risk perception. 'Egalitarian' perspectives induce people to think that the risks of nanotechnology will outweigh the benefits, while 'individualistic' and 'hierarchical' worldviews are linked to a more positive attitude towards nanotechnology (Kahan et al., 2009b). Rather than expecting a direct impact of worldviews on risk perception, Jenkins-Smith (1993) proposed that worldviews influence the processing of information regarding a hazard that results in verbal images of that hazard that differ in content and emotional appraisal. Similarly, Peters, Burraston and Mertz (2004) found that the relationship between worldviews and risk perception was mediated by different affective responses to the risk.

Other studies investigate the role of more specific worldviews. A study by Rohrman (1994) focused on two specific facets of worldviews, people's occupational and political affiliations. By combining these two facets he developed four different groups designated as 'technological', 'ecological', 'monetarian' and 'feminist' and investigated their impact on risk perception in Germany, New Zealand and Australia. Particularly in the case of technological risks, 'ecological' and 'feminist' orientations were linked to higher risk perceptions, whereas respondents with 'technological' orientations were found to give the lowest risk ratings.

Another line of research focuses on the role of motivational values for people's assessment of risks. According to Schwartz and Bilsky (1987) values are concepts and beliefs about preferable end states or behaviors, which go beyond specific situations and which direct the selection and evaluation of behavior and events. Next to the cognitive concept of preferable end states, values also contain an affective and a behavioral component (Rokeach, 1973; Kliebisch, 2002). Based on the work of Rokeach (1973), Schwartz and Bilsky (1987) proposed distinguishing values according to their content and their relations to each other and developed a value classification according to the type of motivational goal the values refer to (Schwartz, 1994). They grouped the values in eleven motivational domains that are further derived from three universal goals referring to needs of individuals as organisms, the requirement of social interaction and of the functioning of social groups (see chapter 5.2 for more details on the Schwartz value classification).

Sjöberg (2000b) investigated the perception of 22 risks related to health, environment and economy related to a number of general value scales. In addition to items from the Schwartz value scales (Schwartz, 1992), he included also Kahle's list of values (Kahle, Beatty and Homer, 1986). Based on the work of Maslow (1954), Feather (1975) and Rokeach (1973), Kahle, Beatty and Homer (1986) developed a list of the core American values. In order to investigate the impact of cultural values on consumer behavior, Kahle's list of values incorporates nine consumer-related instrumental and terminal personal values. Sjöberg (2000b) concluded that the Schwartz value scale predicted best people's risk perceptions. However, similar to studies using Dake's worldview scales (Dake, 1991), the explained variance of the Schwartz value scales is rather small.

Stern, Dietz and Kalof (1993) adapted and expanded the Schwartz model in order to explain differences in environmental concern based on people's values. They distinguished three types of value orientations that they found to have an effect on people's willingness to take political action and pay increased taxes to protect the environment: the 'socio-altruistic value orientation' that is characterized by taking care of other human beings' welfare, concern for nonhuman species and the biosphere called the 'biospheric value orientation', and an 'egoistic value orientation', where a person's self-interest is the main focus. Stern, Dietz and Kalof (1993) proposed that value orientations also contribute to the predictive power of risk perception studies because altruistic and egoistic values as well as environmental values determine the acceptability of risks. Environmental concern was further related to a smaller likelihood of eating genetically modified food (Sparks, Shepherd and Frewer, 1995). Furthermore, in a study about the perception of gene technology, Siegrist (1998) found that 'ecocentristic' and 'anthropocentristic' values are important predictors for people's assessments. People with 'ecocentristic' values were found to have negative attitudes towards gene technology, whereas 'anthropocentrism' was related to more positive attitudes towards it.

In addition, Nordenstedt and Ivanisevic (2010) found that the four higher order value domains (openness to change, self-transcendence, conservation and self-enhancement) by Schwartz (1992) were predictive for the assessment of many of the nine different kinds of hazards in three countries. In a study about the assessment of 24 different ecological risks, the Schwartz value scale and the 'New Environmental Paradigm' were found to be influential predictors for people's risk perceptions (Slimak and Dietz, 2006). The 'New Environmental Paradigm' scale was developed by Dunlap and Van Liere (1978) and investigates people's beliefs about the effects of human intervention in nature.[7] People's views on nature interference were found to be an important predictor for their attitudes towards nanotechnology in food (Vandermoere et al., 2009; 2010). They found that more holistic views about the relation between people and the environment increase the likelihood of being negative rather than positive toward nanotechnology.

2.4.3.2 Religiosity and Spiritual Beliefs

Regarding religiosity, results do not show a consistent pattern. Researchers investigated spiritual beliefs and/or religiosity as factors in mainly technological risk perception, because it is suggested that very religious or spiritual people perceive some forms of technological innovation as human beings claiming to play God by exercising power over creation and/or tampering with nature. Whereas Hossain et al. (2003) did not find any relationship between people's religious beliefs and attitudes to food gene technology, they found an inverse relation between levels of religiosity and attitudes towards nanotechnology (Brossard et al., 2009; Scheufele et al., 2009). Vandermoere et al. (2010) further distinguish traditional religiosity (whether the person is member of a church or religious organization), individual religiosity (self-assessed importance of religion in a person life), and spiritual beliefs (belief in good or any sort of spirit). In their study about attitudes towards nanotechnology in food and food packaging in Germany, they found no effect of traditional religiosity and only a minor effect of individual religiosity. They suggest that views on nature and the relationship between human beings and nature mediate the effect of religiosity. In a

7 The New Environmental Paradigm scale was developed to measure proenvironmental beliefs by means of 12 statements and 15 statements in its revised version on which respondents can agree or disagree (e.g. "Plants and animals have as much right as humans to exist."; or : "If things continue on their present course, we will soon experience a major ecological catastrophe.") (Dunlap et al., 2000).

study in Sweden by Sjöberg and Wåhlberg (2002), New Age beliefs, especially the beliefs in paranormal phenomena and higher consciousness, were related to traditional religious involvement and to relatively higher levels of risk ratings with regard to a wide range of environmental and technological hazards.

2.4.4 Socio-Political Factors

This section describes the impact of the socio-political factors social trust, attitude towards science and technology, and political views on risk perception. It first discusses attitudes towards science and technology as a borderline case between being a socio-psychological factor in terms of being classified as a specific value and a socio-political factor.

2.4.4.1 Attitudes towards Science and Technology

Public opposition towards new technologies is discussed in relation to a so-called technological stigma that is related to high levels of risk perception with regard to technology in general (Gregory, Flynn and Slovic, 2001; Haukenes, 2004). Whereas stigmatization of technology might be a social phenomenon, people differ in their attitudes towards technology and science. This is found to be related to differences in attitudes towards diverse technologies and the perception of technological risks. The majority of the studies that investigate this relationship focused on perceptions of biotechnology or gene technology.

According to Urban and Hoban (1997), negative views about technology did explain high levels of risk perceptions with regard to biotechnology. This correlation has been confirmed in a study by Mohr et al. (2007) for the acceptance of genetic engineering. Similar results were found for the application of gene technology in the food domain (Bredahl, 2001; Gaskell et al., 2004; Lähteenmäki et al., 2002; Siegrist, 2003). For instance in the study by Bredahl (2001) that was conducted in Denmark, Germany, Italy and the United Kingdom, general technological attitude was predictive for respondents' attitude towards genetic engineering in food as well as assessments of risks and benefits of genetically modified foods: Positive beliefs about technology were related to a more positive attitude towards genetically modified foods, a lower perception of their risks and a higher perception of their benefits. Similarly, in a study performed in Switzerland by Siegrist (2003), positive views about technology were associated with lower levels of risk ratings and higher levels of benefit ratings with regard to gene technology.

Furthermore, respondents' views about technology and technological progress were important factors in explaining attitudes towards nanotechnology and its risk and benefit assessments (Cobb and Macoubrie, 2004; Macoubrie, 2006; Siegrist et al., 2007). This has also been proven for the application of nanotechnology in the food domain in a study in France (Vandermoere et al., 2009) and in Germany (Vandermoere et al., 2010). In both countries, respondents with a positive attitude towards technology were significantly more likely to have a positive rather than a negative attitude towards food nanotechnology.

Moreover, in the above-cited study by Siegrist (2003), a pro-technology attitude was related to lower risk ratings of technological food risks such as food irradiation, antibiotics in food or genetically modified foods.

2.4.4.2 Political Views

Only a few studies investigated the role of political leanings for levels of risk perception. In a study by Flynn, Slovic and Mertz (1994), the subgroup of white males that were found to rate all hazards as smaller risks compared to other respondents was also found to be more politically conservative than the remaining sample. Similarly, in the study by Dosman, Adamowicz and Hrudey (2001) in Canada, politically conservative respondents rated risks due to pesticides, food bacteria and food additives as smaller compared to respondents that voted for the reform party. This was also found in Switzerland (Siegrist, 2003), where left-wing political leanings were related to higher levels of technological food risk perception.

2.4.4.3 Trust

Research indicates that social trust is an important factor in explaining differences in people's attitude towards technologies and the evaluations of its risks (Slovic, 1993; Slovic, 1999). The concept of social trust has its roots in socio-political analysis (Frewer, Scholder and Bredahl, 2003). According to Siegrist, Cvetkovich and Roth's (2000: 354), social trust is "the willingness to rely on those who have the responsibility for making decisions and taking actions related to the management of technology, the environment, medicine, or other realms of public health and safety." Already Starr (1969) proposed that people's trust in the management of risk plays an important role for the acceptance of risks. The negative relationship that is generally found between social trust and risk perception is known as the institutional trust hypothesis, which has been broadly confirmed by several studies for different technological hazards (Earle and Cvetkovich, 1995; Siegrist, 2000; Siegrist, Cvetkovich and Roth, 2000; Viklund, 2003). Several studies examining the assessment of nuclear waste repositories or chemical plants found that people with a trusting attitude towards the authorities managing the technology or plant perceived risks to be lower than people not trusting these authorities (Bord and O'Connor, 1992; Drottz-Sjöberg and Sjöberg, 1991; Freudenburg, 1993; Flynn, Burns, Mertz and Slovic, 1992; Siegrist, Cvetkovich and Roth, 2000). Similarly, the higher level of trust in risk management institutions, companies and science involved in gene technology was related to lower levels of risk perception (Poortinga and Pidgeon, 2005; Siegrist, 1999; 2000) and less opposition towards genetic engineering (Hoban, Woodrun and Czaja, 1992). Furthermore, trust in sources that provide information on hazards was found to result in lower levels of perceived risk (Frewer, Howard and Shepherd, 1996; Peters, Covello and McCallum, 1997).

The role of social trust has also been found to be important for the perception of food technologies (Costa-Font et al., 2008 for a review on the factors of genetically modified food acceptance; Eiser, Miles, Frewer, 2002; Frewer, Howard and Shepherd, 1996; Poortinga and Pidgeon, 2005; Siegrist, 1999; Siegrist, 2000; Vandermoere et al., 2010). Vandermore et al., (2009) found that higher levels of trust in governmental agencies increase the likelihood of being supportive for the use of nanotechnology in food-packaging.

According to Luhmann (1989), trust is a means for reducing complexity. According to this hypothesis, it is too time-consuming and complex to assess the pros and the cons in everyday life decision situations. In order to reduce the complex task of responding to risks to a simpler task, people rely on trust in those perceived as being responsible or knowledgeable (Slovic, Fischhoff, and Lichtenstein, 1982; Luhmann, 1989).

This is especially the case when people perceive their knowledge as being inadequate (Siegrist and Cvetkovich, 2000; Earle and Cvetkovich, 1995; Luhmann, 1989; Scheufele and Lewenstein, 2005). Siegrist and Cvetkovich (2000) investigated people's risk and benefit judgments of 25 hazardous technologies and activities and found that negative correlations between trust (limited to questions about trust in authorities regulating each specific technology) and perceived risk were especially strong for hazards for which people indicated to have little knowledge. In the case of lack of knowledge and/or scientific uncertainty about the consequences, evaluating risks and benefits of people is only possible via trust or distrust in those taking the decisions (Japp, 2000; Zinn, 2006b). In this regard, trust is supposed to also have strong emotional components as it is assumed that people trust other people or institutions that are perceived to hold similar salient values. A person's salient values are defined as the person's ideas about the principles and goals that should be followed in a particular situation and that other values might be salient in other situations linked to different meanings for the person (Earle and Cvetcovich, 1995). In order to decide whether or not to trust a person or institution in a particular situation or context, an individual needs proof of the similarity of his or her own salient values and the other person's or institution's salient values. These judgments about salient value similarity and derived trust are however in general an implicit, automatic process based on general agreement and sympathy (Cvetcovich, 1999; Poortinga and Pidgeon, 2004), which is necessary, if trust is to reduce complexity rather than making things more complex (Luhmann, 1989).

3 Gender and Risk Perception

The present chapter gives a detailed overview of the available scientific knowledge on the relationship between gender and/or sex and risk perception. Starting off with a critical assessment of the role of gender in risk research in chapter 3.1, chapter 3.2 presents the empirical results with regard to the impact mainly of sex on risk perception.

3.1 The Role of Gender in Risk Research[8]

There exists a variety of conceptualizations of gender and the relation between sex and gender that are derived from different disciplines such as sociology, psychology or ethnomethodology. Whereas sex is generally used to characterize the biological distinction between femaleness and maleness, gender characterizes the social concepts of femininity and masculinity. Most theorists agree that gender is a system of social practices that produces gender differences and systematic power relations between women and men (Gustafson, 1998).

The most striking difference between conceptualizations of gender can be found in the way gender and especially the relations between sex and gender are defined. In Western society sex is seen as the basis for gender differences. According to the still dominant view, men and women belong to different sex categories based on genetic, anatomic and physiological criteria and these differences are seen as the basis for further behavioral, psychological and social dif-

8 An earlier version of this chapter has been published in German as: Bieberstein, A. (2008). Gendereffekte in der Wahrnehmung von Lebensmittelrisiken: Überblick über und kritische Auseinandersetzung mit geschlechtsspezifischen Unterschieden und Erklärungsansätzen. In: Norman, K. v. und Pesch, S. (eds.): Jahrbuch Junge Haushaltswissenschaft 2007: 85-99 ISBN-10 3-936466-08-4; ISBN-13 978-3-936466-08-9

ferences (West and Zimmerman, 1991). This perspective is shared by biosocial theories that assume a clear distinction between sex and gender, where sex constitutes the limits for the construction of gender (Wharton, 2005).

In this perspective sex, and also race and age, are viewed as ascribed characteristics based on biological items and not influenced by social practices. While concepts of masculinity and femininity may vary across history, so does not the principle of sexual dimorphism.

For other theorists the perception of two sexes is the product of gender distinctions. Connell (1995) and Kessler and McKenna (1978) for example pursue a constructionist approach and deny sexual dimorphism as an objective reality. Sexual dimorphism itself is seen as a social construction, as the process of sex categorization is based on socially agreed upon criteria like genitalia, chromosomes or hormone balance (Wharton, 2005). Here "gender makes women's procreative physiology the basis for a separate (and stigmatized) status, not the other way around." (Lorber, 1991: 356)

There are two important aspects that dominantly influence the role of sex and gender in consumer and risk research: an androcentric perspective and the sameness taboo.

Androcentrism[9] is defined as the practice of defining masculine patterns of life and systems of thought as universal, while considering female ones as deviance. The term has been coined by Charlotte Perkins Gilman by her book "*The Man-Made World or Our Androcentric Culture*" published in 1911 and was especially important for scientific criticism during the 1980s (Gilman, 1911; Gannon, 1999).

Feminist theorists often criticized social research for ignoring gender and thus presenting male experience as universal (Gustafson, 1998). Concerning economic research, this criticism also attacks the neoclassical economic theory with its concept of predefined utility functions that ignored the formation of preferences and thus gender differences in preference formation (Seel, 2004). However, current consumer research and risk perception research is explicitly interested in the formation of attitudes, preferences, and buying intentions, and thus in general takes gender into account. Current research in this field shares the view of feminist theorists who regard gender as "a pervasive filter through which individuals experience their social world, [and thus] consumption activities are fundamentally gendered." (Briston and Fischer, 1993: 519)

However, an androcentric perspective is still dominant even in cases where possible gender differences are considered as is the case in consumer and risk research. As criticized by researchers applying qualitative methods, many quanti-

9 Greek, andro-, 'man, male'

tative studies included risks that were derived from male experiences, and the interrogated women judged these risks higher more because of being less familiar with these risks and less because of general gender differences (Gustafson, 1998). Furthermore, when gender differences in consumer research are presented, it is generally not done gender-neutrally, but suggests that it is women's behavior that deviates from the norm (Briston and Fischer, 1993). This is also the case in risk perception research. Results of gender differences in risk perception are always framed in such a way that it is women who perceive the same risks higher, are concerned by different risks, and ascribe different meanings to some risks. And this is so, even though there exists also studies that show that women are not more risk averse than men (see e.g. for financial risk taking: Schubert et al., 1999).

Research in all disciplines that takes potential gender differences into account is often 'sex difference' research and uses biological sex as an independent variable. This is also the case in most research into gender and risk, especially in research into food risk perception. As a consequence, gender is regarded as an attribute or a sum of stable attributes, as it is the case in individualist approaches in gender theory. Such a research design implicitly suggests that differences between men and women rely on an objective biological basis (Briston and Fischer, 1993). According to Gildemeister and Wetterer (1991) everyday experiences are thus translated into the formation of theory and become the starting point of research, without taking into account that dimorphism itself is the result of its construction. In consequence, an important part of gender theory, namely interactionist and institutionalist approaches, are disregarded. A further consequence of regarding sex as an independent variable is that research is often comparative insofar as it is implicitly assumed that inter-group differences between the group of women and the group of men will be bigger than intra-group differences. According to Hollander and Howard (2000: 340), this comparative approach "may act as self-fulfilling prophecies, predisposing researchers to overlook group similarities and to exaggerate or even elicit information that confirms their preconceptions." Thus other important factors like age, social class and race may be neglected and differences based on gender exaggerated as the assumed inter-group difference demands that "women and men have to be distinguishable."(Lorber, 1991: 1) This is also known as the sameness taboo. As described above, research into risk and gender is dominated by the observation that women in general tend to perceive most risk higher than do men. However, as Davidson and Freudenburg (1996) have shown in their literature review, this is not generally the case, as in some studies the direction of the differences is not consistent and in others, differences are too small to be substantively significant.

3.2 Empirical Evidence on Gender and Risk Perception

The following chapter details the results of previous risk perception studies focusing on the relationship between sex/gender and levels of risk perception. Chapter 3.2.1 presents the results with regard to general technological, environmental and life-style risks, and chapter 3.2.2 focuses on food risk perception.

3.2.1 The Impact of Gender on the Perception of Risk

By now risk research is dominated by the current assumption that women in general perceive many risks higher than men. This is especially the case for technological and environmental risks, where many quantitative studies revealed systematic gender differences, with women being frequently more concerned and less willing to accept risks than men (Brody, 1986; Greenberg and Schneider, 1995; Gutteling and Wiegman, 1993; Kahan et al., 2005; Kasperson et al., 1980; Kleinhesselink and Rosa, 1994; Pilisuk and Acredolo, 1988; Satterfield, Mertz and Slovic, 2004; Siegrist, 1998; Stallen and Tomas, 1988). Notably, earlier risk research showed that fewer men than women were concerned about risks with regard to nuclear power and nuclear waste (Brody, 1994; Kasperson et al., 1980; Kunreuther, Desvousges and Slovic, 1988; MacGreogor et al., 1994; Starr, Langley and Taylor, 2000). Furthermore, Stallen and Tomas (1988) showed women to be more concerned about industrial risks, and several studies indicated similar results with regard to chemical industries and chemical risks in general (Kraus, Malmfors and Slovic, 1992; Slovic et al., 1997; Wester-Herber and Warg, 2002). However, Slimak and Dietz (2006) did not find a gender gap with regard to chemical risk perception. With regard to gene technology, results are generally mixed. In some studies, men were found to be more positive than women (Hoban, Woodrin and Czaja, 1992; Siegrist, 1998), whereas in others, women were more positive about genetic engineering (Evans et al., 1997; Tibben et al., 1993). A study by Siegrist (2000) in Switzerland did not find a significant gender gap with regard to risk perception of gene technology, but found that women evaluated the benefit as lower and trusted institutions using gene technology less than men. Moreover, men are found to be less concerned about risks concerning global warming, climate change and environmental contamination (Eisler, Eisler and Yoshida, 2003; Kahan et al., 2005; Starr, Langley and Taylor, 2000; Stedman, 2004).

Davidson and Freudenburg (1996) reviewed 85 quantitative studies concerning gender and the perception of environmental and technological risks such as nuclear power and waste, gene technology, and environmental contamination. They confirmed the tendency that women show higher concern for technological risks and risks to the environment and that this gender gap is especially strong with regard to nuclear technology and pollution. In all 38 studies investigating nuclear technology and radioactive waste, women exhibited higher levels of concern than men. Furthermore, men were less concerned in 17 of the 19 studies considering other hazards such as toxic chemical waste, groundwater contamination, or genetically engineered organisms, but only in 15 of the 26 studies falling into the category of general environmental concern were women more concerned than men. Davidson and Freudenburg (1996) concluded that gender differences are only consistent and statistically significant in cases where specific risks are addressed or when hazards (even though quite general such as air pollution) are framed as locally effective environmental and health risks. Studies that have taken into account general environmental aspects at the national or even international level got very mixed results, or gender differences were too small to be relevant. More recently, Wiedemann and Eitzinger (2006) analyzed 33 psychometric studies focusing on gender differences with regard to the perception of environmental risks, technological risks and food risks. They found that in 21 of the 33 studies, men were less concerned about the investigated risks, and this gender gap was mostly significant but as already stated by Davidson and Freudenburg (1996) in general quite small.

Other studies investigated people's evaluation of risks such as criminality, car accidents, airplane crashes and fire at home (Brenot, Bonnefous and Mays, 1996; Greenberg and Schneider, 1995; Krewski et al., 2006; Savage, 1993) and life-style risks such as smoking, sunbathing, obesity or unprotected sex (Brenot, Bonnefous and Mays, 1996; Flynn, Slovic and Mertz, 1994; Krewski et al., 2006; Starr, Langley and Taylor, 2000). They found men to rate these risks lower than women. For instance, the study by Krewski et al. (2006) in Canada focused on people's perception of health risks due to the above-mentioned everyday risks and could show that women rated these hazards as higher than did men. In the study by Savage (1993) in the USA, women dreaded the four analyzed hazards airplane and car accidents, fires and cancer more than men, and in the study by Starr, Langley and Taylor (2000) in Australia, women were more likely to perceive most investigated hazards as high risks.

With a focus on risk behavior rather than risk perception, a study by Hersch (1996) in the USA further found men to take higher risks with regard to smoking, not wearing seat belts, tooth-brushing, and checking blood pressure, whereas women less frequently performed physical activities. Byrnes, Miller and Schafer

(1999) conducted a meta-analysis of 150 studies with regard to risk taking and gender. They considered studies investigating self-reported and observed risky behaviors such as smoking, alcohol/drug use, sexual activities, physical activity, and driving, and found that men take greater risks with regard to 14 out of 16 different types of risky behaviors. This tendency is also prevalent in the field of financial decision-making. Women were found to be more risk averse with regard to financial decisions and to perceive risk as higher (Jianakoplos and Bernasek, 1998; Olson and Cox, 2001).This has also been found with regard to contributing to pension assets (Bajtelsmit, Bernasek and Jianakoplos, 1999). A more recent study bridges the two research streams, with one focusing on risk behavior and the other on risk perception: Harris, Jenkins and Glaser (2006) could show women to be less likely to engage in risky behavior concerning gambling (e.g. betting at a horse race), health (such as using sunscreen or wearing a helmet when riding a motorcycle), and recreation (such as mountain climbing), and that this gender gap was mediated by women perceiving the likelihood of negative outcomes as higher and the likelihood of a benefit as lower. Furthermore, women perceived potential negative outcomes as more severe and this partially mediated women's lower likelihood of engaging in risky behavior in gambling and the health domain.

Some of the (fairly few) qualitative studies revealed that women and men do not necessarily worry about the same risks. Larson and Montén (1986; as cited in Gustafson, 1998) for example found that men worry about industrial accidents, whereas women worry more about infectious diseases. Moreover Jacobsen und Karlsson (1996; as cited in Gustafson, 1998) found that men tend to focus on risks around their employment, but women were more concerned about risks concerning the family and other people close to them. Moreover, in a study by Fischer et al. (1991), men were found to be more focused on risks to health and safety, whereas women most frequently mentioned environmental risks. The few qualitative studies that use a constructionist approach and assume that the same risk can mean different things to different people investigate gender differences in the meanings of the same risks (Gustafson, 1998; Jackson, Allum and Gaskell, 2006; Sjöberg, 2000a). In a study by Stern at al. (1993) for example, women seemed to regard nuclear power as primarily an environmental problem, while men perceived it as a mainly scientific and technical matter.

3.2.2 *Gender Differences in Food Risk Perception*

Similar to general risk research, research into food risk perception and gender has been largely dominated by quantitative approaches. A distinction is commonly made between natural (e.g. salmonella, food poisoning), technological (e.g. pesticides, food additives, gene technology), and life-style-related food risks (e.g. high fat diet) (Miles et al., 2004; Roosen, Thiele and Hansen, 2005; Siegrist, 2003).

In a study about the perception of gene technology and other food hazards, Siegrist (2003) found that women showed more concern about natural and technological food risks than men, and in a similar study in England by Miles et al. (2004), men were also less concerned about technological risks, life-style risks, and natural risks (this study also regarded food poisoning etc. as life-style risks). Furthermore, being female was positive related to beliefs in risks of gene technology (a technological food risk) and negative related to beliefs in benefits of gene technology. Whereas results are inconsistent with regard to general gene technology (see above), men are clearly less worried about food gene technology than women. Women were less willing to accept genetically modified foods in the study by Moerbeek and Casimir (2005) and more likely to be highly concerned according to the studies by Krewski et al. (2006), Starr, Langley and Taylor (2000) and Finucane et al. (2000b). Moreover, women were relatively more likely to perceive risks of food gene technology as outweighing the benefits (Hallman et al., 2003).

With regard to pesticides, several studies found that men show less concern than women. In a study by Byrne, Gempesaw and Toensmeyer (1991) pesticide residues were perceived as more dangerous than all other hazards such as irradiation or the use of preservatives, but men were relatively less concerned than women. Similarly, in the studies of Govindasamy et al. (1998), Dosman, Adamowicz and Hrudey (2001), Dunlap and Beus (1992), Knight and Warland (2004), Nayga (1996), and Ott and Maligaya (1989), women exhibited relatively higher concern with regard to pesticide use in food production and were less likely to perceive pesticide use as safe. Furthermore, significantly fewer men were highly concerned about pesticides in food in the study by Finucane et al. (2000b) and by Flynn, Slovic and Mertz (1994). Similar, an investigation in Germany by the German Federal Institute for Risk Assessment in 2009/2010 (Dressel et al., 2010) found that more women than men were concerned about the negative consequences for the environment and human health.

Concerning other technological food hazards such as irradiation, meat from animals that have been raised using antibiotics and hormones, Nayga (1996) found men to be relatively more likely to consider these food production methods as safe. Comparing average risk ratings, women were also relatively more concerned about these three production technologies in a study in the USA by Hwang, Roe and Teisl (2005). However, after running a factor analysis, the authors could show that irradiation and hormones both strongly load on one factor (and also genetic modification), while antibiotics strongly load on another factor. Whereas women were more likely to be highly concerned about the factor comprising irradiation, hormones and genetic modification, men were more likely in the cluster of respondents being highly concerned about antibiotics and pesticides (Hwang, Roe and Teisl, 2005). Similarly, in the two Australian studies by Starr, Langley and Taylor (2000) and Worsley and Scott (2000), more women were highly concerned with regard to food irradiation. In the study by Flynn, Slovic and Mertz (1994) in the USA, more white women than white men rated risks due to food irradiation as significantly higher, and more women perceived this hazard as a high risk than men. In the study by Finucane et al. (2000b) in the USA however, women were more likely to be concerned about hormones and antibiotics in food.

In a study by Buchler, Smith and Lawrence (2010) in Australia and a study by Dosman, Adamowicz and Hrudey (2001) in Canada, as well as in a study in Switzerland by Dickson-Spillmann, Siegrist and Keller (2011), men showed significantly lower risk perceptions for food additives. Similarly, significantly more women were highly concerned about food additives in Australia and New Zealand (Worsley and Scott, 2000). Men were also found to assess the risks due to (chemical) food contaminants (such as dioxin contamination) as relatively lower (Dickson-Spillmann, Siegrist and Keller (2011), Leikas et al., 2007).

In a study about the perception of the 'mad cow disease' in France, Setbon et al. (2005) found that independently of the socio-political context (during and after crisis period), female respondents were more concerned about the investigated 15 health risks (only some of them were food hazards such as food bacteria, chemicals in food). In addition, during the crisis, women perceived the Creuzfeldt-Jakob disease as a higher threat: they predicted a significantly higher number of overall human deaths caused by Creuzfeldt-Jakob disease. Similarly, in a study in England (Harvey, Erdos and Callingor, 2001), in a study in Finland (Leikas et al., 2007), and in a study in Germany (Weikunat et al., 2003), men were less concerned with regard to BSE-related risks.

With regard to natural food hazards, Roosen, Thiele and Hansen (2005) showed that women were significantly more likely to be concerned about natural food risks such as moulds and spoilt foods. In the study by Dosman et al. (2001) in Canada as well as by Knight and Warland (2004) in the USA, women were more concerned about salmonella. Similarly, in Australia Worsley and Scott

(2000) and two US-American studies (Finucane et al., 2000b; Flynn, Slovic and Mertz, 1994) found more women to be highly concerned about bacterial food contamination. Additionally, in the study by Leikas et al. (2007) in Finland, men assessed the health risks due to EHEC-bacteria lower than women. No gender difference was found in the study by Buchler, Smith and Lawrence (2010) in Australia.

Concerning risks of a high fat diet or 'unhealthy' nutrition, results are more mixed. Whereas Knight and Warland (2004) found men to be less concerned about fatty food, women and men did not differ significantly in their risks ratings concerning cardiovascular diseases as a result of a high fat diet in the studies by Leikas et al. (2007) and Worsley and Scott (2000).

More generally, some studies investigated people's general confidence in food and approach to food safety. They found that women are less confident about the safety of food (Berg, 2004; De Jonge et al., 2004; Miles et al., 2004) and perceive food safety in food-shopping as more important (Lin, 1995).

In conclusion, women tend to perceive many food risks higher than do men. This concurs with specific technological and environmental risks and local risks for which a systematic gender gap has been confirmed in the literature review by Davidson and Freudenburg (1996). However, as noted in a study about different kind of health risks (life-style risks, technological risks etc.) Lemyre et al. (2006) noted that the magnitude of the gender gap varies greatly for different types of risks. This is probably also the case for food-related hazards. The first aim of this thesis is thus to provide a systematic review of the literature with regard to food risk perception and possible gender differences in chapter 4, taking into account the size of the gender gap according to different types of food hazards.

3.3 Approaches to Explaining the Gender Gap in Risk Perception

There exist a number of hypotheses trying to shed light onto and explain the gender gap in risk assessment. One of the earlier hypotheses referring to biological explanations suggests that women are more concerned about (health) risks as they give life and tend to be the ones responsible for raising children (Steger and Witte, 1989). Biological explanations referring to reproduction and caregiving have however been criticized and refuted by studies focusing on socio-political reasons or gender role explanations (Davidson und Freudenburg, 1996; Flynn, Slovic and Mertz, 1994; Gustafson, 1998; Slovic, 1999). Today, this biological explanation is generally framed in terms of differing roles due to different underlying socialization processes of women and men. That women and men are socialized to different social roles is especially evident within occupational structures and division of labor, where for a long time women have been assigned the role of the caregiver and discouraged in their access to technological and scientific domains (Blocker and Eckberg, 1989).

Some authors presented, discussed and in some cases tested some hypotheses that help to take a first look behind the scenes of gender differences in risk perception (Davidson und Freudenburg, 1996; Flynn, Slovic, and Mertz, 1994; Gustafson, 1998; Slovic, 1999). These hypotheses are subsumed in the following under 'social roles and gender roles', 'familiarity hypothesis', 'power and status' and 'gender inauthenticity', and are discussed against the background of general theories of gender.

3.3.1 Social Roles and Gender Roles

Many authors suggest that gender differences in risk perception can be attributed to different social roles for men and women in society (gender roles) (Davidson and Freudenburg, 1996; Eagly, 1987; Howard and Hollander, 1996; Slovic, 1999). While some scientists focus more on women's general socialization to care, nurture and maintain life (Gilligan, 1982; Zelezny et al., 2000), Davidson and Freudenburg (1996) talk more about the effective social roles and everyday activities. Linked to the idea that women are socialized to care, it is suggested that they are more concerned about health and safety issues for their families and the community, which might in turn explain womens' higher levels of perceived risk. In their literature review, Davidson and Freudenburg (1996) reviewed the literature also for the different existent hypotheses underlying the gap in risk assessment. They found that the gender gap in technological and environmental risk perception was (partially) mediated by women's higher sensitivity for health and safety issues in all studies that took health and safety sensitivity into account. They conclude that women systematically express greater concerns for environmental risks as they still have the main responsibility in caregiving and nurturing, and that the less the gendered division of labor is prevalent in a household, the less likely are gender differences in risk perceptions. A similar finding is reported by Bord and O'Connor (1997): Men compared to women indicated significantly lower levels of concern for two environmental problems, global warming and hazardous chemical waste sites. However, when they included 'health-risk perception' with regard to the two hazards, the gender effect disappeared. Similarly, men's more positive attitude towards gene technology in food was related to their relatively lower levels of concern about long-term health effects in Qin and Brown (2007). Despite these consistent findings, results from studies considering race and gender strongly question the hypothesis that women's stronger sensitivity is related to caregiving responsibilities. Socialization for nurturing and caregiving cannot explain why white males differ from non-white males, non-white women and white women in the levels of risk perception (Flynn, Slovic and Mertz, 1994). This is further discussed in section 3.3.3.

Very similar to this hypothesis is an explanation derived from the 'economic salience hypothesis', according to which men are socialized economically to care for the family and to be the 'breadwinner' (Blocker and Eckberg, 1989; Davidson und Freudenburg, 1996; Gilligan, 1982). This hypothesis builds on a negative relationship between caring for the environment on the one hand and economic issues on the other hand. It would explain why men, who are often still the primary breadwinners of private households, concentrate on economic issues. Another hypothesis close to the 'gender role hypothesis' suggests that traditional gender roles are intensified by parenthood. It assumes that women becoming mothers take even more caregiving activities relative to men and men as fathers focus even more on their role as breadwinners. This is why women in their role as mothers are even more concerned about environmental risks.

Some quantitative studies that investigated the influence of socioeconomic variables on risk perception included not only the variable 'sex' but also variables such as the level of employment, level of household work activities, number and age of children, and level of child-rearing involvement etc. Results do not show a consistent picture, with some studies finding significant influences of these variables and others not. In a study investigating the determinants influencing an individual's attitude towards the importance of food safety in grocery shopping, Lin (1995) found that people who were employed full-time or part-time perceived food safety issues as less important than people who were fully committed to household work activities. In the above-cited study by Roosen, Thiele and Hansen (2005) a negative relation was found between household work responsibilities and the probability of being concerned about natural food risks, but a positive correlation with the probability for being worried about technical food risks. In Dosman, Adamowicz and Hrudey (2001), however, the level of housework responsibility did not significantly influence the perception of natural and technical food risks.

Concerning the 'parenthood effect', results are also mixed. Whereas Dosman, Adamowicz and Hrudey (2001) found no significant influence of the level of child-rearing activities, they revealed that, with increasing number of children in the household, health risk perceptions of the respondents increase especially concerning food additives. Moreover, according to Hamilton (1985), the age of the children also plays an important role, and respondents with younger children are shown to be more worried about environmental risks. Furthermore, Davidson and Freudenburg (1996) in their literature review found that most studies investigating parenthood effects were able to confirm mother effects; no single study was able to reject it, but they were not able to find verification for the existence of father effects.

3.3.2 Familiarity Hypothesis

The 'familiarity hypothesis', also known as the 'knowledge deficit hypothesis', suggests that knowledge about science and technology or about hazards relate to lower levels of risk assessment with regard to technological risks. In other words, for a long time, lay people's inability to understand complex scientific information has been seen as a reason for the gap between expert and lay risks judgments (Bettman et al., 1987; Cross, 1998). Related to this hypothesis, some authors suggest that men are more familiar with science and technology or particular hazards, and this mediates the gender gap in risk perception (Slovic, 1999). Whereas some studies found that women indicated relatively less familiarity with issues of science and technology (Bieberstein et al., 2011; Bord and O'Connor, 1997; European Commission, 2006), results did not support the negative relationship between risk perception and knowledge (Hoban, Woodrum and Czaja, 1992; Schan and Holzer, 1990) or did not mediate the gender gap in risk assessment (Bieberstein et al., 2011). Studies that compared risk evaluations of male and female scientists found, similar to investigations with lay people, men to be less likely to perceive the investigated chemical risks as moderate or high risks (Slovic et al., 1997) and found men to show lower risk ratings with regard to nuclear technologies (Barke, Jenkins-Smith and Slovic, 1997). In the study by Savage (1993), women dreaded hazards linked to plane accidents, fire at home, car accidents, and stomach cancer more than men and this was not related to lower levels of knowledge. Furthermore, even though some studies reported a positive relationship between self-assessed knowledge and actual knowledge (see for instance Cole et al., 2010), gender differences in self-assessed knowledge with regard to science and technology are also probably due to a gendered construction of science and technology (Faulkner, 2000; Fox and Keller, 1985; Henwood, Parkhill and Pidgeon, 2008) that leads women to underreport their scientific knowledge regardless of actual knowledge levels.

3.3.3 Power and Status

Other important hypotheses are derived from the widely known study by Flynn, Slovic and Mertz (1994) about gender, race and risk perception. They found that gender differences can be explained by differences in levels of power and control, taking socio-political factors into account.

They investigated data on the perception of environmental health risks of 1275 white and 214 non-white persons and found that gender differences can only be found between white women and white men and not between non-white women and non-white men. Only the risk perception of white men differed significantly from the other three groups insofar as the group of white men perceived risks as smaller and were more willing to accept risks. When they analyzed the group of white men more closely, they found that the lower average of risk perception in the white male group was due to about 30 percent of them who perceived the hazard items as extremely low risks. The other 70 percent of the white male group judged the risk items similar to the other subgroups. Furthermore, the white male subgroup with extremely low risk perception had higher education, was more conservative and had anti-egalitarian attitudes, higher levels of societal trust and higher incomes. From this finding they derived the hypotheses that risk perception is linked to power. They suggest that white males perceive lower risks, as they are predominantly the ones who are involved in decision-making, controlling and managing of public life activities. Out of their position of power they have more trust in institutions as they manage these institutions, and they benefit more from new technologies. Similarly, Marshall (2004) investigated the 'white male' effect in a strongly polluted area and found that differences between women and men and between whites and non-whites are mainly caused by extremely low levels of risk ratings among white males and extremely high levels of risk ratings among non-white females.

Based on these results, socio-political factors such as power, social trust, and status, but also value orientations are put forward as important determinants in risk perception and acceptance.

3.3.3.1 Social Trust

According to the 'institutional trust hypothesis', social trust is negatively related to levels of risk perception and has been empirically confirmed by several studies (Earle and Cvetkovich, 1995; Siegrist, 2000; Siegrist, 2002; Visschers et al.,

2007). According to Siegrist (2000) and Earle and Cvetcovich (1995), individuals who want to decide whether or not to trust a person or institution in a particular situation or context make a judgment about the similarity between their own salient values and the other person's or institution's salient values. Value similarity and thus trust is supposed to link people with common social identities together (Poortinga and Pidgeon, 2004). Gender is one of the most important social identities. This might have important consequences especially with regard to the assessment and acceptance of technological risks. As public authorities, especially those involving science and technology but also politics, are stereotypically perceived as male-dominated (Faulkner, 2000), it might be that values of men relative to women are more consonant with the practice and ideology of institutions that are responsible for the management of technological risks (Bieberstein et al., 2011). And indeed, according to the literature review by Davidson and Freudenburg (1996), the level of social trust can be assumed to be a significant reason for the gender differences in environmental concern and risk perception. They report that in many studies, men were found to have higher levels of trust in institutions involving public authorities, science and technology, which in turn leads to men's relatively lower risk ratings with regard to environmental and technological hazards. Furthermore, Siegrist (2000) showed men to have relatively higher levels of trust in institutions and authorities responsible for genetic engineering, and this partly mediated the gender gap in levels of risk perception with regard to gene technology. However, Siegrist (2000) did not find any differences between women and men in the causal model explaining the relation between risk perception, benefit perception, social trust, and acceptance of gene technology. Trust in science and research did not mediate the gender gap in food nanotechnology risk perception in a study in Germany (Bieberstein et al., 2011). But the same study suggested a different causal relationship between self-assessed knowledge, social trust and risk perception for women and men: regardless of levels of knowledge, trust was an important determinant of risk perception for women, while for men the importance of trust for levels of risk perception varied with knowledge levels. According to Luhmann (1989), trust is a means of reducing complexity and becomes especially important when people perceive their knowledge as being inadequate in a given situation (Siegrist and Cvetkovich, 2000; Earle and Cvetkovich, 1995). Assuming lower levels of self-assessed knowledge by women, they hypothesized that women would rely more strongly on trust in institutions and public authorities for their evaluations of risks that could be confirmed in food nanotechnology.

In the above-cited study by Qin and Brown (2007) investigating determinants of attitude towards food gene technology, the authors suggest that women's higher levels of trust in environmental groups is linked to their more negative attitude towards gene technology in food. Their study points to the question of who holds power in society. Whereas institutions involving science and technology as well as politics are perceived as male-dominated (Faulkner, 2000), environmental groups are often headed by women. Similar to this and related to trust and the underlying value similarity between institutions managing technological hazards and the population, men seem to perceive themselves as better represented by the practices and values of these institutions. Frewer (1999) for instance found that women were more likely to demand more public involvement in the risk management process whereas in Flynn, Slovic and Mertz's (1994) study, the 30 percent of white males with low risk judgments had a negative attitude towards public involvement in decision processes.

3.3.3.2 Benefit Perceptions and Perceived Vulnerability to Risk

Related to the idea of unequal power relations and mainly white males holding influential positions in politics and industry, Flynn, Slovic and Mertz (1994) further suggested that (white) men as a consequence benefit more from various technologies or perceive these technologies as economically profitable (Marshall, 2004) and thus perceive risks as lower. And indeed, Alhakami and Slovic (1994) found that people's risks and benefits ratings are interdependent and the perception of benefits has a strong influence on people's acceptance of risks. Moreover, in a study by Siegrist (2000), women perceived benefits of gene technology as lower, and according to a study by Frewer, Howard and Shepherd (1996), gender differences in the acceptance of gene technology disappeared when respondents were confronted with specific applications and their benefits. In addition, it is further assumed that perception of low personal benefits in combination with a perception of being affected by the potential harm of a hazard or a technology is responsible for differences in risk perception (Marshall, 2004). Perceived vulnerability and exposure was found to be lower for men than for women in the study by Savage (1993). Furthermore, in the study by Bord and O'Connor (1997), gender differences in expected health risks explained the gender gap in environmental risk perception.

A hypothesis linked to the idea of unequal power relations and perceived vulnerability is derived from criminology studies that suggest that women are socialized to worry and to perceive the world as a risky place (Baumer, 1978; Riger, Gordon and LeBailly, 1978). From early childhood onward, women are subject to warnings regarding sexual violence by their social environment, leading to their increased sensitivity to risk. This fear of violence is often seen as a form of social control and male dominance over women (Gustafson, 1998) that may lead women to perceiving themselves as vulnerable in many domains of life.

3.3.4 Values and Worldviews

As outlined in chapter 2.4.3, values and worldviews are important factors for people's perceptions of risks and technology acceptance, and especially studies about the so-called 'white male effect' have become prominent for giving further insights into the interaction between gender and worldviews with regard to their role in risk perception. Based on the findings by Flynn, Slovic and Mertz (1994), further evidence for the so-called 'white male' effect was provided some years later in the US study by Finucane et al. (2000b). Similarly to the first study, significantly fewer white males rated every hazard as highly risky and mean risk ratings of the white males significantly differed from the ones by white females, non-white females and non-white males. Also, non-white females were found to rate many of the interrogated hazards highest compared to the other groups. This study further considered questions on worldviews and trust and showed that white males were more likely to endorse 'hierarchical' and 'individualistic' worldviews and were found to give less support to 'egalitarian' and 'fatalistic' worldviews than the other groups. White males further reported higher trust towards technology management. Palmer (2003) could replicate the 'white male' effect for technological and health risks, but not for financial risks. She investigated risk ratings of Taiwanese-Americans, Caucasians, Hispanic-Americans, and African-Americans considering health risks, technological risks, and financial activities. She found Caucasian males and Taiwanese males to exhibit lower levels of risk ratings than the other groups for technological and health risks, but not for financial activities. However, Taiwanese males often showed similar or lower levels of risk than white males, and both groups were more likely to be supportive of 'individualistic' worldviews and less of 'egalitarian' worldviews. Based on these findings, Kahan et al. (2007) proposed that differences in risk perception based on gender and race are an artifact of people's cultural and gender identities that people try to protect. They assumed that different gender roles are connected to different types of worldviews. For instance, in 'hierarchical' worldviews rights and obligations are organized along the lines of age, gender and race whereas in 'egalitarian' worldviews these ascriptions are less dominant (Rayner, 1992; Kahan et al., 2007). Among other, they investigated the interactive effect of gender and worldviews with regard to the perception of environmental risks and risk due to abortion. They found that with increasing levels of 'hierarchical' worldviews versus 'egalitarian' worldviews, males dismissed environmental risks more than females but no differences exist between women and men with increasing levels of 'individualistic' versus communitarian worldviews. Kahan et al. (2007) explain that acknowledging the existence of environmental risks (such as risks due to nuclear power) questions the power of leading governmental and industrial bodies held by mainly 'hierarchical' white males. As a consequence, these risks pose a threat to the identity of 'hierarchical' males but not 'hierarchical' females, whose gender role is linked to motherhood and domestic activities. An inverse picture emerged with regard to the risk due to abortion. 'Hierarchical' females perceived the risk due to abortion as being stronger compared to 'hierarchical' men, but no differences between 'individualistic' women and men existed. According to their findings, gender differences are thus mainly a product of different roles ascribed to women and men in hierarchical worldviews.

In addition to the effect of 'identity threat', differences in value activation are important. Trying to understand gender differences in environmental concern, Stern, Dietz and Kalof (1993) found that women and men hold the same values, but women more strongly anticipated possible threats that were linked to their values. They showed that women and men did not differ in the importance they put on socio-altruistic, egoistic and biospheric values, but women were more likely to consider an environmental problem as having consequences for personal wellbeing, the wellbeing of society, and nature. Thus for women, socio-altruistic, egoistic and biospheric values are more likely to be activated as a consequence of an environmental hazard. According to Dietz, Stern and Guagnano (1998), people sometimes even behave in contradiction to their values as certain contexts and situations activate other values being pursued in this specific situation. Similarly, Finucane et al. (2000b) found that differences in risk perception based on race and gender varied according to the type of hazard that might be related to risk contexts. In the context of hazards it thus depends what types of values are activated, and this further depends on the type of hazard and context. Regarding food risks, a person's approach to technology, food, and life-style are supposed to be important for understanding a person's perception of food hazards (Roosen, Thiele and Hansen, 2005). These approaches are further embedded in social systems and some of them may be highly gendered such as technology and science.

3.3.5 Gender Inauthenticity

Similar to the idea of 'identity threat' or 'identity-protective cognition' (Kahan et al., 2007; Kahan, 2009a) is the concept of 'gender inauthenticity'. It was introduced to research into technological risk perception by Henwood, Parkhill and Pidgeon (2008) drawing upon work by Fox-Keller (1985) and Faulkner (2000).

According to Faulkner (2000), engineering and science are symbolically associated with 'masculinity'. Hence, certain types of technology are constructed in different ways by some women and men. As a consequence of this gendered construction of science and engineering, men's or women's gender identity is related to science and technology in opposite ways: women would risk 'gender inauthenticity' by expressing technological knowledge and being positive and confident about science and technology, while men risk undermining their masculine gender by being skeptical, mistrusting, and showing lack of technological knowledge (Henwood, Parkhill and Pidgeon, 2008). Theories around the 'identity threat' can be seen as a formulation of the interactionist approaches in gender theory. Interactionist approaches focus on social relations and interactions, which are supposed to be important for the production of gender differences and inequalities. Here people's behaviors vary according to social contexts. According to Wharton (2005), women for example may behave in a caring way in the presence of people who expect women to behave like this or in social contexts where the traditionally gendered division of labor expects women to take caregiving activities. The most familiar interactionist approach is the idea of 'doing gender' by West and Zimmerman (1987) based on ethnomethodological views. For them gender is neither a person's attribute nor the sum of characteristics, nor a role, but gender is "the product of social doings" (West and Zimmerman, 1991: 16). Sex categorization and its largely unquestioned acceptance as natural in Western societies are seen as a social construction itself. 'Doing gender' means creating differences between men and women that in turn reinforce the perception of the naturalness and objectivity of these differences (West and Fenstermaker, 1995). Women's and men's behavior as a consequence of trying to avoid 'gender inauthenticity' can be seen as a consequence of internalized behavioral expectations and a form of 'doing gender' that stabilizes their own gender identity and sex categorization.

The concept of 'gender inauthenticity' is not only important with regard to technology but also in a context of food. Women are found to have a more 'virtuous' relationship towards food (Beardsworth et al., 2002), and food plays an important role in women's health concepts (Fagerli and Wandel, 1999), whereas men judge the role of physical training as more important to health (Setzwein,

2004). Furthermore, concerning food-related work, the division of labor is still strongly gendered, with women playing the primary role in purchase decisions, shopping, and preparing meals (Lake et al., 2006). In the study on trust in food in Belgium, Britain and Norway, Berg (2004) found that women had far more often a reflexive relation to food than men and were more often sceptical or sensible regarding food safety issues. In contrast, men were much more often found in the group of naïve and unconscious consumers regarding food. Thus, similar to engineering and science, interest in food issues is likely to be more compatible with femininity, while men might risk 'gender inauthenticity' when showing too much interest and involvement in food issues. In addition, certain types of food such as sweets or meat are strongly gendered and the selection and avoidance of these types of foods as well as expressed preferences are conscious or unconscious forms of 'doing or undoing gender' (Prahl and Setzwein, 1999).

3.3.6 Gender Differences in Images and Related Emotions

As explained in more detail in chapter 2.2.2.2, people's mental images and related emotions when confronted with a hazard play a dominant role in their evaluation of the hazard. Whereas to my knowledge no study has so far directly analyzed relationships between gender, mental images, emotions and the evaluation of hazards, several studies have found that women are more able to elicit more and stronger images (see Harshman and Paivio, 1987 for a review of these studies), and women seem to experience related emotions more strongly (George, 1999 as cited in Loewenstein et al., 2001). With regard to emotions, Sjöberg (2007) found that women reported higher levels of negative emotions (fear and anger) with regard to nuclear waste, terrorism, mobile phones, and food gene technology, and relatively lower levels of positive emotions.

Furthermore, the study by Leikas et al. (2007) in Finland found that increasing trait anxiety[10] was related to higher levels of food risk assessments only among men, but not among women, but women assessed risks as higher and more likely and showed somewhat higher levels of trait anxiety. In other words, the level of trait anxiety made no difference among women.

10 Trait anxiety is here defined as an individual characteristic that is linked to the tendency of being anxious relatively often.

4 Systematic Literature Review on Gender and Food Risk Perception

This chapter presents a systematic review on gender and the assessment of food risks. After detailing the objectives in section 4.1, the applied methodology is discussed in section 4.2, and results are presented in section 4.3. The chapter ends with a discussion of the findings in section 4.4.

4.1 Objectives

In order to reveal possible patterns with regard to the gender gap in food risk perception, the existing literature was reviewed by means of a systematic review. A systematic review is a literature review that summarizes and systematizes existent literature that is relevant for the research question. It allows an assessment of whether research findings are consistent with regard to direction and magnitude and can be generalized, or whether findings are limited to a subset of population or a specific context (Mulrow, 1994). No meta-analysis was performed as the reviewed literature applied very different ways of data analysis. Finding a set of studies based on similar methodologies would result in a relatively low number of studies for each of the food hazards.

The systematic review aims to help answering the following questions:

- Does a gender gap exist for all kinds of food hazards? (existence)
- Is the gender gap in the evaluation of food hazards especially large/small for some types of food hazards? (magnitude)
- In the case of a gender gap, do always women judge risks as higher, or are there food risks for which men perceive risks as higher? (direction)

4.2 Methodology

This systematic review comprises quantitative studies that examined the relationship between the evaluation of food hazards and gender. In order to analyze the above-mentioned objectives, results of empirical studies were categorized by the specific kind of food hazard or food technology.

The systematic review comprises several steps:

1. Search of literature for relevant studies and
2. Study selection
3. Categorization of the studies according to food hazards
4. Data analysis and interpretation of the results

The basis of this systematic review was an already existent exhaustive sample of studies investigating the effect of gender on the evaluation of various risks that was created during the design and preparation of this study. The aim was to identify as many quantitative studies as possible that analyzed the effect of gender on the evaluation of food hazards in a systematic way. Based on the existing collection of studies, further research was found by means of a snowballing technique using the reference section of identified papers. Moreover, homepages of identified key researchers in the field of (food) risk perception such as Paul Slovic, Michael Siegrist and Lynn Frewer etc. were used in order to gain further information on relevant publications or relevant journals. Similarly, a further search strategy was browsing through journals identified as publishing relevant articles such as 'Risk Analysis', 'Journal of Risk Research', 'Appetite', 'British Food Journal' or 'Personality and Individual Differences' and 'Health, Risk & Society' etc. In addition, by means of a range of search terms such as 'risk perception', 'food hazard', but also using the hazards themselves like 'gene technology' or 'pesticides', several articles were searched in electronic databases (Social Science Citation Index, ECONLIT, PsycArticles). Search for literature was not restricted to food hazards, as there were a couple of articles investigating food hazards and not food-related hazards together. In the beginning key-word groups such as 'gender and risk perception' were also used, but as studies in general include information about respondents' sex and also often report sex-related results in tables without explicitly mentioning these results in the abstract and text, this strategy was only used as a starting point. Additional unpublished work or studies not published in peer-review journals (so-called gray literature), such as the studies of governmental agencies, insurance agencies and dissertations, were searched via the internet in general, by reading-through relevant homepages (such as the homepage of the German Federal Institute for Risk Assessment, or of the European Commission) and by search tools of university libraries. Literature search was performed between March and August 2010 including studies that were published between 1978 and 2010. Altogether, 196 studies that investigated risk perception were found.

Of the 196 studies, 132 studies had to be excluded as they either did not investigate food hazards or did not report any results with regard to gender. Some of the remaining 64 studies investigated the perception of more than one food hazard. While not allowed in meta-analysis since studies investigating several food hazards would have a relatively stronger weight on the results, all data points are included for the systematic review. It was assumed that studies investigating several food hazards might give a more accurate picture of how hazards are perceived in relation to each other, which was considered of interest for this study trying to get a detailed picture of the gender gap in the perception of different kind of food hazards.

Thus, 64 studies including 123 research results were included for the systematic review. Studies were categorized according to type of food hazard, yielding nine different kinds of food hazards: bacteria/moulds, BSE, food additives/contaminants, gene/bio-technology, hormones/antibiotics, irradiation, nanotechnology, pesticides, and unhealthy diet. For 108 of 123 data points, it was possible to group them into one of the mentioned hazards, whereas 10 studies (with 15 results) investigated people's perception of food safety in general terms or indicated results only as a combined factor of several food risks.

Similar to De Silva et al. (2005), studies were categorized in five groups:

1. Women judge the risk as much higher than men (F>>M)
2. Women judge the risk higher than men (F>M)
3. Women and men judge the risk similarly (F≈M)
4. Men judge the risk higher than women (M>F)
5. Men judge the risk much higher than women (M>>F)

In order to be able to take as many studies as possible into account, results from bivariate as well as multivariate analysis are taken under consideration. For the categorization of the studies, differences in mean risk perceptions, percentages, correlation coefficients, as well as coefficients derived from studies using multivariate methods (e.g. regression coefficients, analysis of variance) were used. Differences in mean risk perception, differences in percentages of women and men, correlation coefficients, and regression coefficients had to be significant at the 5% level in order to be taken into consideration for group (1), (2), (4) or group (5). In cases where the gap between the perception of women and men was smaller than 0.05 (mean risk perception or percentage of women/men in high risk groups), or correlation or regression coefficients were between ±0.1 in absolute value or not significant, the studies/data points were classified into group (3). When the gap between perceptions or attitudes of women and men was greater than 0.30 or correlation or regression coefficients were greater ±0.4 in absolute value and significant, results were grouped into group (1) or group (5) respectively. Results from multi-nominal models were grouped by considering proportionate change in odds (odds ratio) or changes in probabilities (if indicated).

Appendix A1 presents the included studies and indicates the grouping of each result. In some cases, the gender gap was significant, but no effect size was indicated. These results were classified in group (2) or group (4) respectively. In Appendix A1 these results are indicated as group (2a) and (4a).

4.3 Results

Most studies were conducted in the USA and Canada and in northern and western European countries. There exist a few studies covering Asian regions such as in China, but in most terms these studies focus on more general questions with regard to risk perception, and used combined risk perception factors including food and non-food hazards. Studies that were included in the systematic review comprise nearly the last two decades and date from 1990 to 2009 (time of data collection)[11]. The majority of the studies investigated respondents' levels of worry or risk ratings with regard to a food hazard by means of Likert scales. In addition, studies that investigated attitude or acceptance of a food technology or in a few cases respondents' general willingness to consume or purchase a product were also considered. This was done in order to be able to consider a broader range of studies and to create a bigger data base. It was assumed that general acceptance or attitude can be regarded as proxies for risk perception or risk per-

11 Literature research included studies that were published between 1978 and 2010, however between 1978 and 1990 no study exists that reported results about the perception of food hazards and gender.

ception also as proxy for general attitude, as scientific evidence on the direction of the influence between attitude and risk perception is not clear. However, studies examining people's willingness to pay for specific products or to avoid a technology were not considered here, as risk perception can be considered as a determinant for willingness to pay rather than a proxy.

Table 3 presents the results of the systematic review. The majority of the results are found for gene technology (27) followed by pesticides (17), food bacteria/moulds (16) and risks due to an unhealthy diet (15). This can be explained by the enormous research interest in investigating public opinions about food gene technology during the last 15 years.

Table 3: Number and Percentage of Studies in Each of the Groups per Food Risk

	(1) F>>M[1]	(2) F>M[2]	(3) F≈M[3]	(4) M>F[4]	(5) M>>F[5]	All
Bacteria/moulds	1 (6.25)	7 (43.75)	7 (43.75)	1 (6.25)	-	16
BSE	-	5 (71.4)	2 (28.6)	-	-	7
Food additi-ves/contaminants	-	10 (90.9)	1 (9.1)	-	-	11
Gene technology	-	19 (70.4)	8 (29.6)	-	-	27
Hormo-nes/antibiotics	-	4 (100)	-	-	-	4
Irradiation	-	3 (75.0)	-	1 (25.0)	-	4
Nanotechnology	-	5 (62.5)	3 (37.5)	-	-	8
Pesticides	-	14 (82.4)	3 (17.6)	-	-	17
Unhealthy diet	-	9 (64.3)	5 (35.7)	-	-	14
General food safety	-	9 (60.0)	5 (33.3)	1 (6.7)	-	15
All	1 (0.8)	85 (69.1)	34 (27.6)	3 (2.4)	-	123 (100)

[1] F>>M Women compared to men perceived risks as much higher

[2] F>M Women compared to men perceived risks as higher

[3] F≈M Women and men perceive risks as similar

[4] M>F Mencompared to women perceive risks as higher

[5] M>>F Men compared to women perceive risks as much higher

Source: Own illustration.

In general, the magnitude of the gender gap is small, with standardized coefficients only once exceeding ±0.4 and small differences in mean risk perceptions or small differences in percentage of women and men indicating that risks are high. Across all types of food technologies or potential food hazards, the majority of the results (85 out of 123 = 69.1%) indicate that women perceive risks as higher or are less willing to accept them than men. Only in three cases (2.4%) (one study investigating worry about food bacteria, acceptance of irradiated beef, and another study investigating risks perception as a combined factor of pesticides and antibiotics), were men found to be more concerned. In 34 of the 123 included results (27.6%), no gender gap exists.

The highest percentage of similar perceptions for women and men are found for food bacteria (43.7%) and risks due to food nanotechnology (37.5%). The gender gap is most consistent with regard to hormones and antibiotics where all study results (100%) indicate women to be more concerned. Also, for food additives/contaminants, 90.9% of the results indicate men to be less worried, followed by pesticides (82.4%), irradiation (75%), BSE (71.4%), and gene technology (70.4%).

The category 'general food safety' classifies studies, that asked about consumers' perception of food safety in general terms or studies that report results concerning a combined factor of several food risks together. In 60.0% of the results women are more concerned, in 33.3% no gender gap exists and in 6.7% men are more concerned than women.

Overall, except for nanotechnology, in 70 to 100% of the results related to technology-based food hazards, women perceived risks as higher than men, whereas with regard to life-style risks such as an unhealthy diet or natural food hazards such as food bacteria, results with regard to women's and men's perceptions are more balanced.

4.4 Summary and Discussion

Similar to the results of the literature review about gender and environmental and technological risk perception by Davidson and Freudenburg (1996), the findings here show a consistent gender gap also in the case of food hazards, with men being mostly less concerned. However, the review by Davidson and Freudenburg (1996) also revealed that gender differences in risk perceptions are only consistent and statistically significant in cases where specific risks are addressed or when they are framed as locally effective environmental and health risks. Food risks, as investigated here, can all be classified as specific and locally effective risks, as opposed to national and global subjects such as food security. Additionally, similar to the findings by Davidson and Freudenburg (1996), the magnitude of the reported gender differences in risk ratings and levels of acceptance are small except for one single case.

Except for the case of nanotechnology, the gender gap is most consistent with regard to technological food hazards, which points to a gendered construction of food hazards especially in the case of technological hazards.

Technological food hazards compared to natural food hazards and lifestyle food hazards are generally the ones that provoke highest concern among consumers (Federal Research Centre for Nutrition and Food, 2008; Miles et al., 2004). Some explanations relate to people's perceptions of greater control and knowledge with regard to natural and lifestyle food risks (Miles et al., 2004). The gender gap seems to be most consistent for the most dreaded hazards in general. Thus, both women and men tend to be worried about the technological food hazards, but overall men in the majority of the studies seem to be somewhat less worried. This is likely to be related to a gendered construction of technology and engineering (Faulkner, 2000) resulting in women's more pessimistic approach to technology in general. And according to the findings by Fox and Firebaugh (1992), women's more negative attitudes towards technology were due to women's relatively lower perceptions of the utility of technology. This might also be the reason in the case of food technology. Furthermore, women seem to have a relatively stronger preference for the naturalness of food, which is perceived as opposed to technology (Lookie et al., 2004).

The case of food nanotechnology is interesting insofar as public knowledge about it can be regarded as rather low (Vandermoere et al., 2010) and people's prior beliefs as well as conceptions of the technology are likely to play an important role. Early attitudes about food nanotechnology are likely to be strongly dependent on people's general attitudes towards science and technology, which can explain the gender gap in the recent stage of low concrete public knowledge about nanotechnology. With increasing public knowledge, the gender gap might be attenuated. On the other hand, it is possible that with increasing public awareness and discussion about food nanotechnology, views become more polarized and initial views are fortified as suggested by Frewer et al. (1998) and Frewer, Scholderer and Bredahl (2003).

With regard to risks due to food contamination, moulds, salmonella or other bacteria, results are more balanced, with a high percentage of the studies indicating no gender gap. As seen above, perceived higher personal control is proposed as reason for consumers' overall lower levels of risk perception (Miles et al., 2004). If this is the case, a less prevalent gender gap may indicate that perceived personal control is more important for women with regard to risk perception in general, or that women perceive personal control stronger with regard to 'natural' food risks compared to 'technological' food risks.

The gender gap with regard to risks due to an unhealthy diet is somewhat less evident than for technological food risks, but still considerable. Here, the often reported stronger focus on health with regard to food by women (Fagerli and Wandel, 1999; Lookie et al., 2002; Setzwein, 2004), as well as a close link between attractiveness and weight especially for young women (Beardsworth et al., 2002; Chaiken and Pliner, 1987), are likely to play a role here.

Moreover, the results of the category 'food safety' are similar to the average distribution of the results in the five groups (see the last row of table 3) which is not surprising as this category includes several studies that considered several food hazards together.

Overall, a consistent gender gap exists also in the case of food hazards, with men being mostly less concerned than women, but differences are rather small and much more prevalent in the case of technological food hazards compared to natural or life-style food hazards.

Limitations of the systematic review are related to a probable underrepresentation of the so-called gray literature. Moreover, even though a comprehensive review including all relevant studies was the basic objective of the systematic review, some relevant studies might be missing. This is due to the fact that empirical risk research is a very dynamic and interdisciplinary field that is published also in journals of very diverse disciplinary background. It is likely that studies that investigated risk perceptions with regard to different kinds of hazards including food hazards have not been found, since these studies did not mention food hazards in keywords, abstracts or headings and might be published in journals outside the social science literature. A clear strength of this review is the rigorous application of a 5% significance level for the results being included as indicating a gender gap, but that also meant that studies that did not report level of significances were excluded from the review.

5 The Means-End-Chain Theory

This chapter outlines the methodological background of the empirical investigation in chapter 6. It describes how people's knowledge structures can be modeled, explains why the MEC theory was selected as basis of the data collection and presents the MEC model in detail.

5.1 Models for Presenting Knowledge Structures

Different models have been developed for presenting knowledge structures. The two most important ones are the model of cognitive or semantic networks (network models) (Quillian, 1968; Anderson, 1983; Grunert, 1990) and the means-end chains (MEC) developed by Gutman (1982) and Olson and Reynolds (1983).

According to network models, knowledge structures are also called schemata. Schemata are abstract, organize cognitive processes and are linked to verbal and visual concepts in memory and can be applied to persons (schemata regarding another person or self-schemata), issues and events (Kroeber-Riel, Weinberg and Gröppel-Klein, 2009; Kuß and Tomczak, 2007). Network models organize schemata in semantic networks that are composed of nodes (=attributes, events, concepts) and linkages connecting the nodes (knowledge as a node-link structure) that show the type and strength of association (Cowley and Mitchell, 2003). They allow explaining the type and form of a present knowledge structure, its development and changes (Trommsdorff and Teichert, 2011).

The MEC theory presupposes that knowledge is organized hierarchically and that the evaluation of a product or an issue is based on its relation to principal life values. Thus its principal assumption is that self-relevant product meanings determine consumer choices (Olson, 1995). Unlike network models, the means-end-chain theory thus aims at uncovering not only people's cognitive structures but also their basic motives. This means that MEC models pursue a twofold view: a cognitive structure view and a motivational view (Grunert and

Grunert, 1995). The MEC theory has been developed for advertising research to explain subjective product perceptions in revealing the relationship between attributes (concrete and abstract attributes) that the consumer associates with a product (the means), via consequences (functional and psychosocial consequenes) perceived by the consumer to the attainment of basic life values (instrumental and terminal values) (the ends) (Gutman, 1982; Olson and Reynolds, 1983). The MEC theory focuses on the relationship between an object in question, e.g. a hazard and the person, and allows us to explore the conscious and unconscious rationales of people's risks evaluations. Network models on the other hand focus on the associative relationships between concepts. Compared to the MEC models, they stay mainly at the attribute level, but in a much more detailed manner. The network models thus present the 'horizontal space' around a concept (hazard), whereas means-end chains represent the 'vertical space'.

This thesis builds on the MEC theory as methodological background as its objective is not only to uncover people's knowledge structures and associative networks with regard to the food hazards, but also to understand consumers' motivational basis with regard to their perception of these food risks. Thus, the MEC theory is described in more detail in the following section.

5.2 Historical Background of the MEC Theory

Current MEC research is mainly based on the models proposed by Gutman and Reynolds (1979) and Olson and Reynolds (1983). They were mainly developed in marketing research to be able to understand consumer decision-making (Olson and Reynolds, 2001). However, these models can be regarded as a further development of former MEC models (Herrmann, 1996; Kliebisch, 2002) which are described in the following paragraph.

The means-end-chain theory is based on work by the social-psychologist Tolman (1932), who was one of the first to be interested in consumer's motives behind the choice of certain products. He was interested in the "why of consumption". Tolman (1932) found the basic idea of the MEC theory that products are the means in order to reach higher life goals and values, the so-called ends (Kliebisch, 2002; Ter Hofstede et al., 1998).

Influenced by the ideas of Tolman, Rosenberg (1956) developed a model of attitude formation. He assumed a relationship between individuals' attitudes towards an object/issue and their beliefs about that object/issue. The model theorizes that individuals' evaluation of an object/issue is a function of two cognitive factors: a) the perceived instrumentality of the object helping to achieve a value and b) the importance of that value (Tuncalp and Sheth, 1975).

The model is operationalized in the following notation:

$$(1) \quad A_{ij} = \sum_{k=1}^{n} x_{ik} * y_{ijk}$$

where

A_{ij} refers to the attitude or affect of individual i towards object j

x_{ik} refers to the relative importance of a value k for individual i, often called value importance

y_{ijk} refers to individual i's perceived probability that the object j supports or blocks the attainment of a value k, often called perceived instrumentality (Kliebisch, 2002).

Due to Rosenberg's focus on cognitive structures determining people's attitudes, his model is often cited as the beginning of the MEC theory (Kliebisch, 2002; Kroeber-Riel, Weinberg and Gröppel-Klein, 2009).

The work by the psychologist Milton Rokeach can be regarded as a further milestone in the development of the MEC theory (Kliebisch, 2002). Rokeach (1973) developed a classification system of values, the Rokeach Value System in order to measure people's values (Solomon et al., 2010). According to Rokeach (1973) a value is "(…) an enduring belief that a specific mode of conduct or end-state of existence is personally or socially preferable to an opposite or converse mode of conduct or end-state of existence (…)." (Rokeach, 1973: 5) People thus use values in order to orient themselves in their environment, as they represent relatively stable concepts and beliefs about preferable end states or behaviors (Grunert and Juhl, 1995; Rokeach, 1973). In addition to this cognitive concept of preferable end states, values also contain an affective and a behavioral component (Rokeach, 1973; Kliebisch, 2002). Rokeach (1973) distinguishes 18 instrumental and 18 terminal values.

Instrumental values are defined as ways of behaving (modes of conduct) that further produce terminal values. Examples of instrumental values are 'acting independent', 'being broad minded' and 'showing self-reliance'. Terminal values are preferred end-states of being that human beings aim to achieve in life, such as 'peace' and 'happiness' (Peter and Olson, 2010; Veludo-de-Oliveira et al.,

2006). The full list of Rokeach's value classification is given in Appendix B 1. Instrumental and terminal values are linked hierarchically with instrumental values being pre-stage to terminal values (Rokeach, 1973; Kuß and Tomczak, 2007).

Furthermore, Rokeach (1973) splits the instrumental values into moral (e.g., tolerant and responsible) and performance-oriented values (e.g., intellectual and logical), and the terminal values into personal (e.g., inner harmony and mature love) and social values (e.g., peaceful world and beauty) (Rokeach, 1973). Referring to Rokeach (1973), Schwartz and Bilsky (1987) made a distinction between values according to their content and their relations to each other, and developed a value classification according to the type of motivational goal the values refer to (Schwartz, 1994). As mentioned above, they propose that all values are derived from three universal goals that refer to needs of individuals as organisms, the requirement of social interaction and the functioning of social groups. These values were further grouped in eleven motivational domains. With the exception of spirituality, which is not culturally universal, these motivational domains can further be organized along two bipolar concepts: the first bipolar concept focuses on the opposition of 'self-enhancement' on the one side and 'self-transcendence' on the other. The second dimension contrasts 'openness to change' and 'conservation value'. Figure 3 illustrates the motivational domains alongside their bipolar conceptualizations.

Figure 3: Motivational Domains of the Schwartz Value Survey

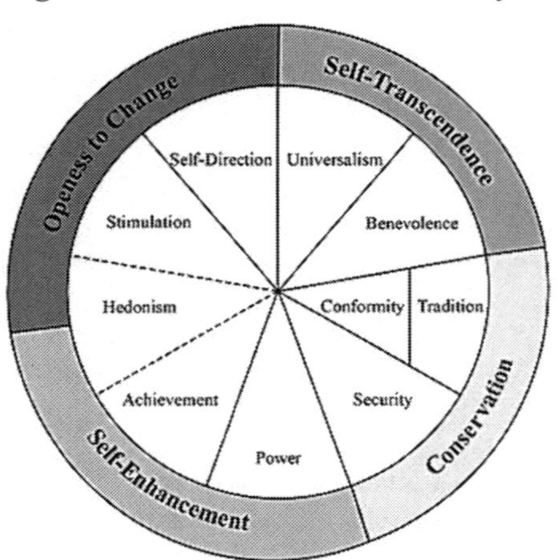

Source: Schwartz (1992): 45.

Additionally, based on the idea of hierarchically organized values by Rokeach (1973), Howard (1977) developed a model to explain the relationship between values, attitudes and the choice of product classes and brands. Whereas the choice of product classes is determined by terminal values, instrumental values are responsible for the choice of brands. Similarly, Vinson, Scott, and Lamot (1977) model the relationship between values and attitudes/evaluations, but make a distinction between global and domain-specific values: global values are central and stable beliefs not dependent on the situation or context, whereas domain-specific values are more dynamic and refer to different domains in people's life such as consumption or social life (Kliebisch, 2002).One of the first attempts to link product characteristics with people's benefit perception of that product was made by the advertising practitioners Young and Feigin (1975). They developed a paper-and-pencil interview procedure that can be regarded as an early version of the hard-laddering method used to construct MEC with large samples (Botschen and Thelen, 1998). On the basis of this interview procedure, Young and Feigin (1975) elicited product-related and psychological or emotional benefits (Kaciak and Cullen, 2005) and constructed the so-called *Grey Benefit Chain,* which presents the most important benefits chains people link to a specific product in question.

5.3 The MEC Model of Gutman and Reynolds (1979) and Olson and Reynolds (1983)

The most commonly used MEC model is based on approaches by Gutman and Reynolds (1979), further developed by Gutman (1982) and Olson and Reynolds (1983). Its objective is to theoretically model the relationship between consumer behavior and their values (Veludo-de-Oliveira, Akemi and Cortez, 2006). Based on the model of Howard (1977), Gutman and Reynolds (1979) proposed a third variable mediating between the product attributes and people's values that they called 'function' or 'benefit'. Gutman (1982) called this mediator the 'consequences' and thus formed the basic model of an MEC chain with three levels of abstraction: the attributes, the consequences, and the values. Hereby, consumers evaluate product attributes according to their consequences that in turn help to achieve life values. The basic MEC model is presented in Figure 4.

Figure 4: Basic Model of an MEC

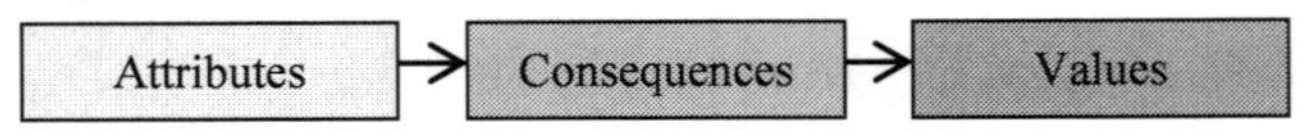

Source: Gutman (1982); Olson and Reynolds (2001).

The MEC model does not consider the product attributes as relevant in themselves, but links their relevance to consumer's perceptions that they lead to desired consequences, which in turn enhance the consumers' personal values. Thus, the model helps to describe how and why products are important in people's lives as consumers choose products that are linked to desirable consequences that lead to their life goal and values (Gutman, 1982, Claeys, Swinnen and vanden Abeele, 1995; Nielsen, Bech-Larsen and Grunert, 1998; Olson and Reynolds, 1983). According to Gutman (1982), the MEC theory is based on four assumptions about consumer behavior:

a. Values, defined as desirable end-states of existence have a strong impact on an individual's decision making
b. People group objects/products into classes according their ability to satisfy their values
c. Every action leads to a consequence
d. Individuals learn that a specific action leads to a specific consequence (Gutman, 1982)

During the last 30 years, two different approaches to the MEC theory have arisen that complement rather than exclude each other (Costa, Dekker and Jongen, 2004; Grunert and Grunert, 1995):

The *motivational perspective* is based on classical approaches aiming at understanding consumer's motivations behind their choices and very closely linked to motivation research.

The *cognitive-structure view* proposes that MECs are excerpts of consumers' cognitive structures (Hermann, 1996) that are relevant in consumption situations. It is assumed that MECs model the organization of consumers' consumption-related knowledge and make it possible to show which parts of the cognitive structures are activated in specific situations (Grunert and Grunert, 1995; Köhler and Junker, 2000).

In both perspectives, an MEC is considered as consumers' knowledge about attributes, consequences and values that are distinguished according to different levels of abstraction and organized hierarchically from lower to higher abstraction levels, with attributes being the most concrete and tangible, and values being the most abstract concepts (Olson and Reynolds, 1983; Olson and Reynolds, 2001).

Following the ideas of Gutman and Reynolds (1979) and Gutman (1983), Olson and Reynolds (1983) proposed a finer distinction with regard to the levels of abstraction and therefore a more complex MEC with six chain levels (Botschen, Thelen and Pieters, 1999). They recommend distinguishing between concrete and abstract attributes, functional and psychosocial consequences, and between instrumental and terminal values:

Concrete and abstract attributes

"Attributes are perceived qualities or features of products or services." (Reynolds and Olson, 2001: 93) They are at the lowest abstraction level in the MEC and are the most concrete characteristics of products or services (Ter Hofstede et al., 1998), including physical and abstract properties. As already mentioned, attributes are distributed along a continuum starting from concrete to more abstract ones (Lin, 2002). Concrete attributes refer to perceptible physical, chemical or technical characteristics of a product such as price and color (Olson and Reynolds, 1983; Vriens and Hofstede, 2000). Abstract attributes on the other hand are the more abstract and less tangible features of products such as style or perceived value (Botschen et al., 1998; Reynolds and Olson, 2001).

Functional and psychosocial consequences

Consequences reflect what a product or service can (or cannot) provide for the consumer based on the product's/service's attributes (Gengler, Mulvey and Oglethorpe, 1999; Ter Hofstede et al., 1998) and explain why a consumer evaluates an attribute positively or negatively (Reynolds and Whitlark, 1995). Desirable consequences are benefits that the consumer tries to gain when choosing a product, whereas undesirable consequences constitute risks consumers try to avoid (Peter and Olson, 2010). Consequences are less directly perceptible, but are a result of purchasing, choosing and consuming the product and thus associated with a combination of several attributes (Olson and Reynolds, 2001; Gutman, 1982; Vriens and Hofstede, 2000).

Whereas functional consequences are in generally directly experienced after the consumption or choice of the product (Olson and Reynolds, 2001; Valette-

Florence and Rapacchi, 1991), such as convenience and taste, psychosocial consequences are produced by the former ones. Psychosocial consequences have a stronger emotional aspect specifying why the functional consequence is of importance for the consumer and relates to how a product makes the consumer feel (Peter and Olson, 2010). For instance, wearing a certain kind of jeans that fits very well might make the consumer feel more attractive, which is related to a psychological consequence. On the other hand, psychosocial consequences also relate to social consequences focusing on the relation of the consumers with other people, such as being respected or liked by others.

Instrumental and terminal values

Values are people's principal life goals and needs (Valette-Florence and Rapacchi, 1991; Ter Hofstede et al., 1998). They are the highest-order goals people try to achieve in their lives and thus guide people's decisions and behavior (Valette-Florence and Rapacchi, 1991). They are considered to be relatively stable (Vries and Hofstede, 2000) and are at the highest, most abstract level in the chain. Values are regarded as intangible and subjective.

As already seen in section 5.2 values are classified in different ways. In relation to the MEC theory Rokeach's (1973) distinction between instrumental and terminal values is usually applied.

5.4 The Relationship between the Self, Situation and Involvement

Whereas in the beginning the sole focus of MEC theory was to describe consumers' product and brand perceptions, Walker and Olson (1991) showed that an MEC may also reveal the relationship between consumers' product knowledge and self-knowledge, insofar as they regarded the end (the psychosocial consequences, the instrumental values and the terminal values) of an MEC as consumers' self-schema, and the means (the concrete attributes, the abstract attributes, and the functional consequences) as consumers' product knowledge. This relationship is depicted in Figure 5. According to Walker and Olson (1991), a consumer's self-knowledge or self-schema is a network of interrelated meanings about oneself (self-meanings), which are organized hierarchically in memory.

Figure 5: Relationship between Product Knowledge and Self Knowledge

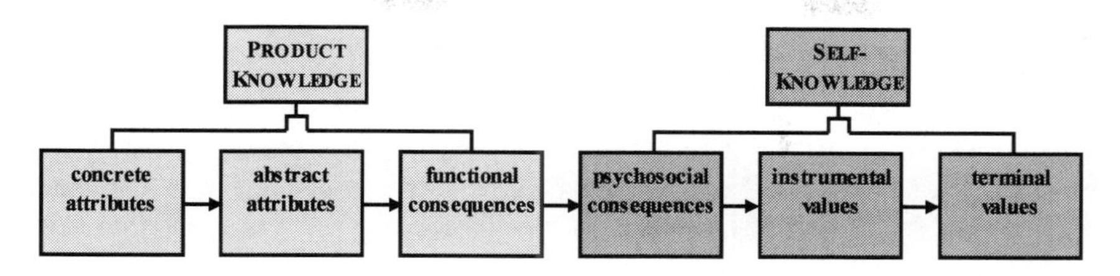

Source: Walker and Olson (1991: 112).

The self-schema includes different kinds of self-related knowledge such as body image (beliefs about one's body), knowledge about one's behavior, episodic knowledge (knowledge about life events), and concepts about one's goals and values (Peter and Olson, 2010; Markus and Nurius, 1986). Furthermore, people have multiple selves that are associated with different social roles, such as the working self or the parent self (Walker and Olson, 1991). These self-meanings form a person's identity and influence a person's behavior across different situations. At the highest level of abstraction are a person's values, which Walker and Olson (1991) defined as being part of an individual's 'core' self. They further assume that while the basic values that a person holds are relatively stable, different aspects of a person's self-schema are activated in different situations (Walker and Olson, 1991). That means that knowledge that is related to a specific social role is only activated and thus relevant in some situations but not in others. Hence, the ends in an MEC represent the activated aspects of consumers' self-schema determined by the choice situation or stimuli. And only these activated self-meanings influence consumers' behavior in that specific choice situation. In other words, the decision situation critically determines which parts of the self-schema are activated in working memory and influence people's choices (Kihlstrom and Cantor, 1984; Reynolds and Whitlark, 1995; Walker and Olson, 1991).

The part of an individual's self-schema that is activated is strongly related to the individual's involvement regarding the situation or product (Celsi and Olson, 1988). Involvement is a motivational state that refers to people's perceptions of relevance or importance with regard to an object, event or action. It exerts a strong influence on consumers' behavior (Kapferer and Laurent, 1985; Krugman, 1966; Mitchell, 1979; Richins and Bloch, 1986; Rothschild, 1975), since involvement determines consumers' affective and cognitive processes

(Peter and Olson, 2010; Sørensen, Grunert and Nielsen, 1996). The cognitive basis of involvement is linked to people's MEC knowledge about the important consequences and values associated with the product or event in question and the strength of the relationship between product knowledge and self-knowledge (individual's needs, goals and values) (Celsi and Olson, 1988). In the study by Walker and Olson (1991), they found that consumers' involvement was greater in the choice situation where consumers' self-related knowledge was activated. Thus consumers' involvement regarding a situation or product depends on how strongly the product knowledge is connected to central aspects of the consumers' self (Celsi and Olson, 1988; Fotopoulos, Krystallis and Ness, 2003). Furthermore, the affective aspect refers to people's affective responses such as emotions and feelings linked to the activated MEC knowledge. Whereas the activation of relatively unimportant consequences is linked rather to weak emotions, the elicitation of strongly self-relevant values is accompanied by strong emotional reactions (Celsi and Olson, 1988; Peter and Olson, 2010). To sum up, involvement towards a product or event is expressed in the extent that self-relevant consequences and values are activated and in the strength of consumers' affective reactions to it.

Based on the work by Bloch and Richins (1983) and Celsi and Olson (1988), Peter and Olson (2010) developed a model of consumer involvement. An extract of their model is shown in Figure 6.

Figure 6: Antecedents of Consumer Involvement

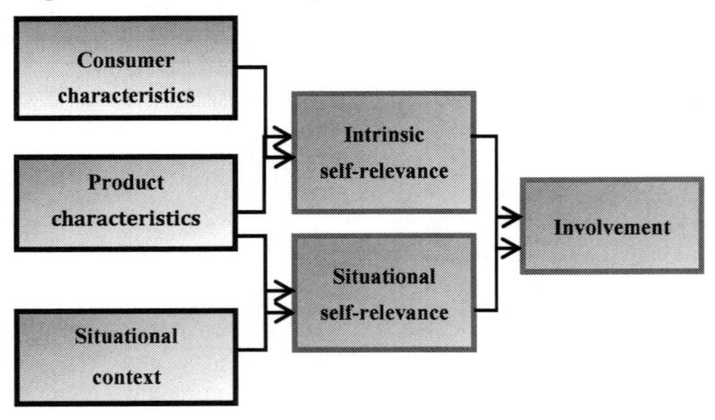

Source: Adopted from Bloch and Richins (1983); Peter and Olson (2010).

Involvement is determined by 'intrinsic self-relevance' and 'situational self-relevance'. Both are responsible for the activation and generation of MEC linking product knowledge with self-knowledge. 'Intrinsic self-relevance' is a factor of consumer characteristics and product attributes. Consumer characteristics include people's values, goals or personality traits, and social roles. These individual characteristics affect what kind of product/event-related consequences and values are perceived as important (Bloch and Richins, 1983). With regard to the product characteristics (such as price, color, perceived risks and benefits), perceived risks of products are supposed to strongly increase consumers' involvement, according to Peter and Olson (2010).

Product characteristics also determine the 'situational self-relevance' (Celsi and Olson, 1988; Peter and Olson, 2010). The 'situational self-relevance' is further influenced by the situational context. The situational context refers to the physical environment such as temperature, the way a product is presented or a sales promotion as well as social environment such as the presence of friends when doing shopping. The situational variables activate relevant MEC only temporarily as they are dynamic and subject to frequent change. In contrast, 'intrinsic self-relevance' relates to people's stored knowledge in long-term memory that is built on past experiences and fairly constant. This knowledge refers to people's knowledge about the relationship between objects/events and their ability to provide important self-relevant consequences and to meet consumers' core values (Celsi and Olson, 1988). It is assumed that more involved consumers have a stronger motivation to process information, often a higher level of knowledge, and have more complex knowledge structures than less involved consumers (Celsi and Olson, 1988; Grunert and Grunert, 1995; Mulvey et al., 1994; Petty, Cacioppo and Schumann, 1983). Based on this, it is assumed that for highly involved consumers more information is activated with regard to an object/event, which is expressed in a higher number and different kinds of attributes (Lastocicka and Gardner, 1978; Sørensen, Grunert and Nielsen, 1996).

Furthermore, high involvement is linked to the activation of MECs with a higher proportion of more abstract elements such as 'psychosocial consequences', 'instrumental values' and 'terminal values' compared to the product-related elements such as 'concrete and abstract attributes' and 'functional consequences' (Sørensen, Grunert and Nielsen, 1996). Hence, the strength expressed in the number of cognitive links between the attributes to the consequences and values is likely to vary with involvement. Moreover, it is assumed that the shorter the path between a less abstract concept such as an abstract attribute and a higher order element such as an instrumental value in the MEC, the more important this attribute is for the consumer. In other words, an abstract attribute is more important when it is directly linked to an instrumental value without intermediation through other elements (Bech-Larsen and Nielsen, 1999; Gutman, 1982).

This idea can be related to the spreading-activation theory according to Anderson (1983) that explains the retrieval of stored information. As explained in section 5.1, knowledge is stored in the form of a hierarchically organized network of associations among concepts. When a concept is processed in the working memory, information can be retrieved in the long-term memory by spreading activation (Anderson, 1983). This means, that when the activation of the first concept is strong enough, it is transferred to the related concept (Cowley and Mitchell, 2003). Thus, the shorter the path from an attribute to an important consequence or value the higher is the probability that this consequence or value will be retrieved.

Generally, food shopping behavior is regarded as an activity of low involvement, as it is considered as an everyday decision based on habits (Grebitus, 2008). However, due to the emergence of several food scandals during the last 15 years and increasing consumers' interest in healthy food-styles, consumers' involvement with regard to food hazards might be relatively high. Furthermore, as mentioned above, the perception of risks is assumed to strongly increase people's level of involvement (Peter and Olson, 2010).

6 Uncovering Women's and Men's Cognitive Structures: an MEC Approach

Against the background of the systematic review of the results of quantitative studies about gender and judgments about food hazards presented in chapter 4, this section further investigates consumers' knowledge structures that underlie consumers' assessments of food hazards.

6.1 Background and Objectives

The aim of this chapter is to investigate whether women and men attach different meanings to food hazards. For this purpose three different kinds of food hazards were selected. Based on the findings regarding the pattern of the gender gap as well as the findings in previous studies suggesting a natural-technological distinction (Roosen, Thiele and Hansen, 2005; Siegrist, 2003), a natural food hazard (mycotoxins) and a technological food hazard (pesticides) were selected. As the third hazard, a less well-known food technology – irradiation – was chosen. Previous research, indicate that people make sense of unknown things by relating it to more known things (Visschers et al., 2007). It was assumed that the more unknown an issue, the more important become general attitudes and values for people's judgments about the issue. Thus, gender stereotypes expressed in differences in general attitudes, e.g. with regard to technology, or in the approach to food might be especially important in the case of an unknown food hazard.

Moreover, all three selected hazards are among the food hazards that are perceived as relatively risky in relation to others in Germany according to a study by the Federal Research Center for Nutrition and Food (2008). In this study, respondents ranked pesticides at the top of 14 interrogated food hazards, with 77.6% of the respondents assessing pesticides as the riskiest food hazard. Similarly, in a study of the Federal Institute for Risk Assessment (Dressel et al.,

2010) about German consumers' perception of pesticides, 80 % of the respondents evaluated pesticides as a high or very high risk. Mycotoxins were placed at rank five (with 65.8% assessing risks due to mycotoxins in food as severe) and irradiated food at rank six (with 53.6% assessing risks due to food irradiation as severe). As this thesis aims at exploring the meanings women and men attach to food hazards, it was considered as appropriate to select hazards that are of relevance for consumers with regard to risk perception.

Focusing on the meanings women and men attach to these three different food hazards, a twofold approach is chosen for this chapter:

First, women's and men's most salient concepts with regard to the hazards are investigated. Salient concepts are the first associations to be activated when a person is confronted with a stimulus and from these concepts or images other cognitions in memory are activated (theory of spreading activation). These 'top of mind' cognitions are considered to be especially important in response-oriented studies (Wiedemann and Balderjahn, 1999), as in quantitative risk-perception studies and they may thus strongly influence consumers' risk evaluations. Furthermore, risk perception is found to be strongly influenced by affect (Loewenstein et al., 2001). The vividness or emotional intensity of the first images that consumers have in mind when they are verbally confronted with a hazard is likely to influence their cognitions and judgments about the stimulus (Jackson, Allum and Gaskell, 2006). Thus, it was investigated whether there are gender differences in the vividness of the most salient associations.

The second part of the analysis focuses on women's and men's motivational factors. According to the means-end-chain theory, knowledge is organized hierarchically in memory and the evaluation of an issue/object is based on how the issue/object is perceived to be related to principal life values (Olson and Reynolds, 1983). While a person's basic values are assumed to be relatively stable (Walker and Olson, 1991), different kinds of values and consequences are likely to be activated for different stimuli. It is analyzed whether women and men associate different kind of consequences to the three food hazards and perceive different kinds of values being threatened. Furthermore, the dominant paths (starting from attributes via consequences to values) in the mind of women and men are elaborated. Apart from the content in terms of images, associations, feelings, consequences, and values linked to the food hazards, the structure of women's and men's cognitions is the subject under investigation. More numerous, complex and more abstract cognitive structures point to a higher level of involvement for the object or issue in question, as explained in section 5.4.

6.2 Methodology

Section 6.2 describes in detail the design of the study and the analysis of the data.

6.2.1 Sample Selection and Data Collection Procedure

A sample of 34 women and 35 men was recruited and invited to participate in a study about nutrition behavior in Munich, Germany in March 2011. Decisions on size and composition of the sample were based on an extended literature review of empirical studies focusing on cognitive structures by means the laddering interviews[12] (e.g. Fotopoulos, Krystallis and Ness, 2003; Zanoli and Naspetti, 2002). One important criterion for laddering interviews is that the interviewees are willing to talk about the issue in question and have at least some knowledge about it, in order to be capable of expressing ideas about the issue or object (Köhler, 2000; Reynolds et al., 2001; Vannoppen et al., 1999). In our study, the respondents had to be interested in food and nutrition issues. Furthermore, as the stimulus of the interviews was Italian herbs, respondents who never consume Italian herbs were excluded during recruitment. The female and male samples were randomly selected based on the quota method allowing a participants selection representative of age, income, education and employment status. To ensure that possible differences between the two sub-groups are not caused by the samples' socio-economic structure, it was ensured that the female and male sample were similar in their socio-demographic profile.

The data collection procedure was split into five parts and is depicted in detail in Appendix C1 showing the interview guide:

a. General information and consent
b. Introduction and 'warm-up' laddering task
c. Entry questionnaire and elicitation of relevant attributes
d. The laddering interviews
e. Exit questionnaire

---

12 A laddering interview is a specific form of an indepth interview which will be explained in detail in 6.2.3.1

At the beginning, interviewees were asked to read general information about the study, were invited to ask questions, and signed the consent. Then, respondents were acquainted with the interview procedure by means of a 'warm-up' task, as the interview format used has been found to produce more reliable results if respondents are already familiar with the method (Breivik and Supphellen, 2003). The main focus of the entry questionnaire were the four different types of Italian herbs that were used as stimuli in order to elicit attributes related to the different kind of food hazards. The products were related to either one of the different food hazards 'mycotoxins', 'pesticides' or 'irradiation', with a fourth alternative as reference product containing none of the mentioned food hazards. The choice of the stimuli is discussed in 6.2.2. The different Italian herbs and the questionnaires are outlined in Appendix C 2 and Appendix C3. Respondents had to rank the four different kinds of herbs according to the likelihood that they would purchase the product. Subsequently, for each of the four herbs, the interviewees had to write down their spontaneous associations, thoughts, or feelings. In order to obtain information about respondents' overall affect, they were asked to rate how good or bad they felt about each of the products on a 5-point scale ranging from 1='very bad' to 5='very good'. Furthermore, respondents' activated emotions were measured by means of the Consumption Emotion Set (CES) according to Richins (1997). She developed an inventory in order to measure emotions that are relevant in the consumption domain. Her inventory comprises 13 dimensions such as anger, peacefulness, or shame. Each dimension comprises a set of sub-dimensions; e.g. 'shame' is a factor that is composed of the items 'embarrassed', 'ashamed', and 'humiliated'. For the purpose of this study, only the three dimensions 'worry', 'anger' and 'contentment' are relevant. 'Worry' consists of the items 'nervous', 'worried' and 'tense'. 'Anger' comprises the feelings 'frustrated', 'angry' and 'irritated', and 'contentment' the items 'contented' and 'fulfilled'. For example, the respondents were asked to rate on a 5-point scale the extent to which the product makes him or her angry or produces contentment, from 1='not at all' to 5='very much'. Finally, the interviewees had to assess the risks and benefits due to regular consumption of each product on a 5-point scale (from 1='not risky at all/not beneficial at all' to 5='very risky/very beneficial'). It was assured that interviewees did not page backward to check and revise assessments already made.

The risk and benefit assessment was the basis of the elicitation procedure, which is described in detail in 6.2.2.2. After the elicitation of the relevant concepts, the laddering interviews were conducted (see 6.2.3.1).

Finally, the interviewees had to fill in the exit questionnaire focusing on their socio-economic background (age, education, occupational status, household income, size of household and presence of children in the household) and more general questions such as respondent's 'attitude towards science and technology', 'reflexivity with regard to food choice', and 'trust in food'. 'Attitude towards science and technology' was measured on a 10-point scale that ranged from 1 ('the world is a lot worse off because of science and technology') to 10 ('the world is a lot better off because of science and technology'). 'Food reflexivity' and 'trust in food' were measured according to Berg (2004) with two questions: 'Food reflexivity' was described with the question '*To what extent do you choose foods that you consider to be healthy in your everyday diet?*' and 'trust in food' was described with the question '*To what extent are you confident that the foods you buy are not harmful for yourself or your family?*' For both questions, the scale ranged from 1= 'a very large degree' to 5='a very small degree' and a 6 as a 'don't know' option. Based on the two questions, Berg (2004) developed a consumer typology that distinguishes between sensible (reflexive trust), skeptical (reflexive distrust), naïve (non-reflexive trust) and denying (non-reflexive distrust) consumers. The typology was operationalized by coding the answers '1' and '2' as reflexive and trusting and '3', '4' and '5' as non-reflexive and low trust. The four different consumer types are formed by combining the different groups.

At the end, interviewees were debriefed and thanked. For those participants who wished to have more information about food irradiation, a one-page information sheet was handed at the end. Before starting data collection, the questionnaires, the elicitation, and laddering procedure were pretested and revised. The complete procedure lasted between 50 and 120 minutes and each person was paid €15 for his/her time. The data of the questionnaires were analyzed by IBM SPSS Statistics 19.

6.2.2 Choice of Stimuli and Elicitation Technique

The following section details the choice of the stimuli (6.2.2.1) and the choice of the elicitation technique (6.2.2.2).

6.2.2.1 Choice of Stimuli

Previous research has shown that the choice of the stimuli and the context has a strong influence on the reliability and predictive ability of the elicited cognitive structures for consumers' decisions (Bredahl, 1999; Reynolds and Gutman, 1988). The MEC theory explicitly acknowledges that the kinds and importance of elicited attributes are context dependent, which is seen as a major advantage of the MEC theory compared to other models trying to understand consumer behavior (Asselbergs, 1993 as cited in Costa, Dekker and Jongen, 2004; Grunert and Grunert, 1995; Olson and Reynolds, 2001). Working with a specific product and a specific decision situation is seen as essential in order to be able to understand results from laddering interviews adequately (Bredahl, 1999; Reynolds and Gutman, 1988). According to Reynolds and Gutman (2001), laddering works best when respondents make their associations while thinking of a real situation. Furthermore, the use of a set of alternative products for the elicitation task, not only the object of interest (Costa, Dekker and Jongen, 2004), is recommended in order to increase the realism of the interview.

In contrast to most of the MEC studies, this study's focus is not on different types of products and related consumers' purchase motives, but on consumers' assessments of different kind of food hazards. Thus, suggestions with regard to products and context have to be adapted to the objectives of this study. Following suggestions by Bredahl (1999), who elicited consumers' cognitive structures with regard to genetic engineering, we also linked our food hazards to a specific product in order to increase realism and reliability. Furthermore, in an MEC study by Miles and Frewer (2001) on five different food hazards, they were not able to distinguish between attributes and consequences. They assumed that one of the reasons might be that they did not link the hazards to specific products and that the questions about e.g. the hazard 'BSE' in general were too abstract and not linked to a specific context.

For this study, Italian herbs with differing characteristics were selected. Each of the three different food hazards or technologies 'mycotoxins', 'pesticides', and 'irradiation' are relevant with regard to herbs or spices. Moreover, it was expected that a relatively large share of the German population consumes Italian herbs compared to other herbs. Compared to other products, Italian herbs as stimuli worked well during pretests. Four different product profiles were developed for the Italian herbs:

- **A:** Conventionally produced Italian herbs that might contain mycotoxins, free of pesticides
- **B:** Conventionally produced Italian herbs that might contain pesticides, free of mycotoxins
- **C:** Irradiated Italian herbs, free of mycotoxins, free of pesticides

- **D:** Conventionally produced Italian herbs, free of mycotoxins, free of pesticides

With regard to the situational context, respondents were asked to imagine that they were in a supermarket and wanted to purchase Italian herbs. The four different herbs were presented to them with an indication of the different characteristics (e.g. 'might contain pesticides'). Respondents were further told that product characteristics are not necessarily written on the products themselves, but e.g. another person would explain to them the differences between the herbs. Next, the participants were asked to rank the Italian herbs according to the likelihood of purchase. This choice situation and especially the comparison between different product alternatives, which were comparisons between different food hazards in this study, should help to activate the more relevant cognitions linked to a real situation. Compared to general questions about what people think when they hear e.g. 'BSE' as in the study by Miles and Frewer (2001), the purchase situation context is supposed to increase consumers' perceived self-relevance of the topic, and the ranking task already implicitly forces respondents to make a first evaluation of the food hazards. More important for this study, however, is the risk and benefit evaluation of each of the different Italian herbs. As this thesis aims to gain a deeper understanding for differences in perceptions of food hazards, the real starting point of the attribute elicitation is participants' assessments of the risks and benefits on a scale ranging from 1 ('not risky at all/not beneficial at all') to 5 ('very risky/very beneficial'). It is expected that this procedure will help to elicit people's cognitions that are relevant when they are asked to judge different kind of risks, as it is the case in most quantitative studies.

6.2.2.2 Elicitation Technique

Different techniques exist for eliciting attributes used as the starting point for the laddering interviews. These techniques differ mainly in the cues that are presented to respondents (Steenkamp and Van Trijp, 1997) and in the structure of eliciting the attributes (Breivik and Supphellen, 2003). These differences can be ascribed to different approaches to the way that knowledge is organized in memory (Breivik and Supphellen, 2003). Several elicitation techniques are proposed in the literature; these can be divided into three main types of techniques (Costa, Dekker and Jongen, 2004; Grunert and Grunert, 1995; Reynolds and Gutman, 2001; Steenkamp and van Trijp, 1997):

1. Techniques based on different sorting methods (triadic sorting and free sorting; hierarchical dichotomization)
2. Techniques based on ranking methods
3. Direct elicitation techniques (direct/free elicitation; picking from attribute lists)

In sorting methods, participants are asked to group objects that are alike in some important characteristics and different from others. This is done exactly in free sorting, whereas other sorting methods are somewhat more restrictive. When *triadic sorting* is used, respondents are presented with triads of product alternatives, and respondents are asked to indicate which pair of the three products are similar and at the same time different from the third with regard to an important aspect. This procedure is repeated for different triads until the important attributes according to which consumer distinguish objects, products, or brands are elicited. *Triadic sorting* is based on Kelly's (1955) personal construct theory. The theory proposes that consumers ascribe meaning to the world around them by means of constructs, and he developed the so-called repertory-grid method in order to reveal people's constructs. A construct is a characteristic (descriptive factor) that distinguishes two objects from a third. These constructs are supposed to constitute people's relevant attributes.

Hierarchical dichotomization on the other hand is inspired by the schema theory (Cantor and Mischel, 1979) and presupposes that knowledge is organized hierarchically and dichotomously in memory. Participants are asked to split several product alternatives into dichotomous subsets during several sequences based on the perceived similarity or dissimilarity and they should term the attributes that guide their partitioning (Coxon, 1982).

When using ranking techniques, respondents are asked to rank objects according to preference or likelihood of purchase for a specific context. Participants are then asked for the reasons of their ranking in order to uncover participants' perceptions of distinctions between the objects (Sørensen and Henchion, 2011) and to elicit the relevant attributes for these distinctions.

Regarding direct elicitation techniques, respondents are asked to indicate for a specific context, most often a product choice situation, the attributes influencing their choice. In the case of *attribute lists*, participants can choose from proposed attributes, whereas in the case of *direct* (also called *free*) *elicitation*, respondents should name the relevant attributes freely (Steenkamp and Van Trijp, 1997). The *free elicitation* technique is based on the spreading activation theory (Anderson, 1983), which does not presuppose a specific conceptualization of knowledge organization in human memory, but simply assumes that the activation runs from one memorized concept to the next, depending on the strength of the activation of the former one. Accordingly, *free elicitation* assumes that participants will mention the attributes with the highest degree of activation, that are at the same time the most relevant attributes with regard to the object and context (Breivik and Supphellen, 2003; Grunert and Grunert, 1995).

A few empirical studies exist that compare different elicitation techniques with regard to the elicited attributes (Bech-Larsen and Nielsen, 1999; Breivik and Supphellen, 2003; Kanwar, Olson and Sims, 1980; Lines, Breivik and Supphellen, 1995; Steenkamp and van Trijp, 1997). Method effects were investigated for the number of elicited attributes (Bech-Larsen and Nielsen, 1999; Steenkamp and van Trijp, 1997; Kanwar, Olson and Sims, 1980), level of abstraction (Bech-Larsen and Nielsen, 1999; Steenkamp and van Trijp, 1998), subjective importance of attributes (Bech-Larsen and Nielsen, 1999; Breivik and Supphellen, 1995), variability of attributes (Bech-Larsen and Nielsen, 1999; Lines, Breivik and Supphellen, 1995), predictive ability of elicited attributes (Bech-Larsen and Nielsen, 1999; Breivik and Supphellen, 2003; Lines, Breivik and Supphellen, 1995), and time requirement (Bech-Larsen and Nielsen, 1999; Steenkamp and van Trijp, 1997). In general, more complex procedures such as triadic sorting were found to be more time-consuming and thus liable to decrease participants' level of attention than simple procedures such as picking from an attribute list or free elicitation (Bech-Larsen and Nielsen, 1999). Furthermore, in Steenkamp and Van Trijp's study, free elicitation produced a higher number of attributes and more abstract attributes than sorting methods (Steenkamp and van Trijp, 1997). However, this was not confirmed by the study of Bech-Larsen and Nielsen (1999), where sorting methods generated the highest number of attributes, and techniques did not differ in the proportion of abstract attributes they generated. However, in both studies, free elicitation techniques generated a lower number of concrete attributes than ranking or sorting methods (Bech-Larsen and Nielsen, 1999; Steenkamp and van Trijp, 1997). Similarly, the ability of the elicitation method to produce attributes important for product choice (predictive ability) was found to be strongest for ranking techniques in the study by Lines, Breivik and Supphellen (1995), but not in the study by Bech-Larsen and Nielsen (1999) or the study by Breivik and Supphellen (2003). Method effects are not consistent, and some of the studies state that differences due to the application of different techniques are quite small. All reviewed elicitation techniques seem to perform well with regard to the elicitation of the most relevant attributes (Breivik and Supphellen, 2003; Bech-Larsen and Nielsen, 1999; Steenkamp and van Trijp, 1997). Furthermore, some authors admit that differences in elicited attributes may be related to different product categories rather than to the applied methods themselves (Bech-Larsen and Nielsen, 1999; Breivik and Supphellen,

2003). They thus conclude that the choice of the method should be directed by the objective of the study, and, if possible, simple methods should be preferred as they are less exhausting for the participants.

Sorting methods are seen as useful when the aim is to elicit the whole range of cognitive structures and the focus is on tangible differences between objects. However, due to this exhaustive technique, sorting methods are also found to generate unimportant attributes (Bech-Larsen and Nielsen, 1999). Ranking procedures are assumed to be closest to consumers' decision-making in real-life situations (Sørensen and Henchion, 2011) and are often suggested when the aim is to understand people's preferences among several alternatives. In contrast to free elicitation, which mainly produces abstract attributes, ranking methods allow the generation of concrete as well as abstract attributes (Grunert and Grunert, 1995; Reynolds and Gutman, 2001). Particularly the concrete attributes are seen as determinant for the distinction between objects, which makes the ranking procedures interesting in terms of predictability of choice among alternatives (Reynolds, Gutman and Fiedler, 1985). Furthermore, regarding predictability, attribute lists are seen as the most appropriate (Bech-Larsen and Nielsen, 1999). Studies with an explorative purpose and studies that aim to understand how people compare fairly abstract objects should favor direct elicitation techniques (Bech-Larsen and Nielsen, 1999; Costa, Dekker and Jongen, 2004). Especially, free elicitation has the advantage that it puts no constraint on respondents' answers, and thus results are less subject to bias from the interviewer (Miles and Frewer, 2001). It is therefore expected that free elicitation is strongest in generating the attributes perceived as most important by the respondents (Bech-Larsen and Nielsen, 1999). However, as seen above, free elicitation fails in producing concrete attributes (Bech-Larsen and Nielsen, 1999; Böcker et al., 2005; Steenkamp and van Trijp, 1997).

As the purpose of this study was to elicit women's and men's cognitive structures relevant to the evaluation of different kinds of food hazards, the free elicitation technique was used. Working with food hazards as abstract objects as well as the explorative objective of this study makes this technique an appropriate tool. Particularly for studies with a focus on evaluation (like this study), Breivik and Supphellen (2003) suggest the use of direct elicitation techniques because it saves time and it is much easier for participants to understand and handle. Food hazards themselves are already characteristics/attributes of food products. As such, it was expected that mainly abstract attributes and consequences would be generated during elicitation. Thus, the disadvantage of free elicitation (neglecting concrete attributes) was not seen as a problem in this study. Moreover, as free elicitation is based on the idea of the spreading activation theory (Anderson, 1983), elicited attributes are the ones with the strongest activation and thus the most important ones (Bech-Larsen and Nielsen, 1999), especially with regard to response-oriented tasks in quantitative risk evaluations. In other words, attributes and consequences produced during free elicitation might be the ones activated when people are asked to assess risks with Likert scales in quantitative studies. However, the same issue also involves the potential risk that only the most relevant attributes are elicited, which impedes a detailed picture of participants' cognitive structures. Letting people make comparisons between objects as done in sorting and ranking procedures is likely to generate a broader range of attributes. For this reason, the choice of the stimulus is of special importance in free elicitation techniques. Furthermore, direct elicitation methods were found to work better the second time the participants were confronted with them. Thus, warm-up tasks are recommended to avoid method effects due to task ambiguity (Breivik and Supphellen, 2003). As a warm-up task, participants were asked to imagine that they want to buy a new car and they were asked what aspects they would consider to be important and why.

As laddering interviews and thus elicitation procedures were done for all three food hazards for each respondent, subjects were first asked to rank the products, according to the likelihood of purchase. Food hazards can be regarded as fairly abstract issues for consumers, not always linked to very specific knowledge for each hazard. It was expected that the ranking task could help respondents to make distinctions between the different hazards and to elicit more hazard-specific concepts later. However, in contrast to ranking elicitation techniques, subjects were not asked for the reasons for their rankings. Thus, in this study, the ranking task was only used as a first stimulus in order to make participants aware of the three different food hazards and helping in a first evaluation. As explained above, this task was linked to a choice situation of Italian herbs in a supermarket that respondents were asked to imagine.

In a second step, participants noted their associations, thoughts and feelings for each of the products before moving on to the third step, the real attribute elicitation. As in quantitative risk perception studies, interviewees were asked to assess the risks and benefits of each of the products on a Likert scale ranking from 1 to 5 (see above). Then they were asked about what they considered and what came to mind when doing the evaluations. Participants' answers were tape-recorded and noted by the interviewer and used as starting points for the laddering interviews afterwards. When this was done for the three products A, B and C (D was only the reference product), the interviewer selected only the attributes and consequences that were related to the food hazards and sorted them according to each hazard. The concepts noted were presented to the participants and they were asked for clarification if necessary as described by Miles and Frewer (2001). As such, attributes and later the derived ladders no longer refer to the products but only to each of the three food hazards. As sometimes a few different attributes are elicited, not all can be laddered usually due to time constraints. Reynolds and Gutman (2001) proposed letting respondents order elicited words and phrases according to perceived importance and then laddering only the top three concepts. However, as this was found to be very time-consuming and often perceived as irritating and difficult by respondents, they were finally just asked which of concepts they wanted to start the interview with. Nevertheless, it is expected that all important concepts were laddered, as generally not more than three to four different concepts were elicited. The first three to four concepts are supposed to be the most important ones in free elicitation techniques.

6.2.3 Laddering

The laddering technique was originally developed in clinical psychology by Dennis Hinkle (1965) in order to elicit belief structures, but is now used in many other fields such as consumer research, architecture and information technology (Veludo-de-Oliveira, Akemi and Cortez, 2006). It is the most prominent method for studying people's values according to the motivational approach in the MEC theory (Costa, Dekker and Jongen, 2004; Reynolds and Gutman, 1988) and has been introduced in marketing and consumer research by Gutman (1982) and Reynolds and Gutman (1988). The laddering method aims to elicit consumers' attribute-consequence-value chains that they link with a certain object. On the basis of the elicited attributes, laddering mainly consists of a specific interview procedure using series of direct probes, typically the 'Why is this important to you' question, which allows researcher to uncover people's MECs step by step (Reynolds and Gutman, 1988). The laddering technique is composed of three main elements:

1. Laddering interview
2. Content analysis
3. Analysis of the hierarchical value maps (HVMs)

6.2.3.1 Laddering Interview

Depending on the extent of standardization, one can distinguish soft laddering and hard laddering. The soft laddering interview is a one-to-one in-depth interview method (Gutman, 1982). The previously elicited attributes are the starting point for the laddering technique as in general the most important attributes are 'laddered' in asking the respondent questions like "Why is this important to you?" to develop the 'chain' or 'ladder' from concrete attributes to more abstract structures, i.e., the consequences and values. In soft laddering interviews, respondents' natural flow of speech is not restricted and ladders are constructed only after the interviews. Respondents are allowed to fork ladders by generating more than one attribute, consequence, or value, depending on the underlying concept, and can go back and forward in their chains without having to follow a strict bottom-up path (Costa, Dekker and Jongen, 2004; Russell et al., 2004a). By contrast, hard laddering methods use paper-and-pencil or computerized questionnaires and employ a-priori lists from which respondents choose their attributes, consequences, and values (Russell et al., 2004a). Participants are asked to produce their MEC in increasing abstraction levels from the attributes at the bottom and the values at the top (Costa, Dekker and Jongen, 2004).

Table 4: Overview of Soft and Hard Laddering

Soft Laddering	Hard Laddering
▪ Gives a more detailed and broader picture of people's cognitive structures ▪ Recommended for complex and abstract issues ▪ Appropriate for issues of high or low-involvement ▪ Applied mainly in motivational MEC approaches ▪ Very time-consuming ▪ Only small samples ▪ Interviewer effects due to the face-to-face situation and reconstruction of the ladders by the interviewer	▪ Focus on the important linkages between pre-determined concepts ▪ Recommended for concrete products ▪ Appropriate for issues with medium involvement ▪ Less time-consuming ▪ Appropriate for larger samples ▪ Interview effects due to a priori lists

Source: Own illustration based on Botschen and Thelen, 1998; Costa, Dekker and Jongen, 2004; Grunert and Grunert, 1995; Russell et al., 2004a.

Whether hard or soft laddering is more appropriate depends on the research question. Table 4 gives an overview of the strengths and weaknesses of the two methods and their usefulness with regard to research objectives.

Two studies compared the effects of different laddering techniques on the elicited cognitive structures (Botschen and Thelen, 1998; Russell et al., 2004a). In both studies, soft and hard laddering methods generated similar consequences and values, and some of the most important links were the same. However, soft laddering produced more complex hierarchical value maps (the aggregated individual ladders) and more abstract MECs, meaning that more consequences and values were elicited (Botschen and Thelen, 1998; Russell et al., 2004a). According to Russell et al. (2004a), soft laddering is thus especially useful when a very broad and detailed picture of people's cognitions is the aim of the study and is appropriate for uncovering complex underlying motivations and values. Soft laddering is thus recommended for studies following the motivational approach of the MEC theory. Hard laddering allows investigation into the strength of the relation between pre-determined concepts. This is useful when research is done on a very specific subject with the focus of getting to know the most important associations and strong linkages (Grunert and Grunert, 1995). As soft laddering allows reseachers to identify a more subtle and broader range of people's cognitions including weaker associations and linkages, it is further recommended when the research object is fairly complex and abstract (Asselbergs, 1993 as cited in Costa, Dekker and Jongen, 2004; Grunert and Grunert, 1995; Miles and Frewer, 2001; Reynolds and Gutman, 2001). This is the case e.g. for general public issues such as food hazards (Miles and Frewer, 2001). In contrast, hard laddering is sufficient when working with concrete products.

Furthermore, Grunert and Grunert (1995) suggest that participants' levels of involvement and experience with the subject or product be considered when choosing the laddering method. According to them, when people are supposed to have low involvement and little experience or high levels of involvement and much experience, soft laddering should be used. When average involvement is expected, hard laddering techniques are more appropriate (Grunert and Grunert, 1995).

In addition, the two methods differ implicitly on the assumptions regarding the retrieval of information. The soft laddering task and the related memory processes are those of the spreading activation theory (Anderson, 1983; Grunert and Grunert, 1995). The laddering question 'Why is this important to you?' activates a construct in memory and this activation spreads to other related concepts. The consequences and values for which the activation was strong enough are retrieved. The strength of activation depends on how often linkages between concepts have already been used. In contrast, hard laddering presents people with the attributes, consequence and values on lists from which they have to choose, and it is expected that choices of these cues tend to be based on familiarity (Grunert and Grunert, 1995).

Another advantage of soft laddering is that it supports participants' natural flow of speech; however, this also makes the method very time-consuming and interviews must be conducted with quite small samples. Hard laddering, by contrast, due to its questionnaire-based approach, is less time-consuming and can be carried out with large samples of more than 50 subjects.

Both methods entail potential interview(er) biases due to their way of administering the data collection. Hard laddering uses a priori lists, with the risk that elicited concepts are only those given on the lists and/or that respondents choose concepts that they would not select without being reminded by the list presented to them. It is thus expected that soft laddering generates people's cognitive structures more accurately (Russell et al., 2004a). In this regard, soft laddering has the advantage of eliciting respondents' relevant constructs and not the ones regarded as important by the researcher. Moreover, the validity of the generated data is threatened by strategic response behavior on behalf of the participants, where soft laddering, due to the face-to-face situation, has the potential to prevent it (Grunert and Grunert, 1995). On the other hand, biases due to feelings of social pressure to respond to the interviewer's questions in the in-depth interviews are eliminated in the hard laddering procedures (Botschen and Thelen, 1998; Jonas and Beckmann, 1998), and questionnaires make it easier to control the whole data collection format. Furthermore, as soft laddering encourages the natural flow of speech, respondents jump back and forth between levels of abstraction, give several reasons for one concept (forked ladders) and cite redundant information. The interviewer has to reconstruct the ladders after the interview, which increases the possibility of bias (Grunert, Grunert and Sørensen 1995).

There are several reasons why soft laddering was chosen for the purpose of this study: First of all, the study aims at getting a detailed representation of women's and men's cognitive structures with regard to the different food hazards and is strongly interested in the higher-order consequences and values men and women link to these hazards. The motivational objective and this study's interest in subtle differences between the knowledge structures of men and women make the soft-laddering method more appropriate for the study. Second, as this study focuses on the cognitions activated when people are asked to assess risks and benefits of potential food hazards/technologies, soft laddering is supposed to produce a better representation of women's and men's knowledge structures than hard laddering (see above). Third, people's involvement regarding food hazards can be expected to be quite high even though their explicit knowledge might be low, because working with hazards might entail stronger involvement as people tend to try to avoid damage. To ensure that respondents have fairly high levels of involvement regarding our research topic, only respondents interested in nutrition and food issues were recruited. And fourth, as suggested in a previous laddering study focusing on food hazards (Miles and Frewer, 2001), soft laddering is more adequate when working with general and abstract subjects such as food-safety issues.

As laddering interviews were carried out for all three food hazards per participant, the order in which each of the hazards was laddered was alternated. That means that a third of each food hazard was laddered first, another third second, and a third is laddered last. This was done as previous interviews about one hazard might have an impact on the elicited concepts in the subsequent interview.

Appendix D1 depicts the frequency of the laddering order in percentages. The distribution is not fully balanced as in some cases only one or two of the hazards were laddered due to time constraints when already the first and/or second laddering interview was very time-consuming. As in the case of the attribute elicitation technique, the laddering procedure needs a warm-up procedure since the series of repetitive 'Why is this important to you?' questions may induce the participants to give strategic answers when the procedure becomes too obvious for the respondent (Botschen, Thelen and Pieters, 1999; Veludo-de-Oliveira, Akemi and Cortez, 2006). Thus, the particular character of the laddering method was explained to the interviewees at the beginning and the above-mentioned warm-up task concerning car purchase decisions was also continued for the laddering procedure. As a consequence interviewees understand that the kinds of questions and the way of being interrogated are part of the specific interview technique used and independent of given answers.

As seen before, differences in participants' MECs might also be due to an interviewer effect. It was tried to minimize this effect by working with trained interviewers. Interviews were conducted by three interviewers. They were given a thorough introduction to the theory behind laddering and the objective of the research as suggested by Reynolds, Dethloff and Westberg (2001). Furthermore, interviewers were trained in the laddering technique and practiced the method several times before starting the data collection. Problems encountered during this training phase were discussed.

The attribute perceived as most important, or rather the ones respondents wanted to start with, posed the starting point of the laddering interview. The interviewer asked respondents why this attribute is perceived as important with regard to the assessment of the food hazard in question. The respective responses were the basis for the next 'Why is this important to you?' question. As such, the interviewer tried to uncover participants' MECs from the elicited attribute to the consequences and the values. All interviews were tape-recorded and these recordings constituted the basis of the subsequent data analysis.

Figure 7 presents the different elements of an MEC and illustrates them by means of examples.

It is important to note that a chain from attributes through consequences to values elicited from a single person is usually called a 'ladder', whereas the term MEC is used for ladders aggregated across individuals (Wiedemann and Balderjahn, 1999). Furthermore, an individual ladder does not always cover all abstraction levels, and each of the elements can contain more than one cognitive concept (Olson and Reynolds, 1983; Böcker et al., 2005).

Figure 7: An Example of an MEC for Pesticides

cA	aA	fC	pC	iV	tV
	unnatural	negative health	low performance	self-direction	happiness
no labeling		not enough information	no control	freedom of choice	
		emission in soil		responsibility	preservation of the earth

cA: concrete attribute; aA: abstract attribute; fC: functional consequence; pC: psychosocial consequence; iV: instrumental value; tV: terminal value

Source: Own example presented according to Olson and Reynolds (1983).

The 'Why is this important to you?' question is not always appropriate depending on participants' answers, and thus Reynolds, Dethloff and Westberg (2001: 106) propose a few alternative probes such as 'How does that make you feel?', 'Why is that a negative to you?' or 'Why do you want that?'. In contrast to typical MEC studies, the study object was not a product, but different food hazards. Thus, the kind of questions to help respondents to walk up the ladder had to be slightly different. Based on a similar study focusing on concerns about animal welfare by Köhler (2005) and according to suggestions by Reynolds, Dethloff and Westberg (2001) for negative ladders, the following probes were used next to the 'Why is this important to you?' question:

- 'Why do you want to avoid that?'

- 'Why are you concerned about that?'
- 'How does that make you feel?'

When one MEC, from the attribute to the consequences and/or values, was completed, the interviewer asked the participants for further reasons, why they mentioned this attribute and if possible continued that path. This was done by the 'Is there another reason why this attribute is important to you?' question. Due to the natural flow of speech in soft laddering interviews, respondents often cited several reasons/consequences at one time that were then laddered subsequently. When the respondent had nothing left to add, the interviewer started to ladder the second attribute and then the third and last attribute was laddered.

Often participants are not able to verbalize thoughts and feelings or are blocked and cannot state a reason why something is important or concerning. Reynolds and Gutman (1988; 2001) and Reynolds, Dethloff and Westberg (2001) suggested several solutions to deal with these kinds of problems, e.g.:

- *Reiteration of the situational context or alternative scenario*: reminding the respondent of the context/specific situation based on which they should elicit their MEC or asking the participants to imagine a similar situation relevant to the research object in question.
- *Postulation of the absence of an object or state of being*: the participant is asked to describe feelings and consequences due to the absence of the object of state of being.
- *Negative laddering*: asking the respondent why they want to avoid doing certain things and feelings, especially in situations where respondents feel unable to verbalize why they behave a certain way.
- *Third person probe*: ask interviewees about other people's feelings in a similar situation. This is especially useful for sensitive topics that people feel uncomfortable discussing.
- *Redirecting techniques*: the interviewer can use silence in order to give the respondent the possibility to think about more cognitions or the interviewer repeats what the interviewee has said and asks for clarification.

However, sometimes it is necessary for the interviewer to just note the problem in order to consider this during data analysis, or to return to that ladder later, as participants who feel forced to answer might generate irrelevant and artificial ladders. Quite often, the interviewee generates non-concrete or abstract attributes but directly cites consequences, or the respondent directly ladders from an attribute to a value. In these cases, reverse or backwards laddering is employed by asking e.g. 'What characteristic of irradiation makes you feel concerned about your health?' or 'In what way does naturalness (abstract attribute) enhance you quality of life (terminal value)?' This is done in order to elicit complete ladders on all abstraction levels.

The interviewer stopped further probing into a ladder when participants started to give circular answers or when they were unable to verbalize more concepts even after the above-mentioned techniques (Fotopoulos, Krystallis and Ness, 2003). To ensure that all aspects mentioned were laddered, the interviewer made notes during the interview, which was especially necessary when interviewees forked ladders and the interviewer had to resume started ladders after some time.

6.2.3.2 Data Analysis

The audio tapes were transcribed and recordings as well as transcribed text documents were archived together in order to ensure easy access to full context information at any time. The availability of context information, also called indexicality, allows the researcher to better capture the 'right' meaning of the interviewees' answers. This is on the one hand an advantage of the soft laddering approach, but also a necessary prerequisite as ladders are reconstructed after the interviews (Costa, Dekker and Jongen, 2004; Fotopoulos, Krystallis and Ness, 2003; Grunert and Grunert, 1995). As developed by Gengler and Reynolds (1995), data analysis includes three main steps:

1. Content analysis (data reduction and categorization of relevant ideas found in the ladders into summary codes)
2. Creation of the implication matrix (aggregation of the most important individuals' concepts and the linkages between them)
3. Construction of the hierarchical value maps (graphical representation of the MECs of a group of individuals based on the implication matrix)

These steps are described in the following.

Content analysis

To be able to create HVMs for groups of respondents, every in-depth interview has to be analyzed using content analysis. The first step of the data analysis, the content analysis, is a qualitative one and constitutes the core of the MEC study, as it converts qualitative (interview) data into quantitative nominal data (Costa, Dekker and Jongen, 2004; Reynolds and Gutman, 2001). According to Mayring (2010), the objective of content analysis is to analyze textual documents or transcribed interviews systematically. This is done according to explicit rules based on the methodology of content analysis and based on the theories that are the foundation of the study. That means that all statements in a text or interview, that are relevant with regard to the study's theory and its related hypotheses are important (and only those) (Reynolds and Gutman, 2001). The purpose of content analysis is to reconstruct the relevant aspects of a text or communication by reducing the complexity and amount of information (Costa, Dekker and Jongen, 2004; Geis, 1992). This is done by developing a category system that classifies meaning into broader and more abstract categories (Mayring, 2010; Brosius, Koschel and Haas, 2009).

The content analysis of this study was done similarly to previous MEC studies (e.g. Costa, Dekker and Jongen, 2004; Fotopoulos, Krystallis and Ness, 2003; Wiedemann and Balderjahn, 1999) and according to suggestions by researchers doing methodological research about the laddering method (Grunert and Grunert, 1995; Reynolds and Gutman, 2001; Reynolds, Dethloff and Westberg, 2001). The initial task of the content analysis is the reduction of the data of the transcribed interviews by cutting them into separate phrases and deleting irrelevant elements. This procedure demands a thorough review of respondents' verbatim statements in order to filter out the statements representative of what the participant wanted to express (Veludo-de-Oliveira, Akemi and Cortez, 2006). Moreover, at this stage, elements relevant for the study's objective have to be identified while redundant and unimportant information has to be deleted. In this study, each of the three interviewers did this for the interviews she had conducted, as it was supposed that the respective interviewer would best be able to assess the relevance of interviewees' statements.

The next step is the coding, which consists in the development of a set of summary labels for the relevant elements at each level of the MEC (Reynolds, Dethloff and Westberg, 2001). The aim is that all codes reflect the important elements under study mentioned by the participants. Synonymous statements by respondents are grouped together under a code with the aim of generating a system of idiosyncratic concepts (Reynolds, Dethloff and Westberg, 2001; Veludo-de-Oliveira, Akemi and Cortez, 2006). Next, these codes are classified under the different abstraction levels: attributes (concrete and abstract), consequences (functional and psychosocial), and values (instrumental and terminal) (Reynolds and Gutman, 2001). This was done in several iterative steps: on the basis of 13 interviews, two different coders developed a first code book. This was done with the aid of a literature-based code book developed by the coders from categories found in laddering studies about food choice and technology/hazard perception. Furthermore, at this stage contextual information is important to ensure that codes reflect respondents' statements accurately (Costa, 2003). Contextual information is often one of the elements that were deleted in the first data reduction phase; however, it is often very important in order to classify the extracted 'chunk of meanings'. In order to increase the availability of contextual information and thus its consideration in the coding process, the deletion of non-relevant information in the text database was done by using the MS Word Track Changes function that allows one to read deleted elements while at the same time marking them as canceled. Following Fotopoulos, Krystallis and Ness (2003), this first coding was performed by using keyword-in-context lists aiming at higher inter-subjectivity and transparence and by inserting the codes directly in the transcribed interviews. An example of a typical documentation of the interviews is given in Appendix D2. Based on these 13 first coded interviews, the two coders developed a first code book. Code books and keyword-in-context lists were compared by the two coders and classifications were discussed until they reached a consensus and a common code book was created (Costa, Dekker, Jongen, 2004; Bech-Larsen, 1996; Grunert and Grunert, 1995). Based on this code-book, all interviews were coded by means of the keyword-in-context procedure. When necessary, new codes were added. Once all interviews were coded in this way, the subsequent coding procedure was done by means of LadderMap™ software developed by Gengler and Reynolds (1993). LadderMap™ supports the reviewing and revision of the content analysis and helps to increase the intersubjectivity (Grunert and Grunert, 1995). It allows the printing of a lexical listing that contains a list of all attributes, consequences, and value codes, with the verbatim statements classified under these codes (Gengler and Reynolds, 1995; Lastovicka, 1995). These lexical listings were cross-checked by both coders and when necessary discussed until coders reached agreement. In this iteration phase the LadderMap™ software is very helpful as the classifications can be changed on the basis of the code book, and the software automatically readjusts the individual ladders according to changes made (Costa, 2003; Gengler and Reynolds, 1995). The following iteration procedure focuses on the reduction of the numbers of identified codes by combining similar labels in order achieve a number of 50 to 60 summary codes as suggested by several authors

(Gengler and Reynolds, 2001; Grunert and Grunert, 1995; Reynolds and Gutman, 2001).

As this study focuses on possible hazards, negative statements were dominant. As a consequence, participants mainly cited negative consequences or how a hazard might prevent them from reaching certain values, even though sometimes framed in a 'positive' way, due to the dominance of the 'negative laddering' format of the in-depth interviews. Thus, in most cases, seemingly opposite elements such as 'tasty' and 'not tasty' were combined under one code. However, this was not advisable for all cases, as there exists a couple of positive ladders with the meaning that e.g. irradiation helps to prevent vitamin damage, and as a consequence food is considered to be healthier. For the evaluation of a technology or potential hazard it makes a considerable difference if a ladder is positive or negative. Hence, as in a study by Zanoli and Naspetti (2002), for each food hazard the positive ladders were entered in a separate database during the third iteration phase when working with the LadderMap^{TM} software in order to be able to interpret the meaning of the chains.

During all iteration procedures, the underlying theories and related hypotheses have to be kept in mind. As noted above, this is especially important during the first step when identifying the 'chunk of meanings' to ensure that elements relevant for the research question are extracted. However, this is also necessary during the subsequent coding iterations when combining or splitting codes. For example, for the research question it might be important to distinguish between concerns about family welfare and the person's own welfare. That means that for the coding it is important to filter out not only one of the 'welfare' statements and omit the other one during the first data reduction. For the same reason it is not advisable to combine 'family welfare' and 'personal welfare' under a common code during later iterations. The final set of codes should accurately reflect the participants' statements while being broad enough to comprise a number of similar but different statements, and codes should be clearly distinguishable (Mayring, 2010).

Based on the final code book, a third coder was trained, who then coded a random sample of the transcribed interviews for testing inter-rater reliability. Very short interviews were first excluded and then for each food hazard a sample of 15 interviews was randomly selected without replacement. In other words, each identification number could be selected only once for one of the three hazards. This was done to ensure that the coding by the third coder was based on a relatively large number of different respondents with differing verbalization styles. Reliability is calculated in order to test the quality of coding with regard to its objectivity. Inter-rater reliability refers to the consistency in measurements performed with the same methods but by different researchers. For the purpose of this study, the reliability of the code-book and thus the quality of coding is tested (Brosius, Koschel and Haas, 2009; Früh, 2007). The index of reliability according to Perrault and Leigh (1989) was measured. In behavioral science, Cohen's kappa[13] (Cohen, 1960) is often used, which estimates a measure of agreement between two raters while checking for agreements one would expect by chance. However, Cohen's kappa has also been criticized for taking marginal distributions between categories associated with each of the two raters as given (Grayson and Rust, 2001; Perrault and Leigh, 1989; Tanner and Young, 1985). Perrault and Leigh (1989) developed another index of inter-rater reliability that does not depend on marginal frequencies and that is specifically advisable for applications in consumer research and marketing. Their index $\mathbf{I_r}$ is operationalized as follows:

$$\boldsymbol{I_r} = \sqrt{\left(p_a - \frac{1}{c}\right)\left(\frac{c}{c-1}\right)}$$

when $p_a \geq (1/c)$. If $p_a < (1/c)$ I_r is set to 0.

c refers to the number of coding categories and

p_a refers to the proportion of agreements between the two raters (Grayson and Rust, 2001; Perrault and Leigh, 1989).

The index of inter-rater reliability for the mycotoxin interviews was 0.86, for the pesticides 0.82 and for irradiation 0.85. All disagreements were discussed until consensus was reached and coding was adapted accordingly.

The final code book referring to all food hazards together and to positive and negative ladders has been translated into English and is depicted in Table 10 in section 6.3.2 presenting the results of the content analysis.

The implication matrix

The second step of the analysis of laddering data is considered as the bridge between the qualitative and quantitative elements of the laddering technique, as

---

13 Cohens Kappa is measured in the following way: $K = \frac{\Pr(a)-\Pr(e)}{1-\Pr(e)}$ where Pr(a) refers to the proportion of agreements among raters and Pr(e) refers to the probability of agreement among raters that happen by chance (Cohen, 1960; Grayson and Rust, 2001).

the codes from the qualitative content analysis are aggregated across all individual ladders (Devlin and Birtwistle, 2003; Veludo-de-Oliveira, Akemi and Cortez, 2006). An implication matrix is a square matrix that consists of columns and rows equivalent in number to the number of codes. The matrix displays the number of times each code is linked to another code in such a way that in all cases one code (row) precedes another code (column) (Reynolds, Dethloff, Westberg, 2001; Reynolds and Gutman, 2001). These connections between pair of codes can be direct or indirect. Direct linkages refer to relationships among adjacent codes, where one code directly precedes another code without another element in between. Indirect relations refer to a connection between a pair of codes with intermediary elements. Whereas direct connections represent cause-effect relationships between elements, indirect relationships reveal fairly general associations between elements (Veludo-de-Oliveira, Akemi and Cortez, 2006; Reynolds, Dethloff, Westberg, 2001; Reynolds and Gutman, 2001). In the matrix, the cells present the number of times all row codes lead to all column codes, where the number of direct connections is displayed to the left of the slash and the total number of direct plus indirect connections between the same pair of codes to the right of the slash.

Table 5 gives an excerpt of an implication matrix.

Table 5: Example of an Implication Matrix

	Artificial	Health risk	Restriction due to disease	Self-determination
Artificial	0/0	5/7	0/14	0/16
Health risk	0/0	0/0	7/12	3/15
Restriction due to disease	0/0	0/0	0/0	7/10
Self-determination	0/0	0/0	0/0	0/0

Source: Own illustration.

In order to determine the strength of associations, Reynolds and Gutman (2001) suggest considering both types of relations. The implication matrices are presented in Appendix D3 to Appendix D10[14].

Construction of the hierarchical value map

The final analysis of the laddering data is in general done at the aggregate level in the form of a hierarchical value map (HVM). A HVM is a graphical representation of the most frequently mentioned attributes, consequences, and values, and the connections in between for groups of respondents (Bredahl, 1999). The HVM depicts the reconstructed MEC from the aggregate data of the implication matrix. As previously mentioned, the term 'ladder' is generally used in this context to describe the individual chains elicited during the interviews, whereas 'chain' is used for the aggregated ladders of groups of respondents. The HVM is constructed by establishing step by step the chains from the implication matrix considering the connections among elements (Reynolds and Gutman, 2001; Wiedemann and Balderjahn, 1999). The HVM can depict indirect and direct linkages. It can also focus on direct connections only between elements, depending on what one wants to show. For soft laddering studies this might sometimes be impossible due to the fact that only relatively few participants mentioned each of the direct connections (Costa, 2003; Olson and Reynolds, 2001; Reynolds and Gutman, 1988; Reynolds and Gutman, 2001). In order to be able to interpret the HVM, only relations exceeding a specific strength are mapped. This process of deciding which elements and connections to include is a trade-off between ensuring the interpretability of the map and not omitting too much information from the interviews (Costa, 2003). As a general guideline, the HVM should represent at least 70% and on average 75 to 85% of the original individuals' ladders (Fotopoulos, Krystallis and Ness, 2003; Gengler and Reynolds, 1995; Reynolds, Dethloff, Westberg, 2001; Reynolds and Gutman, 2001). In order to cope with these requirements, the choice of the cut-off point plays a key role. The cut-off point is defined as the number of times a connection between a pair of elements (either direct or indirect linkages) has to be mentioned in order to be presented in the HVM. As a general rule of thumb, Reynolds and Gutman (1988; 2001) propose a cut-off point between 3 and 5 for 50 to 60 participants. They recommend playing

14 For mycotoxins and pesticides two implication matrices (one for women and one for men) were created. For irradiation four implication matrices (one with negative ladders and one with positive ladders for women and one with negative ladders and one with positive ladders for men) were created.

with differing cut-off levels in order to select the best solution regarding ease of interpretation and amount of information stored. Another suggestion is to calculate the proportion of links shown in the HVM with differing cut-off points and choose the 'best' solution (Pieters, Baumgartner and Allen, 1995). Other authors simply suggest selecting a cut-off level that produces the most interpretable solution without losing too much information (Audenaert and Steenkamp, 1997). However, Grunert and Grunert (1995) criticize the lack of theoretical and/or statistical criteria for the decision about cut-off levels for laddering data. Accordingly, Leppard, Russell and Cox (2004) suggest a 'top-down strategy' for determining the cut-off level that takes into account the different abstraction levels of MEC. According to them, the number of linkages between different levels of abstractions differs for most participants. Generally, a larger number of links occurs at the lower abstraction levels from attributes to consequence. This can be explained by respondents' increasing difficulties to verbalize more abstract concepts such as values (Leppard, Russell and Cox, 2004), and is rooted in the MEC theory itself that assumes that larger numbers of concrete concepts are linked to relatively smaller numbers of abstract concepts in memory (Veludo-de-Oliveira, Akemi and Cortez, 2006). Therefore, Leppard, Russell and Cox (2004) criticize using the same cut-off point for the different abstraction levels, as links between higher order concepts (psychosocial consequences and values) would be underrepresented in the map. With the 'top-down method', the cut-off point is determined for each abstraction level separately and in several steps. In the first step, the cut-off level for links departing from attributes is determined by the most important linkage (defined as the most often mentioned connection). The same is done for the links departing from consequences to higher order consequences and values. This results in an HVM1 that displays only the most important links and is thus in general clear and simple. In a second step, this process is repeated for the second largest cell entries (the second highest number of times a link was mentioned) for the different abstraction levels. The resulting HVM2 is based on less strong linkages, thus includes additional linkages and contains HVM1. In successively considering less strong linkages and thus selecting decreasing cut-off levels, several HVMs (HVM1, HVM2, HVM3, HVM4 and so on) are generated in the described manner until the HVM becomes too complicated and unclear (Barrena and Sánchez, 2010; Leppard, Russell and Cox, 2004).

Similar to the suggestions by Leppard, Russell and Cox (2004), the cut-off value was chosen separately for the relations coming from each of the levels of abstraction. However, unlike the 'top-down' approach, not the most important links (the highest number of times a link is mentioned, the second highest number of times a link is mentioned etc.) are depicted across all abstraction levels, but differing cut-off points in each level of abstraction were compared to the related relative number of relations that would be presented in an HVM as proposed by Böcker, Hartl and Nocella (2008). They suggest that when comparing HVMs of groups of people, the share of information that is depicted in the HVMs against the total amount of information should be similar. Furthermore, it is suggested that cut-off levels are chosen in a way that HVMs depict a representative amount of information while still assuring the interpretability of the HVMs (Böcker, Hartl and Nocella, 2008; Gengler and Reynolds, 1995). Thus, cut-off values in each abstraction level were selected in a way to depic as much information as possible and to represent similar shares of information in each abstraction level in the women's and men's HVM. This was done for the following reasons: The dominance of health-related concepts results in several equally important relations, especially for relations departing from functional and psychosocial consequences. As a consequence, the strict appliance of the 'top-down' approach by Leppard, Russell and Cox (2004) would lead to an underrepresentation of other relations in those abstraction levels. Furthermore, relations between elements of the same level of abstraction were considered in this study. In other words, linkages between different kinds of functional consequences or between psychosocial consequences were also considered and not only the links in higher abstraction levels. This was decided when looking at the data, as particularly concepts at the level of psychosocial consequences were found to be highly interrelated. Moreover, as the number of women and men in the groups differ for each of the three food hazards, the cut-off is chosen in a way to ensure that in each group a similar percentage had to have mentioned a relation in order to be considered in the HVM. Similarly to the 'top-down' approach, this strategy reduces problems of meaningless data that is linked to absolute cut-off points (Leppard, Russell and Cox, 2004; Russell et al., 2004b).

Several authors suggest appling the principle of non-redundancy when building the HVMs (Grunert and Grunert, 1995; Olson and Reynolds, 1983). The principle of non-redundancy requires that a direct link between non-consecutive elements is only depicted in the HVM if these elements are not linked via an intermediary element. For instance, a direct link from an attribute X to a value Z should not appear in the HVM if there is a link from the attribute X to a consequence Y and this consequence Y is further linked to the value Z. Due to the principle of non-redundancy, some of the direct links are omitted when establishing the HVM as they are considered as redundant. However, in order to ensure that depicted MECs can be interpreted as a valid measure of participants' cognitive structures, elicited ladders have to be fairly homogenous. If it can be assumed that the group of respondents has more heterogeneous cognitive structures, Grunert and Grunert (1995) suggest taking redundant relations into account to avoid misinterpretations. In this study it is assumed that the group of women and the group of men do not constitute homogenous groups, suggesting that next to sex, other determinants influence cognitions with regard to food hazards. Thus, in the cases where a relatively large number of respondents in a group mentioned a direct link compared to the indirect link, the direct link is also depicted.

6.3 Results

Chapter 6.3 has three parts. The first part presents information on the socio-demographic characteristics of the sample and the results of the questionnaires. The second part outlines results of the content analysis of consumers' first associations to the food hazards. The third part presents the results of the laddering interviews. Each part ends with a summary and discussion of the results.

6.3.1 Sample Description and General Product Comparisons

This chapter gives an overview of the sample's socio-demographic profile along with results concerning women's and men's attitude towards science and technology and their approach to food. It also presents respondents' assessments of the products.

6.3.1.1 Socio-Demographic Characteristics and General Attitudes

Table 6 shows the socio-economic profile for women and men. Some differences exist with regard to education, income, the presence of children in the household and food shopping responsibility. A higher share of men indicates 'secondary general school' as their highest level of education and to have a university degree, whereas more women indicate 'grammar school' as their highest level of education. With regard to occupation, the male sample has a higher frequency of students, unemployed respondents, and respondents in fulltime employment, whereas in the female sample a higher share indicates to be housewives or part-time employees. Further, the share of women with children living in their household is twice as high as that of men. Differences with regard to food shopping responsibilities are rather small with women bearing more often the main responsibility for food shopping.

Table 6: Socio-Demographic Characteristics of the Sample (by Gender)

	Women; N=34; 49.3%		**Men; N=35; 50.7%**	
	Frequency	**Percent**	**Frequency**	**Percent**
Age				
20-35	9	26.5	10	28.6
36-55	13	38.2	14	40.0
56-77	12	35.3	11	31.4
Education				
Secondary general school	6	18.2	10	30.3
Intermediate secondary school	12	36.4	11	33.3
(Specialized) Grammar school	11	33.3	5	15.2
University (of applied studies)	4	12.1	7	21.2
Income[1]				
Low	8	25.0	9	26.5
Medium	18	56.25	17	50.0
High	6	18.75	8	23.5
Occupation				
Student	3	9.4	6	18.2
Househusband/Housewife	7	21.9	0	0
Unemployed	0	0	3	9.1
Retired/Pensioner	6	18.8	7	21.2
Fulltime employment	7	21.9	14	42.4
Part-time employment	9	28.1	2	6.1
Other	1	3.1	1	3.0
Children living in household				
Yes	16	48.5	8	22.9
No	17	51.5	27	77.1
Food shopping responsibility				
Main responsibility	26	76.5	22	62.9
Shared responsibility	3	8.8	4	11.4
Not responsible	5	14.7	9	25.7

[1]low: <€600 to €1200; medium: €1201 to 3000; high: >€3001;

Source: Own illustration.

In contrast to previous studies (Fox and Firebaugh, 1992; Trankina, 1993; Bieberstein et al., 2011), no differences exist between women's and men's attitudes towards science and technology, with both groups being fairly positive about it. Consistent with previous studies, women consider health aspects in their everyday food choice significantly more than men (significant at 5%), and women also report less confidence in the safety of food; however this is not found to be significant (see Table 7).

Table 7: Attitude towards Science and Technology and Approach to Food Split by Gender

	Gender	N	Mean (Stdv.)	Sig.*
Attitude towards science and technology[1]	Women Men	34 34	7.03 (1.678) 7.09 (2.391)	Ns.
Health reflexivity[2]	Women Men	34 34	1.76 (0.654) 2.21 (0.687)	P<0.05
Trust in food[3]	Women Men	33 33	3.21 (0.696) 2.94 (0.704)	Ns.

[1]Attitude towards science and technology was measured on a 10-point scale that ranged from 1 (the world is a lot worse off because of science and technology) to 10 (the world is a lot better off because of science and technology); [2]Health reflexivity was measured on a 5-point scale that ranged from 1 (a very large degree) to 5 (a very small degree); [3]Trust in food was measured on a 5-point scale that ranged from 1 (a very large degree) to 5 (a very small degree); * According to Mann-Whitney-U-tests; Ns. = non significant

Source: Own illustration.

Figure 8: Consumer Typology According to Berg (2004)

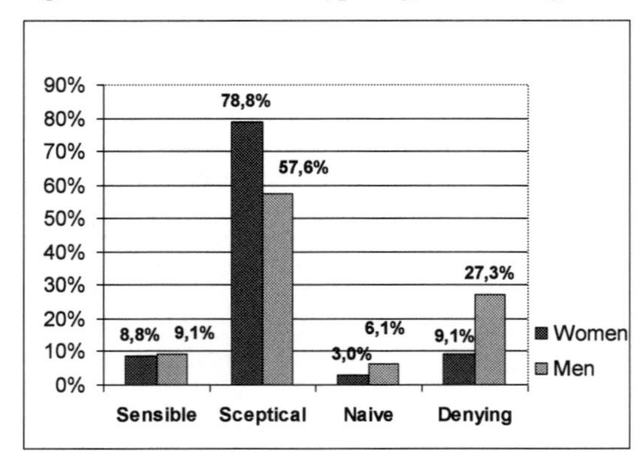

Source: Own illustration.

Comparing the frequency of women and men with regard to the four consumer types according to Berg (2004), a considerably higher share of women is part of the group of 'skeptical' consumers (high reflexivity and low trust), whereas relatively more men are in the groups of 'naïve' (low reflexivity and high trust) and 'denying' (low reflexivity and low trust) consumers (see Figure 8). The share of 'skeptical' consumers is largest for both women and men, followed by a considerable share of 'denying' consumers among men (27.3%) but not women (9.1%).

6.3.1.2 Across-Product Comparisons and General Evaluations of Products

Table 8 depicts the results for the ranking of the four Italian herbs (A, B, C, and D) according to likelihood of purchase for women and men separately. As a reminder, product A relates to the product that 'might contain mycotoxins', product B 'might contain pesticides', product C is 'irradiated' and product D is the reference group without any relation to a food hazard. As expected, all men and 93.8% of women indicate that they would most probably purchase product D. Product C is most frequently mentioned as second alternative (rank 2) by both women and men, but by a far larger share of men (61.8%) than women (43.8%). However, with regard to product C, the group of men and even more the group of women is split, with 29.4% of men and 40.6% of women selecting it as a last alternative, indicating very heterogeneous attitudes towards irradiation in both groups.

Table 8: Percentage of Men and Women that Ranked Each Product at Position One to Four

		1st rank	2nd rank	3rd rank	4th rank
Product A:	Men	-	26.5	41.2	32.3
Mycotoxins	Women	3.1	18.7	46.9	31.3
Product B:	Men	-	11.7	50.0	38.3
Pesticides	Women	3.1	34.4	37.5	25.0
Product C:	Men	-	61.8	8.8	29.4
Irradiation	Women	-	43.8	15.6	40.6
Product D:	Men	100	-	-	-
Ref. product	Women	93.8	3.1	-	3.1

Source: Own illustration.

Product B is ranked at the third position by most men (50.0%), but only 37.5% of women. The share of women ranking product B as second and third is quite similar, also indicating heterogeneous attitudes with regard to pesticides in the female sample. Most women (46.9%) as well as most men (41.2%) selected product A at the third position. Comparing shares and ranks between product A (mycotoxins) and B (pesticides), men seem to be somewhat less reluctant towards mycotoxins, with 26.5% selecting product A as second alternative compared to 11.7% selecting product B as second alternative, and 41% selecting product A as third rank compared to 50% selecting product B as third rank. Overall, women seem to be somewhat more favorable towards pesticides, with 18.7% selecting product A as second alternative compared to 34.4% selecting product B as second alternative, and 46.9% selecting product A as third rank compared to 37.5% selecting product B as third rank.

Table 9 presents the results for the affective and risk-benefit evaluation for the products, with the total number of women and men responding to each of the questions, the mean and standard deviations (in parentheses). With regard to products A and B, spontaneous affect is rather negative to neutral, with women being somewhat more negative than men about product A (mycotoxins) (2.03 compared to 2.26), and men being somewhat more negative than women towards product B (pesticides) (2.03 compared to 2.29). For both women and men, overall spontaneous affect with regard to product C (irradiation) is almost neutral, with men being more positive than women.

For the emotions 'contentment', 'anger' and 'worry', which are composed of two to three items, Cronbach's α for each of the emotions related to each product is indicated below Table 9. Compared to the reference product D (for which both women and men indicate high contentment and almost no anger and worry), for women and men contentment is rather low with regard to products A, B and C, while anger and worry is neutral to high for products A, B and C. Women and men award similar ratings with regard to 'contentment', 'anger' and 'worry' in most cases; however for product A (mycotoxins), men indicate higher levels of 'anger', with a mean of 3.40 for men and 2.96 for women. Furthermore, for product C men indicate higher levels of 'contentment' (1.90 compared to 2.21) and lower levels of 'worry' (3.03 compared to 2.79).

Except for product D, risk ratings are quite high and benefit ratings quite low for both women and men, and no gender differences exist for product A and B. However, for product C, men perceive lower levels of risk than women (3.65 compared to 3.11) and higher levels of benefit (2.06 compared to 2.60).

*Table 9: Affective and Risk/Benefit Evaluation of Products A, B, C by Gender and by Product**

	Product A: Mycotoxins[1]		**Product B: Pestici-des**[2]		**Product C: Irradia-tion**[3]		**Product D: Reference product**[4]	
	N; Mean (stdv.)		**N; Mean (stdv.)**		**N; Mean (stdv.)**		**N; Mean (stdv.)**	
	Women	**Men**	**Women**	**Men**	**Women**	**Men**	**Women**	**Men**
Affect (1=very bad to 5= very good)	34; 2.03 (0.870)	35; 2.26 (0.780)	34; 2.29 (0.906)	35; 2.03 (0.923)	34; 2.24 (0.987)	35; 2.69 (1.323)	34; 4.21 (1.067)	35; 4.46 (1.010)
Contentment (1=not at all to 5= very much)	33; 1.73 (0.894)	35; 1.87 (0.926)	33; 1.79 (0.884)	35; 1.84 (1.056)	33; 1.90 (1.100)	35; 2.21 (1.159)	33; 4.24 (0.936)	35; 4.30 (0.972)
Anger (1=not at all to 5= very much)	33; 2.96 (1.127)	34; 3.40 (1.088)	33; 3.01 (1.295)	35; 3.11 (1.032)	33; 3.03 (1.273)	35; 3.01 (1.195)	33; 1.22 (0.670)	35; 1.25 (0.720)
Worry (1=not at all to 5= very much)	31; 3.14 (1.125)	34; 3.35 (0.957)	32; 3.16 (1.247)	35; 3.06 (0.957)	31; 3.03 (1.172)	35; 2.79 (1.286)	33; 1.26 (0.564)	35; 1.31 (0.747)
Risk rating (1=not risky at all to 5=very risky)	34; 3.85 (0.958)	35; 3.80 (0.759)	34; 3.71 (0.938)	35; 3.86 (0.944)	34; 3.65 (1.178)	35; 3.11 (1.143)	34; 1.34 (0.691)	35; 1.37 (0.646)
Benefit rating (1=not beneficial at all to 5= very beneficial)	34; 2.03 (0.904)	35; 2.26 (0.919)	34; 2.00 (1.101)	35; 2.09 (0.981)	34; 2.06 (1.127)	35; 2.60 (1.311)	34; 4.12 (1.175)	35; 4.26 (1.120)

[1] Cronbach's **α** Consumption Emotion Scale (CES): Contentment A (α=0.579), Anger A (α=0.710), Worry A (α=0.731)

[2] Cronbach's **α** CES: Contentment B (α=0.529), Anger B (α=0.814), Worry B (α=0.814)[3] Cronbach's **α** CES: Contentment C (α=0.662), Anger C (α=0.815), Worry C (α=0.857)

[4] Cronbach's **α** CES: Contentment D (α=0.760), Anger D (α=0.896), Worry D (α=0.714)

* According to Mann-Whitney-U-tests no significant differences were found between women and men.

Figure 9 further presents the average differences between the risk and benefit ratings for each of the four products and split according to gender. Across products A, B, and C and across gender, risks are perceived to be higher than benefits. In the case of product C compared to products A and B, a higher share of women (14.7%) and an even higher share of men (37.1%) perceive benefits of the product to outweigh the risks. For product C, the group of men seems to be fairly equally split between those perceiving benefits to be higher than risks (37.1%), those perceiving benefits to be equal to risks (20.0%), and finally those indicating risks outweighing benefits (42.9%). For products A and B for both women and men, a small share of respondents perceive benefits to outweigh risks, a somewhat higher share of respondents indicates benefits to be similar to risks, and a relatively high share of respondents perceives risks to outweigh benefits. For women, this pattern also emerges for product C, but in a somewhat more moderate manner.

Figure 9: Percentage of Respondents in 'Risk- Benefit' Groups by Gender

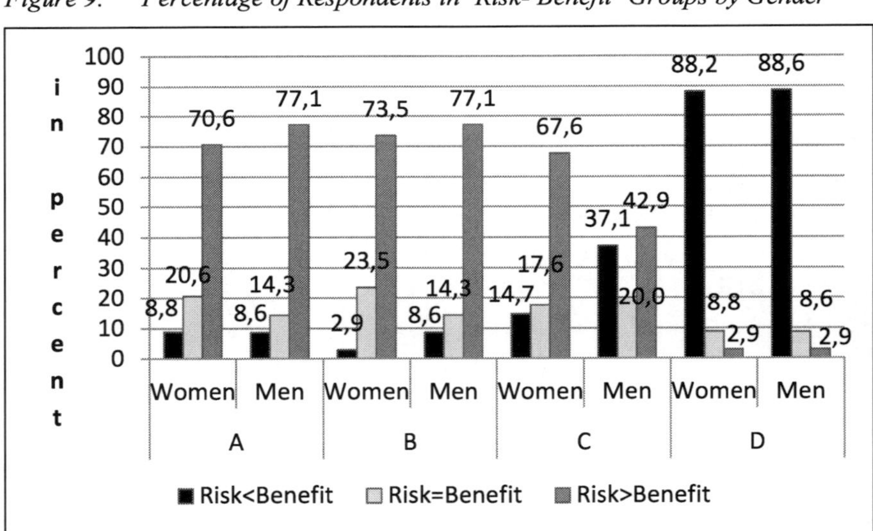

Source: Own illustration.

6.3.1.3 Summary

Different from previous findings, women and men do not differ in their general attitude towards science and technology. Regarding women's and men's approach to food, women are found to have a significantly more reflexive approach to food and clearly more women are 'skeptical' towards food safety, while more men are in the group of 'denying' consumers.

Men are clearly more positive than women regarding product C (irradiation), with higher levels of positive feelings (affect and emotion), a lower level of 'worry', a lower level of risk perception, and a higher level of benefit judgment. Perception of product B (pesticides) is similar for women and men, and also for product A (mycotoxins) no clear gender differences exist, with men being somewhat more positive about it and evaluating benefits as higher than women, but men show also stronger feelings of 'anger' than women.

With regard to products A (mycotoxins) and B (pesticides) risks outweigh the benefits for the majority of women and men. This is also the case for product C (irradiation) for women. In contrast, for product C (irradiation), the male sample is quite equally split into those that perceive risks to outweigh benefits, those that perceive risks to be equal to benefits, and those that perceive benefits to be higher than risks.

6.3.2 'Top of Mind' Associations

This section will present the content analysis of the in-depth laddering interviews. Table 10 presents the content codes alongside with explanations and examples that are the results of the content analysis of the first associations as well as the complete laddering interviews. These codes were used to analyse the very first associations of respondents. As in the starting elicitation procedure of the very first associations respondents were asked about their general thoughts, associations and feelings, not only attributes, consequences and values emerge among the content codes, but also general associations (e.g. 'disasters' such as Chernobyl and Fukushima). These are grouped under 'attributes', but a footnote indicates that these concepts are rather general associations that were mentioned during the first elicitation procedures.

Table 10: Summary of Content Codes

Content code	Explanation
Attributes	
Artificial/ not artificial	Not originally inside, chemical, artificial, something that is added
Beneficial/ not beneficial	Unnecessary, not beneficial; necessary; helpful
Conventional production	
Comparison with other hazards[1]	
Disasters[1]	
Free of pesticides/mycotoxins	
Harmful	General statements concerning the hazards' harmful potential: poisonous, dangerous, risky, unhealthy
No labeling	No labeling that product contains mycotoxins, pesticides, irradiation or the amount/degree of it
Irreversible/reversible	
Spreading in nature	Widespread, spreading in nature, unpreventable
Unlikely	Unlikely that mycotoxins, pesticides are in the product
Visible/not visible	Can(not) feel, hear, see or taste it
Functional consequences	
Buy/use	
Buy/use (not)	
Beneficial (not) when harmful	
Benefit reduction due to mycotoxins/pesticides/irradiation	
Economic consequences	Pests cause damage to the economy
Environmental contamination	Negative consequences for nature (plants, soil, water, animals)
Food control	
Food quality	Fresh products, healthy products, negative consequences for the taste, shelf life, appearance
Free of mycotoxins/pesticides	
Health risk	Damage to human body and negative health consequences such as allergies, headache, organ failure, cancer
Health risk (family)	Health risk to children, family and others
No information	Not enough information, want to get information

Content code	Explanation
Functional consequences (cont.)	
Intake in human body	Pesticide intake, irradiation/mycotoxins enter human body
Plant protection	Fighting/elimination of pests, support plant growth
Spreading in nature	Widespread, can be found in many food products, emission in nature, contaminants, unpreventable (irradiation)
Psychosocial consequences	
Anger	Being angry or mad
Anxiety	Feeling of anxiety, fear
Bad feeling	
Burden to others	Other people have to take care for oneself, being a burden for other people
Certainty/uncertainty	(No) traceability of consequence, assessable consequences by consumers and science
Change in mood	Becoming aggressive, unmotivated, lethargic
Consumer's consciousness	Valuation of food, to accept higher food prices for good quality, support small farmers
Consumer expectations	Expectations are met/satisfied
Control/no control by consumers	(Not) being able to control, monitor or take an action and avert something
Deception	Being deceived
Disgust	Feeling of disgust
Enjoyment	Enjoyment, fun related to concrete things such as food
Feeling of guilt	
Feeling of uncertainty	
Freedom of choice	Decision under certainty and full information, freedom of choice due to alternatives
Financial/time burden	Have to see the doctor, buy expensive medicine, societal costs, financial restrictions
Health	Health, preservation of health, self-preservation
Health (children, family, others)	
Healthy diet	Take care of having a healthy diet; importance of a healthy diet
Human beauty	Wanting to look good, having a nice appearance
Inspiration	Get new ideas/impetus, satisfy curiosity
Leisure/education	Time for other things, time with children, leisure activities, get educated

Content code	Explanation
Psychosocial consequences (cont.)	
Naturalness	Preference for naturalness, sustainable, ecological and natural way of living/producing
Performance	Personal performance and achievement potential, being productive at work
Producer's profit	Greed of gain by producers
Regeneration	To regenerate, recharge ones batteries
Restriction due to disease	Restrictions due to health problems, immobility
Shame	Feeling of shame
Social contact/ no social contact	(Don't) meet friends and other people anymore
Social relationships	Being able to have good relationships with other people; having problems with other people
Stigmatization	Being stigmatized
Subsistence	To make ones living (financially but also concerning the organization of personal and family life)
Success	Be successful
Wellbeing (own)	No stress, feeling good
Worry/no worry	To be worried, can(not) eat without worries

Content code	Explanation
Instrumental values	
Benevolence	Taking care of; responsibility for family/children/others; quality of life (children/family); wellbeing (children/family)
Honesty	Being honest; importance of truthfulness
Justice	Reciprocity, justice
Social trust	Trust in producer and food safety management
Responsibility (producer)	Producer has the responsibility
Responsibility (own)	Responsibility for oneself and to act when necessary
Terminal values	
Hedonism	Happiness, enjoyment of happy life, satisfaction; quality of life
Long, healthy life	Becoming old and healthy
Preservation humanity	Preservation of future generations
Preservation of nature	Preservation of the earth, protection of nature

Content code	Explanation
Terminal values (cont.)	
Security	Safety, social security and stability, personal stability and of relationships; inner peace and harmony
Self-direction	Independence, freedom, self-determination; creativity
Self-esteem	Self-confidence, self-affirmation, belief in own worth
Self-fulfillment	Self-actualization, to be able to reach one's goals, to make a contribution, to start a family; self-determination
Sense of belonging	to be part of society, feeling at home
Social recognition	Status, prestige, power
Universalism	Grace of charity, human dignity and equality, unity with nature, broad-minded

[1] The concepts 'comparison with other hazards' and 'disasters' are general associations that were mentioned during the first elicitation procedures when respondents were asked about their general associations as well as their thoughts related to risks and benefits evaluations.

Source: Own illustration.

Regarding the general and very first associations of women and men with regard to the products and the associations related to their risk and benefit ratings, Appendix E4 to Appendix E6 depict the four most important concepts in descending order for each of the products and split according to gender.[15] Except for a few concepts, all concepts mentioned are related to the food hazards, and descriptions as well as discussion of the results thus refer to food hazards and not to the products. In the few other cases that are related to other product attributes such as 'flavor', this is explicitly mentioned. The following descriptions of the elicited associations focus on the top four concepts in the minds of respondents and on concepts (even though not among the top four) where differences between women and men are considerable.

15 Results of Appendix E4 to Appendix E6 are based on detailed tables in Appendix E1 to Appendix E3.

6.3.2.1 *General 'Top of Mind' Associations*

The concepts 'harmful' and/or 'health risk' are among the top four for all respondents asked for their thoughts and associations that come to mind and their feelings for each of the three food hazards. 'Harmful' relates to the general capacity of causing damage and posing a risk, and 'health risk' refers to more specific associations concerning illness and damage to the human body. Moreover, across all three food hazards, a concept related to complete rejection of the product/hazard ('buy (not)')[16] is prevalent among women, but not among men.

Regarding the associations for each of the hazards separately, in addition to the health-related concepts 'harmful' and 'health risk' that are important for women and men, complete rejection of the product due to mycotoxins is also among the top four concepts for both women and men. Furthermore, relatively more men express the unspecific negative feelings 'feelings of uncertainty' (women: 3.6% compared to men: 12.5%) and 'bad feeling' (women: 14.3% compared to men: 37.5%), whereas more women express the emotion 'worry' (women: 10.7% compared to men: 0%). Considering the three affections together, more men express negative affective reactions.

For pesticides as for mycotoxins, the health-related concepts 'harmful' and 'health risks' are equally important for women and men. However, in contrast to mycotoxins, more women spontaneously mention negative affections and emotions ('bad feeling', women: 14.3% compared to men: 3.2%; 'worry', women: 14.3% compared to men: 3.2%) and considerably more women than men clearly reject the product that 'might contain pesticides', with 17.9% of women and 6.5% of men mentioning the concept 'buy (not)'. While important for mycotoxins and pesticides, for both women and men, the health-related concepts 'harmful' and 'health risk' are less strongly linked to pesticides than to mycotoxins. Except for this, for women the very first associations related to mycotoxins and pesticides are very similar, whereas men seem to link more unspecific negative affections to mycotoxins and more concrete concepts to pesticides such as 'intake in human body'.

With regard to irradiation, the feeling of not having enough information ('no information') is dominant for both sexes. There are no considerable differences between women and men with regard to 'bad feeling', 'feeling of uncertainty' and 'worry', which are similarly important for irradiation as for mycotox-

16 In this thesis, negations of concepts are generally built by adding a ('not') after the attribute or verb in order to avoid separation of the same concepts (e.g. 'buy' and 'buy (not)') when being sorted alphabetically in the code book.

ins and pesticides. The attribute 'radioactive' is further important for irradiation across sexes, but mentioned by more women (20.0% of women compared to 14.7% of men). More women link concepts around 'health risk' to irradiation (23.3% of women compared to 14.7% of men) and more women also clearly reject irradiation, with 20.0% of women compared to 5.9% of men mentioning that they would not buy the irradiated product ('buy (not)'). Men more often than women mention concepts that relate to other hazards ('comparison with other hazards', with 3.3% of women and 11.8% of men) or that refer to previous and current 'disasters' such as the nuclear accidents of Chernobyl or Fukushima (women: 10.0% compared to 17.6% of men).[17] Interestingly, some men (14.7%) but not women also mention positive aspects of irradiation considering 'food quality' such as longer shelf-life or the elimination of bacteria or other contaminants.

6.3.2.2 'Top of Mind' Associations Related to Risk and Benefit Evaluation

Regarding the associations that women and men mention when they are asked what they considered when they evaluated the risks of the three food hazards, the health-related concepts 'harmful' and 'health risk' are the most dominant concepts for mycotoxins and pesticides and of similar importance for women and men.

Similar to the very first associations, after the health-related concepts, a considerable share of both women and men mention that they would reject the product due to mycotoxins ('buy (not)'). However, 12.1% of men but only 2.4% of women believe that mycotoxins are 'not always harmful'. Both women and men, but relatively more men (10.3% of women compared to 15.2% of men), are thinking of bad food quality ('food quality (no)') when making a risk judgment for mycotoxins.

Considering pesticides, also the health-related concepts 'harmful' and 'health risk' are dominant for both sexes; however, considerably more women (17.9%) than men (2.9%) mention that there are no health risks or not necessarily health risks due to pesticides ('health risk (no)). More men (20.6%) than women (7.1%) compare pesticides with other (food) technologies/hazards in order to make a judgment. Furthermore, the evaluation of pesticides seems to be influ-

---

17 Data were collected between March 10th 2011 and March 29th 2011. The nuclear accident of Fukushima happened on March 11th.

enced by the perception of not being able to control and avert risks due to pesticides ('consumer control (no)') by more women (14.3%) than men (2.9%).

For the associations taken into consideration when judging irradiation, quite a lot of differences between women and men emerge: Only for women are the health-related concepts 'harmful' and 'health risk' important (37.9% of women and 6.1% of men mentioned 'harmful'; 24.1% of women and 3.0% of men mention 'health risk'). Similarly, a significant share of women (24.1%) but not of men (3.0%) mentions their clear opposition towards the irradiated product ('buy (not)'). While the lack of information ('information (no)') is perceived by both women and men (see above the general associations in 6.3.2.1), only women seem to consider it for their risk evaluations, with 24.1% of women mentioning it also with regard to their risk ratings.

Furthermore, 13.8% of the women but only 3.0% of the men mention that they had the disasters Chernobyl and Fukushima ('disasters') in mind when they made their risk evaluations. For men, no real concentration is observable, with the most important concept 'food quality (no)' being mentioned only by 12.1% of men followed by 'free of mycotoxins' (9.1% of men) that is related to the product C itself, but not to irradiation.

Regarding the associations that women and men mention when they were asked what they had in mind when they evaluated the benefits of the three products/or food hazards, a somewhat different picture emerges: first of all, benefit perceptions seem to be strongly linked to risk perceptions. Many respondents state that as long as there might be a risk, they see no benefit ('not beneficial when harmful') or that the benefit is reduced if there is a risk ('benefit reduction due to (…)). These two concepts are dominant across all three food hazards/products and sexes. 'Not beneficial when harmful' and 'benefit reduction due to (…)' are kept separate, as the first concept relates to a complete negation of any benefit whereas the respondents that mention the second still perceive benefit from the product, but this benefit is reduced due to one or more product attributes. As such, 'not beneficial when harmful' is fairly similar to the complete rejection 'buy (not)'. In the case of 'buy (not)' the reasons are however not clearly stated.

Considering the negation of benefit and complete rejection together, it is stronger for women than men, with 62.9% of women and 37.5% of men mentioning these concepts for mycotoxins (48.1% of women and 21.9% of men mentioned 'not beneficial when harmful'; 14.8% of women compared to 15.6% of men mentioned 'buy (not)'). However, more men (21.9%) than women (14.8%) mention the moderated version 'benefit reduction due to mycotoxins'. Also, more men (9.4% and 9.4%) than women (3.7% and 7.4%) mention the concepts 'health risk' and 'food quality (no)'. Both women and men also mention positive concepts with regard to mycotoxins when they are asked for the benefit ratings: 'Food quality' as related to the positive influence of Italian herbs on taste is mentioned by 18.5% of women and 9.4% of men.

With regard to pesticides, the interrelation between risk and benefit judgments seem to be less strong, or at least less often directly framed as such. 'Not beneficial when harmful' is mentioned by 17.9% of women and 24.1% of men, and 'buy (not)' was mentioned by 10.7% of women and 17.2% of men, indicating a clearer rejection of benefits for product B for men than for women. More women mention the concept 'benefit reduction due to pesticides' (women: 10.7%; men: 6.9%). Only a share of men (10.3%) but not of women indicate that they would buy the product if necessary ('buy'). However, positive aspects of product B regarding 'food quality' and the capacity of product B to 'flavor' is mentioned by 10.7%/10.7% of women but only by 3.4%/0% of men.
Considering irradiation, 'not beneficial when harmful' is similarly important for women (30.4%) and men (33.3%), and even though less important than for mycotoxins, it is more important than for pesticides. However, 21.7% of women, but only 3.3% of men, state that they completely reject the product ('buy (not)') which indicates a stronger rejection by women. In addition, more women indicate that they took health concerns into consideration when making their benefit ratings (13.0% of women compared to 0% of men mention 'harmful'; 13.0% of women and 3.3% of men mention 'health risk'). A similar share of women and men also mention the positive aspects 'free of mycotoxins' (13.0% of women and 13.3% of men) and 'free of pesticides' (13.0% of women and 10.0% of men). Finally, the most important concepts across the three different elicitation tasks are considered (general associations, associations when risks are judged, and associations when benefits are judged). In this case, the percentage of concepts mentioned refers to the relative frequency a concept is mentioned related to the total number of concepts that is mentioned across the elicitation tasks. Before, when the most important concepts were regarded for each elicitation procedure separately, percentages referred to the relative frequency of women or men that mentioned a concept. Respondents sometimes mention the same concepts in two or all three elicitation tasks. Hence, looking only at the share of respondents that mentioned these concepts would not consider that some concepts are mentioned several times.

Table 11 shows the number of different concepts and the total number of concepts at each level of abstraction, and the relative frequency of the total number of concepts at each abstraction level related to the total number of concepts that are mentioned by women or men for each food hazard. Women and men mention between 36 and 40 different kinds of concepts, with functional consequences constituting the biggest shares (43.1% to 56.1%), followed by attributes with shares between 26.1% and 40.9%. For irradiation, the share of attributes and functional consequences is almost identical.

Table 11: Number of Different Concepts, Total Number of Concepts, and Relative Frequency for Each Abstraction Level[1]

	Mycotoxins		Pesticides		Irradiation	
	Women (N=29)	Men (N=33)	Women (N=28)	Men (N=34)	Women (N=30)	Men (N=34)
Emotions	4; 16 (9.8%)	4; 21 (11.4%)	4; 17 (10.9%)	3; 4 (2.8%)	6; 25 (13.8%)	6; 20 (12.3%)
Attributes	10; 45 (27.4%)	8; 48 (26.1%)	11; 48 (31.0%)	10; 50 (34.7%)	14; 74 (40.9%)	13; 58 (35.6%)
Functional consequences	15; 92 (56.1%)	15; 98 (53.3%)	16; 80 (51.6%)	17; 79 (54.9%)	15; 78 (43.1%)	15; 75 (46.0%)
Psychosocial consequences	4; 7 (2.4%)	5; 10 (5.4%)	3; 8 (5.2%)	5; 10 (6.9%)	1; 1 (0.6%)	5; 9 (5.5%)
Instrumental values	3; 3 (1.8%)	3; 5 (2.7%)	2; 4 (2.6%)	1; 1 (0.7%)	0	1; 1 (0.6%)
Terminal values	1; 1 (0.6%)	1; 2 (1.1%)	0	0	3; 3 (1.7%)	0
All	37; 164 (100%)	36; 184 (100%)	36; 155 (100%)	36; 144 (100%)	39; 181 (100%)	40; 163 (100%)

[1]The first number in each cell presents the number of different concepts that were mentioned for a specific abstraction level, the second number presents the total number of concepts that were mentioned and the percentage in parentheses presents the relative importance of each abstraction level in terms of the total number of concepts that were mentioned.

Source: Own illustration.

Clearly, the more abstract levels such as psychosocial consequences, instrumental and terminal values hardly play a role for the first associations, but psychosocial consequences constitute a bigger share with regard to all food hazards for men than for women (see Table 11). After functional consequences and attributes, emotions seem to be important with regard to the most salient associations, with a share between 2.8% and 13.8%. Concerning pesticides, women seem to mention a considerably higher share of emotions than men (women: 10.9% compared to men: 2.8%).

Table 12: Top Four Concepts Across all Three Elicitation Tasks[1]

'Top of mind' associations (all together)					
Mycotoxins		**Pesticides**		**Irradiation**	
Women	**Men**	**Women**	**Men**	**Women**	**Men**
1.Health risk (14.6)	1.Health risk (15.8)	1.Harmful (13.2)	1.Health risk (15.3)	1.Harmful (9.9)	1.No information (8.0)
2.Harmful (14.0)	2.Harmful (12.0)	2.Health risk (11.8)	2.Harmful (13.2)	1.Buy (not) (9.9)	2.Beneficial (not) when harmful (6.1)
3.Buy (not) (9.8)	3.Buy (not) (9.8)	3.Buy (not) (6.6)	3.Comparison with other hazards (6.9)	2.Health risk (9.4)	3.Free of mycoto-xins (6.1)
4.Beneficial (not) when harmful (7.9)	4.Bad feeling (7.1)	4.Bad feeling (5.3)	4.Buy (not) (6.3)	3.No information (8.8)	3.Food quality (5.5)
				4.Radioactive (5.5)	4.Bad feeling (4.3)
					4.Widespread (4.3)
					4.Disasters (4.3)
					4.Health risk (4.3)

[1] Numbers in parentheses depict the relative frequency that a concept is mentioned in relation to all mentioned concepts per food hazard; Source: Own illustration.

Table 12 presents the four most important concepts that are mentioned across elicitation tasks. The health-related concepts 'harmful' and 'health risk' and complete rejection ('buy (not)') are the top three cognitive concepts across all food hazards for women and for mycotoxins and pesticides for men. For mycotoxins and pesticides, the relative share of women and men mentioning these three concepts is similar. For mycotoxins the rejection of benefit due to mycotoxins ('not beneficial when harmful') is more important for women (7.9% of all concepts) than for men (3.8% of all concepts). For pesticides, the share of negative affect and emotions is clearly higher for women than for men (bad feeling: women: 5.3%; men: 1.4; worry: women: 2.6; men: 0.7%). 'Comparison with other hazards' seems to be much more important for men (6.9%) than for women (3.3%). For both women and men, the perception of lacking knowledge and information ('no information') is an important concept with regard to irradiation. Whereas for women only negative aspects of irradiation are among the top four concepts, positive and negative concepts are more balanced for men, with 'free of mycotoxins' (6.1%) and 'food quality' (5.5%) and 'bad feeling' (4.3%), 'not beneficial when harmful' (6.1%) and 'health risk' (4.3%).

6.3.2.3 Summary

To sum up, functional consequences followed by attributes are most important among the first concepts that come to mind when respondents are confronted with food hazards.

Across all elicitation tasks (general, risk, and benefit-related), the health-related concepts 'harmful' and 'health risk' and complete rejection ('buy (not)') are the top three cognitive concepts across all food hazards for women. For men, they are the top three cognitive concepts for mycotoxins and pesticides. With regard to irradiation, the perception of lacking knowledge and information ('no information') is further an important concept for women and men. For women, only negative aspects of irradiation are among the top four concepts, whereas men mentioned positive and negative concepts.

With regard to the very first general associations and feelings linked to each of the food hazards, associations related to mycotoxins are strongly related to health for women and men. Other important concepts are rather unspecific such as the general rejection of the product, and especially men elicit general negative affective concepts. This is similar for women with regard to pesticides, while for men negative affect seem not to play an important role for pesticides.

Regarding associations elicited when asked to rate the risks of the three products, concerns about health are important for women and men with regard to pesticides and mycotoxins, but only important for women with regard to irradiation. Whereas more men than women believe that mycotoxins might not always be harmful, more women than men think that pesticides do not (always) cause health risks. For making a risk judgment, men compare pesticides with other hazards, while lack of control is a major focus of women. For the risk rating of irradiation, women but not men have a clear negative position and have concepts such as health concerns, lack of information and disasters in mind. Men's thoughts tend to be sparse with regard to irradiation.

If one looks at the associations that women and men mention when they are asked, what they had in mind when they evaluated the benefits of the three products, one can clearly see that a considerable share of women and men strongly link benefit judgments to their risk judgments. Many respondents state that as long as there might be a risk, they see no benefit ('not beneficial when harmful') or that the benefit is reduced if there is a risk ('benefit reduction due to (...)). For women, mycotoxins and irradiation seem to more clearly nullify possible benefits of the herbs, whereas for men it tends to be pesticides that have this effect.

6.3.3 Results of the Laddering Interviews

This sub-chapter first gives an overview of some quantitative measures regarding participants' knowledge structures, followed by the presentation of the results of the content analysis of the laddering interviews. Furthermore, the content of the consumers' knowledge structures with regard to the food hazards is graphically presented in HVMs that are further analyzed with regard to their complexity.

6.3.3.1 Variability, Complexity and Level of Abstraction

Before focusing on the results of the content of the laddering interviews, some quantitative measures are described that give an initial picture of women's and men's cognitive structures. As described in more detail in chapter 5.4, the amount and variety of activated information as well as the degree of complexity of the cognitive structures are indicators of a person's level of involvement (Lastocicka and Gardner, 1978; Petty, Cacioppo and Schumann, 1983; Celsi and

Olson, 1988; Grunert and Grunert, 1995). In addition, the proportion of abstract concepts is proposed as a further indicator of involvement (Sørensen, Grunert and Nielsen, 1996).

Table 13: Number of Different Kind of Elements Elicited for Each of the Three Food Hazards per Abstraction Level (by Gender)[1]

	Mycotoxins		Pesticides		Irradiation	
	Wo-men N=29	Men N=26	Wo-men N=28	Men N=33	Wo-men N=31	Men N=29
Attributes	5	5	6	3	7	7
Functional consequences	7	6	10	10	9	9
Psychosocial consequences	35	32	31	34	30	30
Instrumental values	6	4	6	6	4	5
Terminal values	11	10	10	10	11	11
All	64	57	63	63	60	62

[1] Concepts framed in a positive or negative way are considered together here.

Source: Own illustration.

Attributes, consequences, and values elicited during the laddering interviews have been coded for each of the three food hazards. Table 13 shows the number of different kind of concepts (the variety) for each abstraction level and the sum of all. As expected, a relatively low number of attributes for all food hazards is elicited during the laddering interviews. This can be attributed to the fact that the topic of the laddering interviews focused on food hazards and not on products, and the hazards themselves can be regarded as product attributes. In addition, across all food hazards and both sexes, the number of different concepts is highest for the psychosocial consequences. Compared to the food risks mycotoxin and pesticides, irradiation elicite a slightly higher variety of attributes and functional consequences, but a smaller number of psychosocial consequences is elicited from women and men. Comparing the variety of elements, no gender differences emerge for pesticides and irradiation. However, more women than men link a larger number of different concepts to mycotoxins (64 for women, 57 for men), which is especially due to more different kinds psychosocial consequences and values.

In addition to the number of concepts, previous research proposes the number of elicited ladders and average ladder length as measures of complexity of cognitive structures and consumers' involvement (Barrena and Sánchez, 2010; Sørensen, Grunert and Nielsen, 1996; Zanoli and Naspetti, 2002).

Table 14 depicts the different measures. As group size varies for each of the food hazards and between women and men, average numbers of concepts, ladders and ladder length are indicated here.

Overall, both women and men elicite on average the highest number of concepts with regard to pesticides (women: 16.29; men: 17.41), directly followed by mycotoxins for women (15.69) and by irradiation for men (14.81). Women mention on average a higher number of concepts with regard to mycotoxins (women: 15.69; men: 12.26), whereas men elicite a higher number of concepts on average with regard to pesticides (women: 16.29; men: 17.41). With regard to irradiation, the average number of all concepts is somewhat higher for men (14.81) than for women (13.84).

Women compared to men elicite a somewhat higher number of ladders on average with regard to mycotoxins (women: 5.90; men: 5.19) and irradiation (women: 5.74; men: 5.32), whereas men elicite a higher number of ladders on average for pesticides (women: 6.32; men: 6.79). Women and men both elicite the relatively highest number of ladders for pesticides.

With regard to average length of ladders, women elicite significantly longer ladders for mycotoxins (women: 4.11; men: 3.71). Men have significantly longer ladders for irradiation (women: 3.59; men: 3.80) and longer cognitive ladders for pesticides (women: 3.70; men: 3.99), however the difference in ladder length for pesticides is not significant.

The last column of Table 14 (average ladder length to the first value) will be discussed below.

Table 14: Measures of Complexity (Negative and Positive Concepts Together)

		Number of con-cepts[1]	Average number of concepts[2]	Average number of ladders[2]	Average lad-der length[2]	Average ladder length to first value[3]
Mycotoxins	Women (N=29)	64	15.69 (8.120)	5.90 (3.109)	4.11* (1.054)	3.82 (1.210)
	Men (N=26)	57	12.26 (6.729)	5.19 (3.124)	3.71 (1.693)	3.64 (1.253)
Pesticides	Women (N=28)	63	16.29 (6.341)	6.32 (2.932)	3.70 (1.295)	3.76 (0.984)
	Men (N=33)	60	17.41 (8.639)	6.79 (3.847)	3.99 (1.088)	3.95 (1.537)
Irradiation	Women (N=31)	62	13.84 (6.419)	5.74 (2.683)	3.59* (1.814)	3.70 (1.185)
	Men (N=29)	67	14.81 (9.418)	5.32 (3.198)	3.80 (1.112)	3.88 (1.347)

[1] Different types of concepts
[2] Numbers in parentheses are standard deviations
[3] Only ladders are included that reached the value level
[*] Significant differences between women and men at the 10% significance level according to Mann-Whitney U-tests.
Source: Own illustration.

Table 15 presents the average numbers of elements mentioned at each abstraction level and gives an overview of abstraction levels for the three food hazards, split by gender.

Table 15: Total and Average Numbers of Elements Elicited at Each Abstraction Level[1]

		A	fC	pC	iV	tV	Sum of all
Mycotoxins	Women N=29	0.72 (0.922)	2.79 (1.449)	7.55* (4.808)	0.89 (0.976)	3.72 (3.411)	15.69 (8.120)
	Men N=27	0.67 (1.000)	2.45 (1.281)	5.12 (2.913)	0.704 (1.171)	3.34 (3.150)	12.26 (6.729)
Pesticides	Women N=28	1.29 (1.301)	3.32 (1.744)	6.71 (3.137)	1.07 (1.585)	3.89 (3.270)	16.29 (6.341)
	Men N=32	0.81 (1.061)	3.41 (1.583)	7.72 (4.609)	0.97 (1.787)	4.50 (3.612)	17.41 (8.639)
Irradiation	Women N=31	1.39 (1.498)	2.90* (1.513)	5.71 (3.617)	0.71 (0.902)	3.13 (3.041)	13.84 (6.419)
	Men N=31	1.10 (1.076)	3.95 (2.081)	6.07 (4.878)	0.48 (0.677)	3.23 (3.48)	14.81 (9.418)

A= attributes; fC= functional consequences; pC= psychosocial consequences; iV= instrumental value; tV= terminal value;

[1] Numbers in parentheses are standard deviations.

* Significant differences between women and men at the 10% significance level according to Mann-Whitney U-tests.

Source: Own illustration.

Psychosocial consequences with a share of 41% to 48.1% are clearly dominant across all three food hazards followed by the terminal values with a share between 21.8% and 27.2% and functional consequences with 17.8% and 26.6%. With a share between 4.6% and 10.0%, attributes play only a minor role.

Considering mycotoxins, women compared to men mention on average a higher number of concepts (women: 15.69; men: 12.26; see Table 14). However, the share that each level of abstraction holds is quite similar for women and men. With regard to the psychosocial consequences, women give a significantly higher number of concepts (women: 7.55; men: 5.12). Walker and Olson (1991) labeled psychosocial consequences, instrumental values, and terminal values as part of a person's self-concept. Accordingly, the share of these self-relevant concepts against the total number of concepts is calculated. The self-relevant concepts make up 77.5% of women's overall cognitions and 74.6% of men's overall cognitions with regard to mycotoxins. For pesticides, men elicite a slightly higher average number of concepts (women: 16.29; men: 17.41) and the share of psychosocial consequences, instrumental values, und terminal values is higher for men (75.9%) than for women (71.7%), which points to men's higher abstraction level.

With regard to irradiation, the average number of all concepts is somewhat higher for men (14.81) than for women (13.84); however, women have a higher level of abstraction, with a share of 69% of the self-relevant concepts compared to men with a share of 66.1%. Thus, with regard to irradiation, the self-relevant concepts, albeit still dominant, are somewhat less important than mycotoxins and pesticides. In addition, men elicite a significantly higher number of functional consequences than women (women: 2.90; men: 3.95).

Linked to the level of abstraction is the probability that a self-relevant concept is retrieved in memory and thus plays a role for the decision-making process. According to the theory of spreading activation (as explained in chapter 5.4), the shorter the path from the first concept (that a person has in mind about an object or issue) to the self-relevant concepts, the higher the likelihood that the more abstract concepts in a person's memory are activated and thus play a role in judgment. The last column in Table 14 presents the average length of paths from the first concept to the first value mentioned by the respondents. With regard to mycotoxins, women have on average a longer path to the value level than men, but a higher share of ladders reach the value level. For pesticides, men have longer paths until they reach the value level, but a higher share of ladders that reach the value level. With regard to irradiation, men's paths are somewhat longer until the first value is reached.

6.3.3.2 Results of the Content Analysis

For the presentation of the results of the content analysis of the laddering interviews, positive and negative ladders are regarded separately. As detailed in chapter 6.2.3.2, this allows interpretation of the subsequent HVMs and relating the content analysis to HVMs. While negative ladders relate to the hazards' negative consequences and the threat of values and goals, positive ladders relate to the perceived beneficial characteristics and consequences or to the lack of negative consequences. Due to the low number of concrete attributes, concrete and abstract attributes are considered together in the presentation of results.

Negative ladders

Table 16 presents only the most important concepts that were mentioned by at least 25% of the group of women or men and/or constitute at least 2% of the overall concepts for each food hazard (cross in bold/cross in normal text).

It thus takes into account the relative frequency of different individuals that mentioned a concept as well as the relative importance compared to the total number of concepts mentioned (considering multiple mentions of one concept by the same respondent). Tabele 16 is based on detailed tables in Appendix E7, Appendix E9 and Appendix E11, presenting the number of times and share that each concept has been mentioned. Explanation with regard to the meaning of each concept is given in the code book that is depicted in sub-chapter 6.3.2. Regarding content and meaning of the elicited elements, a large number of concepts that are perceived as important by the respondents are similar across the three food hazards and across gender.

The following concepts are perceived as important across all food hazards and by both groups: the functional consequences 'no food quality' and 'health risk', the psychosocial consequences 'health', 'restriction (due to) disease', and 'wellbeing', the instrumental value 'benevolence', and the terminal values 'hedonism' and 'long life'. Thus the threat to the respondent's own health and well-being, as well as threats to the wellbeing of close friends or family ('benevolence'), are dominant cognitive constructs across all food hazards.

Similarly important and elicited by both sexes for two of the three food hazards are the attribute 'harmful' for mycotoxins and pesticides, the functional consequence 'no information' with regard to pesticides and irradiation, the psychosocial consequence 'uncertainty' for pesticides and irradiation, the psychosocial consequences 'pleasure' for mycotoxins and pesticides, and the terminal value 'self-direction' for pesticides and irradiation. The perception of not being satisfactorily informed, the wish for more information ('no information') and the perception of not being able to assess and trace the consequences ('uncertainty') are important cognitions with regard to pesticides (with 28.6% of women and 24.2% of men mentioning 'no information' and 35.7% of women and 36.4% of men mentioning 'uncertainty') and even more important with regard to irradiation (with 43.3% of women and 48.3% of men mentioning 'no information and 33.3% of women and 44.8% of men mentioning 'uncertainty').

Table 16: Important Attributes, Consequences, and Values Elicited for the Three Food Hazards by Gender

	Mycotoxins		Pesticides		Irradiation	
	Women	Men	Women	Men	Women	Men
Abstract attributes						
Artificial			**X**	X	X	
Beneficial (not)			**X**			
Harmful	**X**	**X**	**X**	**X**	X	
Radioactive						X
Functional consequences						
Food control						X
Food quality	**X**	**X**	**X**	**X**	**X**	**X**
Health risk	**X**	**X**	**X**	**X**	**X**	**X**
Intake in human body		X	X	**X**		
No information			X	X	**X**	**X**
Plant protection			X			
Widespread						X
Psychosocial consequences						
Certainty (no)	X		X	X	**X**	**X**
Disgust		X				
Financial/time burden	**X**			**X**		
Freedom of choice	X		**X**		**X**	**X**
Health (own)	**X**	**X**	**X**	**X**	**X**	**X**
Health (family/friends)		X				
Healthy diet		X				
Leisure/education				X	X	
Performance	**X**			X		
Pleasure	X	**X**	X	**X**		**X**
Restriction disease	**X**	X	**X**	X	**X**	**X**
Social contact	X					
Wellbeing (own)	**X**	X	**X**	**X**	**X**	**X**
Worry					X	
Instrumental values						
Benevolence	**X**	X	X	X	**X**	**X**
Terminal values						
Hedonism	**X**	**X**	**X**	**X**	**X**	**X**
Long, healthy life	X	**X**	X	**X**	**X**	**X**
Preservation nature			X			
Self-direction	**X**		X	**X**	**X**	**X**
Self-fulfillment		**X**				

X = concepts that make up at least 2% of overall concepts per food hazard and that were mentioned by at least 25% of the respondents; X = concepts that make up at least 2% of overall concepts per food hazard or that were mentioned by at least 25% of the respondents. Source: own illustration.

While important for pesticides and irradiation, the threat to personal independence, freedom and self-determination ('self-direction') is more strongly linked to pesticides by men and to irradiation by women.

The threat to one's ability to take decisions with full information and certainty or having alternatives ('freedom of choice') is a key concept for women as it is rated as important across all three food hazards, while only playing a role with regard to irradiation for men. Moreover, the attribute 'artificial' is an important concept with regard to pesticides and irradiation in the minds of women, but only linked to pesticides in the minds of men.

In the following, key similarities and differences between the cognitions of women and men are regarded for each of the three food hazards separately.

Mycotoxins

With regard to the most frequently mentioned concepts 'harmful', 'health risk' and 'health', 'no food quality' and 'hedonism', no gender differences emerge except for 'health', which is mentioned by almost all men (92.3%), but only 58.65 of the women. However, a concept similar to health, 'wellbeing', is mentioned by more women (62.1% of women and 42.3% of men). For several cognitive concepts, considerable gender differences exist and for the majority of them, more women mention these concepts: More women than men mention the emotion-related concepts 'anxiety' and 'worry', with 20.7% of women and 11.5% of men eliciting 'anxiety', and 13.8% of women and 3.8% of men mentioning 'worry'. Furthermore, concepts around the ability to relax and regain energy ('regeneration'), burdens and physical restriction due to illness ('financial/time burden' and 'restriction disease'), and the threat to the ability to perform at work ('performance') are mentioned by considerably more women than men (17.2% compared to 0% for 'regeneration'; 24.5% compared to 11.5% for 'financial/time burden'; 44.85 compared to 23.1% for 'restriction disease'; and 34.5% compared to 19.2% for 'performance'). A threat to the health of family members or friends ('health risk family/friends' and 'health family/friends') is perceived as similarly important by women and men, but the instrumental value of responsibility and taking care of the wellbeing of close friends or family ('benevolence') is mentioned by considerably more women (48.3% compared to 23.1%). Additionally, having good social relations with other people ('social relations') and the ability to get to know and meet other people ('social contact') is mentioned by relatively more women (31.0% compared to 15.4% for 'social contact' and 17.2% compared to 0% for 'social relations'). For women, the psychosocial consequence ‘uncertainty’ and the terminal value ‘self-direction’ play a dominant role with regard to all three food hazards, and both are linked to mycotoxins by far more women than men (27.6% compared to 7.7% for ‘uncertainty’ and 37.9% compared to 23.1% for ‘self-direction’).

However, several values are more strongly linked to mycotoxins for men than for women. Relatively more men mention the instrumental value ‘justice’ (15.4% compared to 3.4%) and the terminal values ‘security’ (23.1% compared to 13.8%), ‘self-fulfillment’ (30.8% compared to 20.7%), and ‘universalism’ (19.2% compared to 10.3%), a concept referring to ideas about the unity of human beings with nature and human dignity.

Pesticides

Several of the concepts found to be important across all food hazards such as ‘health risk’, ‘uncertainty’, ‘health’, ‘wellbeing’, ‘restriction (due to) disease’, ‘no food quality’ and ‘benevolence’ are found to be similarly important for women and men with regard to pesticides. For pesticides and the most important values ‘hedonism’ and ‘long life’, women more strongly link the threat to happiness, satisfaction, and quality of life to pesticides (‘hedonism’), whereas for men, the value of being able to live a long, healthy life (‘long life’) and the threat to quality of life and happiness (‘hedonism’) is almost equally important.

When it comes to the most important gender differences, women mention the attribute ‘not beneficial’ relatively more often than men (28.6% compared to 15.2%). For men, the attribute ‘harmful’ is relatively more strongly linked to pesticides, with 54.5% of men and 42.9% of women mentioning that concept. The related functional consequence ‘intake in human body’ is mentioned by more men (30.3% compared to 17.9%). Furthermore, for men, pesticides pose a threat to the ability to perform at work (‘performance’: 33.3% of men and 17.9% of women), to have the capacities and possibilities for leisure activities (‘leisure/education’: 33.3% of men and 17.9% of women), and to meet other people (‘social contact’: 21.2% of men compared to 10.7% of women). For far more men than women, pesticides constitute a financial and time burden (‘financial/time burden’: 39.4% of men and 7.1 of women). However, twice as many women link the constraint to their ‘freedom of choice’ to pesticides (50.0% of women and 24.2% of men). With regard to values, for relatively more men pesticides pose a stronger threat to the self-centered values ‘self-direction’ (39.4% of men compared to 28.6% of women)’, ‘self-esteem’ (21.2% of men and 14.3% of women) and ‘self-fulfillment (18.2% of men and 10.7% of women). A threat to personal and social stability ('security') is perceived by 18.2% of men, but by only 10.7% of women. Furthermore, more than twice as many men mention the instrumental values 'justice' (24.2% of men compared to 10.7% of women) and the importance to trust producers and food safety management institutions ('social trust': 15.2% of men and 7.1% of women). However, a considerable share of women, but not of men, mention their own responsibility and acting when necessary ('responsibility (own)': 17.9% of women compared to 0% of men). Similarly, 'preservation of nature' is linked by twice as many women to pesticides as by men (28.6% of women compared to 15.2% of men).

Irradiation

The concepts 'food quality', 'no information', 'restriction (due to) disease', and 'wellbeing' are similarly important for women and men, and as in the case of mycotoxins and pesticides, women more strongly link concepts related to 'hedonism' than to 'long life', whereas for men, relative frequencies for the two values are equal.

All concepts related to personal health such as 'harmful', 'health risk', and 'health' are linked to irradiation by more women than men ('harmful': 26.7% compared to 17.2%; 'health risk': 80.0% compared to 72.4%; 'health': 56.7% compared to 44.8%). The attribute 'artificial' is mentioned by more women (20.0% compared to 13.8%), whereas the attribute 'radioactive' is mentioned by more men (20.7% compared to 13.8%). Considerably more men link concepts such as unpreventable and widespread ('spreading in nature') to irradiation (17.2% of men compared to 6.7% of women) and believe that irradiated food is tested for its safety ('food control': 13.8% of men and 0% of women). Furthermore, irradiation more often causes negative emotions among women (30% mentioned 'worry' and 23.3% mentioned 'anxiety') than among men (13.8% mentioned 'worry' and 13.8% mentioned 'anxiety'). Financial and time burdens due to illness ('financial/time burden') as well as the ability to take part in leisure activities ('leisure/education') is relatively more important for women, with 16.7% and 26.7% compared to 6.9% and 6.9% of men mentioning these concepts with regard to irradiation. The perception of not being able to assess and trace the consequences of irradiation ('uncertainty') and not being able to take informed decisions or avoid irradiation by choosing other products ('freedom of choice') is linked by a considerable number of women and men, but seems to be more important for men (44.8% of men compared to 33.3% of women mention 'uncertainty' and 44.8% of men compared to 30.0% of women mention 'freedom of choice'). More men than women (27.6% compared to 16.7%) perceive irradiation as a threat to enjoying everyday things ('pleasure'). Moreover, the feeling of being deceived or cheated ('deception') is only important for men (17.2%) but not for women (0%).

While important for both women and men, 'benevolence' and 'self-direction' are mentioned by relatively more women (40.0% compared to 27.6% for 'benevolence' and 43.4% compared to 27.6% for 'self-direction'). 'Self-esteem' is further only considered as important by the group of women, with 20.0% of women but only 6.9% of men mentioning that concept. Thus, the rather egoistic values 'self-direction' and 'self-esteem' as well as the rather altruistic value 'benevolence' is more strongly linked to or threatened by irradiation in women's than in men's minds. However, the altruistic value 'preservation humanity' is perceived as more important by men. Far more men (20.7%) than women (3.3%) link worries about the preservation of future generations to the food hazard/technology irradiation.

Positive ladders

With regard to mycotoxins and pesticides, only very few respondents mention few positive ladders. Four women elicite a total of seven positive ladders and one man mentioned two positive ladders with regard to mycotoxins, the four women also mentioned negative ladders. Similarly, with regard to pesticides, six women elicite a total of 13 positive ladders and four men mentioned four positive ladders, but all of them also elicite negative ladders. Eleven women elicite 16 positive ladders and eleven men mentioned thirty-two positive ladders with regard to irradiation, and ten of the eleven women and nine of the eleven men also mention negative ladders at the same time. Results of the content analysis of the positive ladders are depicted in Appendix E 8, Appendix E 10 and Appendix E 12.

Considering mycotoxins, the concepts 'artificial (not)' are mentioned by two of the four women and 'food quality' by three of the four women. One woman and one man further mention that 'naturalness' is important for them. Somewhat more positive concepts are mentioned with regard to pesticides. Whereas for women a good 'food quality' in terms of a longer shelf life or an attractive product appearance and no risk to health ('health risk (no)') are dominant positive consequences linked to pesticides, men mention the functional characteristic that pesticides are used to protect plants from from pest damages ('plant protection'). With regard to irradiation, about a third of women and men also mention positive ladders next to negative ladders, more of those were however mentioned by men. Due to the lack of knowledge that is indicated by many of the respondents, the cognitive structures are split into two parts: a negative one with the irradiation's harmful potential, and a positive one that is mainly based on the respondents' own assumption of a 'harmful (not)', a natural '(artificial (not)') or especially for men also a 'beneficial' form of irradiation. With regard to functional consequences, the same concepts are perceived as important for women and men; however, more important for men are a positive effect on 'food quality', no 'health risk', and 'plant protection'. What is further noticeable is the dominance of attributes and functional consequences with regard to positive ladders for both women and men. For men only, the higher order concepts 'wellbeing (own)' and the related quality of life ('hedonism') are important. Men but not women mention a high number of different kinds of psychosocial consequences in the positive ladders.

To sum up: with regard to mycotoxins and pesticides, the positive associations are in general only minor side paths next to the dominant negative paths for both women and men; but the positive associations are considerably more frequent among women. For irradiation, another picture emerges, with fairly undecided cognitive structures with regard to positivity or negativity of food irradiation by a third of both women and men. However, men's involvement with regard to the positive aspects of irradiation is considerably stronger.

6.3.3.3 Analysis of the Hierarchical Value Maps

HVMs are created only for negative ladders. For mycotoxins and pesticides, this is due to the low number of respondents that elicited positive ladders. For irradiation, the number of respondents that mention positive ladders is sufficient to create HVMs, but both women and men have heterogeneous ladders with a high majority of relations that are mentioned only once. Thus, also for irradiation, it is not possible to create a readable HVM.

During the following interpretation of the HVMs the presence of so-called key concepts plays an important role. In this context, key concepts are defined as cognitive elements that have several incoming and/or outgoing relations with other cognitive elements.

As noted in chapter 6.2.3.2 the principle of non-redundancy is not strictly applied. Following Grunert and Grunert (1995), if it can be assumed that the group of respondents has heterogeneous cognitive structures, redundant relations should be taken into account to avoid misinterpretations. Looking at the data of this study, some respondents in each subgroup have quite short paths with only few elements before they reach a high abstraction level, while others have many intermediary connections. In this case, complying with the principle of non-redundancy would mean not to consider the shorter and more direct paths. For this reason, strong direct paths that were mentioned by more than six respondents are depicted in the HVMs by means of broken arrows.

For ease of interpretation, the elements 'health risk' and 'health' are interpreted together and named as 'health concerns'. The results for all three food hazards show that the same respondents sometimes seem to link the same consequences to the more specific element 'health risk', and sometimes to the more general concept 'health'. It thus seems that the distinction between these two concepts is for some of the respondents more a result of different verbalization styles (more concrete ones versus more abstract ones), but has no effect on the type of related consequences. However, the distinction between the two concepts is maintained in the HVM in order to be able to distinguish lengths of paths and also to consider those respondents making the distinction between specific health risks and the general concept of health.

Mycotoxins

Table 17 presents the selected cut-off levels for mycotoxins in each level of abstraction along with the percentage of women and men that had to mention that relation and the amount of information that is depicted in the HVMs when applying the selected cut-off points.

Table 17: Selection of Cut-Off Values and Related Information Content of HVM for Each Abstraction Level (Mycotoxins)

Mycotoxins	**Women (N=29)**		**Men (N=26)**	
	Cut-off (% of respon-dents)	% of depict-ed relations all/direct	Cut-off (% of respon-dents)	% of depict-ed relations all/direct
A→C,V;	3 (10.3%)	56.1/70.8	3 (11.5%)	53.3/40.0
fC→C,V;	3 (10.3%)	61.5/62.5	3 (11.5%)	56.8/66.7
pC→pC, V;	3 (10.3%)	33.8/38.3	3 (11.5%)	21.0/27.0
iV→V;	2 (6.9%)	66.6/50.0	2 (7.7%)	57.1/66.7
tV→tV;	2 (6.9%)	57.1/35.7	2 (7.7%)	62.1/66.7
Average		Ø 55.0/51.6		Ø 50.1/53.4
% of all linkages		47.6/47.5		42.4/46.2

A=attributes; C=consequences; V= values; fC=functional consequences; pC= psychosocial consequences; iV= instrumental values; tV= terminal values;

Source: Own illustration.

For instance, a cut-off level of three was chosen for relations from attributes to all consequences and values (A→C, V) for women and men. That means that in this case, in order to be considered in the HVM, at least 10.3% of women and 11.5% of men have to mention a relation coming from an attribute. As a consequence, 56.1% of all relations and 70.8% of all direct relations of women and 53.3% of all relations and 40.0% of all relations of men are depicted in the HVM for relations coming from attributes.

The cut-off values in each abstraction level in the two maps are the same. The cut-off values are three for relations from attributes, functional and psychosocial consequences and two for relations from instrumental and terminal values. The women's HVM represents 47.6% of all linkages and 47.5% of all direct linkages.

For the men's HVM, these are 42.4% and 46.2% respectively. In both maps, the share of depicted relations departing from psychosocial consequences is quite low, with 33.8% for the women's HVM and 21.0% for the men's HVM. This is due to a relatively high number of different psychosocial consequences resulting in a large number of rather weak links departing from psychosocial consequences.

Figure 10 and Figure 11 present the HVMs of women and men for mycotoxins. All concepts that appear in the HVMs are shown alongside the percentage of respondents that mentioned that concept. Furthermore, the arrow thickness indicates the strength of relation between two concepts expressed by the relative frequency of respondents mentioning that relation. The thinnest arrows show the relations made by less than 15% of the respondents, but not lower than the respective cut-off levels of two or three depending on the abstraction level. The medium and thickest arrows show relations that were made by 15% to less than 35% of respondents and by 35% and more of respondents respectively. Appendix F1 also depicts the related number of times that a relation was mentioned.

For instance, in the HVM of women (see Figure 10) 'harmful' is mentioned by 51.7% of women and the thick arrow to 'health risk' indicates that 'harmful' is linked to 'health risk' by equal to or more than 35% of women. Moreover, negative consequences for physical appearance ('bad look') is seen as a consequence of 'health risk', but this link is mentioned by less than 15% of women as indicated by the thin arrow. 'Bad look' poses further a threat to personal 'wellbeing' (as indicated by less than 15% of women) which is further necessary to meet other people ('social contact'). 'Social contact' is further linked to 'hedonism' and thus seen as a precondition for a happy life.

In the HVM of women and men the number of attributes, functional consequences, instrumental and terminal values is similar, but women link a far larger palette of psychosocial consequences to mycotoxins (18 psychosocial consequences for women compared to 12 psychosocial consequences for men). From the functional and psychosocial consequences 18 of 22 consequences reach the value level in the women's HVM compared to 10 of 15 consequences in the men's HVM. This is also due to women's higher variety of psychosocial consequences that are strongly interconnected before many of them reach the value level.

The following summarizes the congruent parts of the two HVMs.

The HVMs share the following chains:

- health risk – health – long life
- health risk – health – hedonism
- health risk – health family/friends
- harmful – health risk – wellbeing
- food quality – disgust – pleasure – hedonism

In both maps, health-related concerns are central. A few paths lead to 'health concerns' (6 for women and 3 for men) and a large number of paths depart from it (10 for women and 14 for men). Concerns related to health are thus key concepts in the women's and men's cognitions with regard to mycotoxins. Except for two chains in the women's HVM and one chain in the men's HVM, every chain is somehow connected to 'health risk' and/or 'health'. Furthermore, women and men share the chain from 'harmful' to 'health risk' to 'health' to 'long life' which in both maps constitutes a dominant chain and a similar health chain ending directly with 'hedonism': 'harmful – health risk – health – hedonism'.

Second, women and men share the chain from 'health risk' to 'health family/friends' and both concepts and the relation between the two are equally important in both HVMs.

Third, the only chain that is completely independent of health concerns is the one starting from 'food quality' to 'disgust' to 'pleasure' and ending in 'hedonism', which is existent in the men's and women's HVMs. This chain is mentioned by a subgroup of women. Most women mentioned the intermediary concept 'wellbeing' between 'disgust' and 'pleasure'.

Fourth, 'hedonism' related to aspects around quality of life, satisfaction, and happiness is a very important key concept in both maps, expressed in the relatively high frequency of respondents in both subgroups who mention that concept, and with eight incoming links in the men's and women's HVMs.[18]

18

→ < 15% of respondents mentioned that relation

→ >= 15% and < 35% of respondents mentioned that relation

→ >= 35% of respondents mentioned that relation

-·-·-·-> Broken arrows indicate direct links mentioned by more than six respondents

Figure 10: *HVM for Mycotoxins (Women; N=29)*

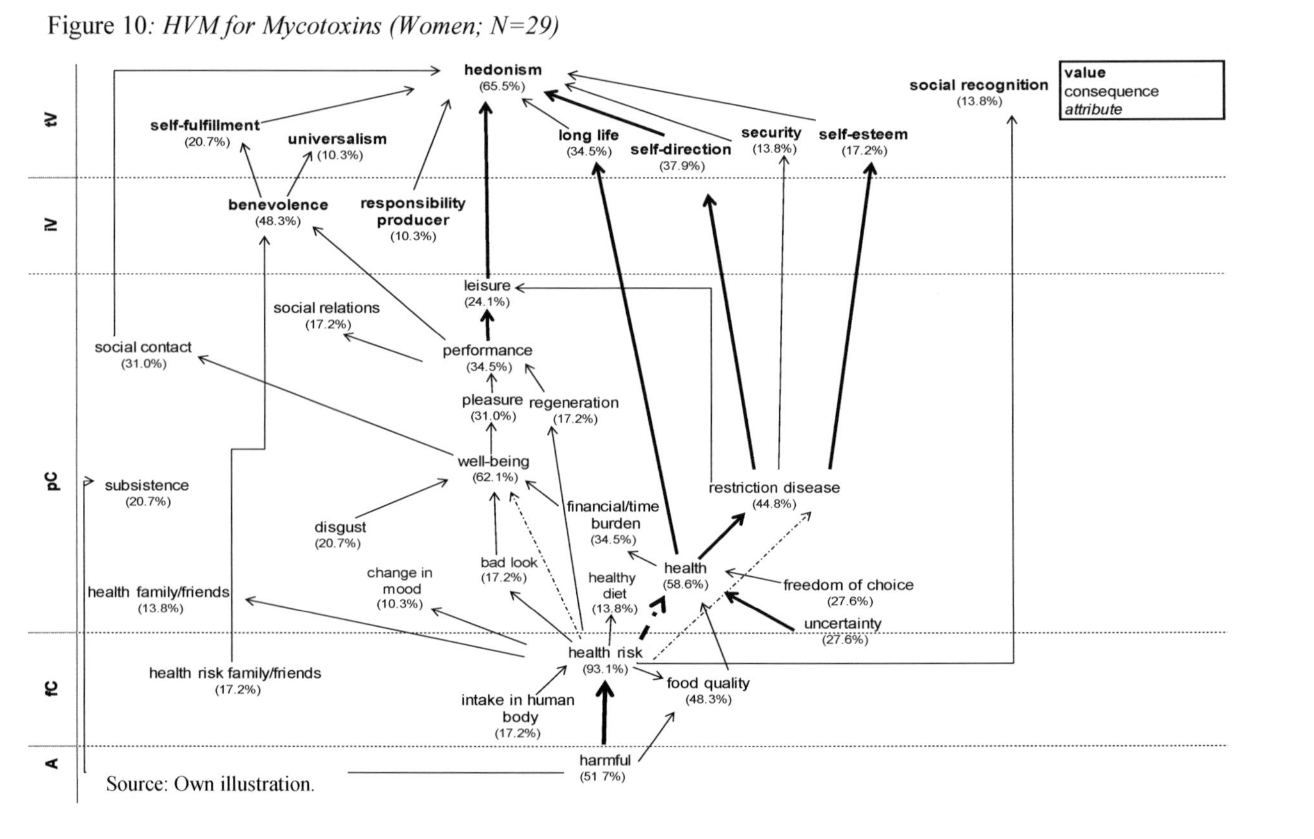

Source: Own illustration.

Figure 11: HVM for Mycotoxins (Men; N=26)

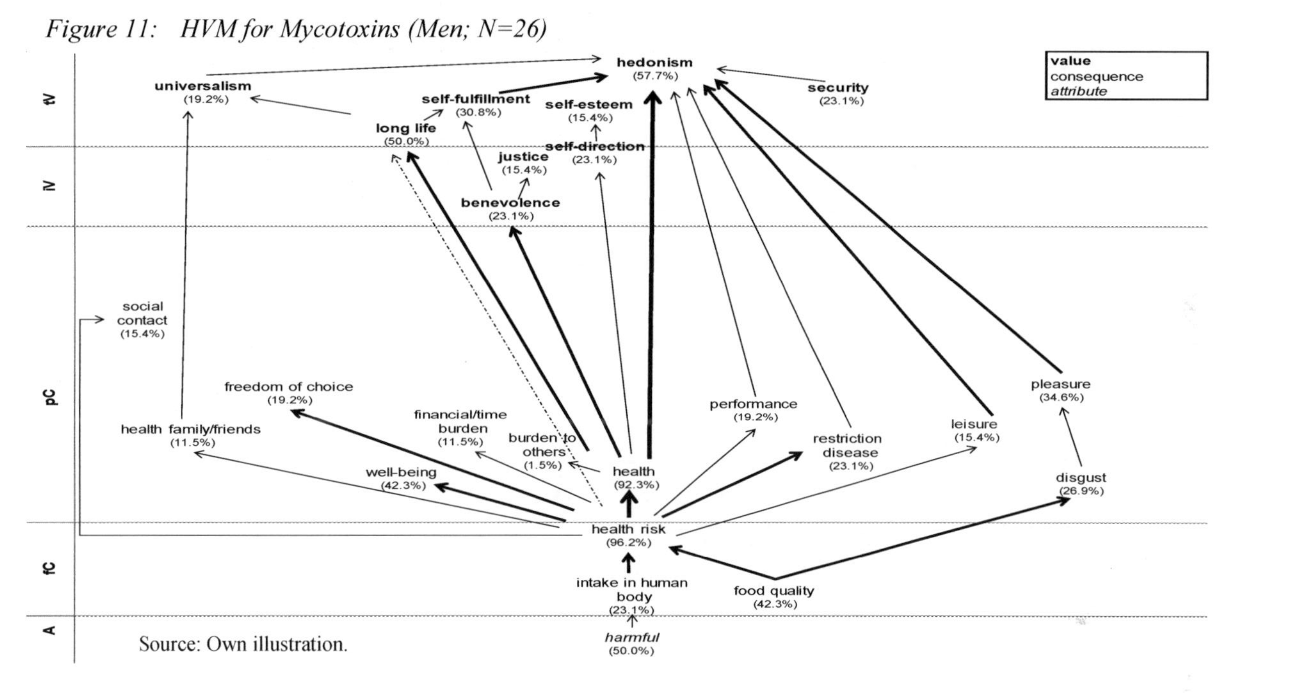

Source: Own illustration.

The following summarizes the key differences between the HVMs of women and men:

The differences between the men's and women's HVMs mostly relate to strong interconnections between the psychosocial consequences in the women's HVM, but not in the men's HVM. In the men's HVM, 'health concerns' constitute the only and dominant key concept, whereas in the women's HVM, several intermediary concepts also play a key role with regard to outgoing paths. Apart from 'health concerns', 'wellbeing' has two outgoing links (one to 'pleasure' and one to 'social contact'), and 'performance' has three outgoing links (one to 'social relations', to 'leisure', and to 'benevolence'). In women's minds, the ability to perform well ('performance') is instrumental to having good 'social relations', having time and money to enjoy 'leisure' time, and taking care of the wellbeing of close people ('benevolence'). 'Performance' and 'benevolence' are also more important in the women's HVM regarding the relative frequency of respondents who mentioned these elements.

A fourth important key concept concerning the outgoing links in the HVM of women is 'restriction disease'. Whereas the men's HVM contains physical restrictions due to illness ('restriction disease') that constitute a direct threat to happiness, quality of life, and satisfaction ('hedonism'), the women's HVM shows restrictions due to illness that primarily pose a threat to 'self-direction', 'self-esteem' and 'security'. The chains 'harmful – health risk – health – restriction disease – self-direction' and 'harmful – health risk – health – restriction disease – self-esteem' are important cognitive chains in the women's HVM. Particulary the threat to 'self-direction' seems to be more strongly linked to mycotoxins in women's minds than in men's, whereas the threat to 'self-fulfillment' is more important in the men's HVM.

Regarding the key differences with regard to the relative frequency of concepts, the concepts 'benevolence', 'social contact', and 'social relations' – all related to the relationships with other people – are perceived to be threatened by women more than men. Similarly, concepts related to personal independence (such as 'financial time burden', 'restriction disease' and 'self-direction') as well as concepts related to performance at work and organization of everyday life (such as 'performance' and 'subsistence') are relatively more important for women than for men. For men, however, mycotoxins seem to be a threat to social stability and harmony ('security') and to 'self-fulfillment'.

Pesticides

Table 18 presents the selected cut-off levels for the HVM of women and men with regard to pesticides. The cut-off values in each abstraction level are the same for women and men. The cut-off values are three for relations from attributes, functional and psychosocial consequences, and two for relations from instrumental and terminal values. Table 18 further indicates the percentage of links depicted in the HVM. The women's HVM represents 38.8% of all linkages and 39.9% of all direct linkages elicited from women. For the men's HVM, these are 42.2% and 43.3% respectively. In both maps, the share of depicted relations departing from psychosocial consequences is quite low, with 24.5% for the women's HVM and 29.9% for the men's HVM. Moreover, in the women's HVM, relations departing from instrumental values are not depicted, as each relation was only mentioned by one participant.

Table 18: Selection of Cut-Off Values and Related Information Content of HVMs for Each Abstraction Level (Pesticides)

Pesticides	**Women (N=28)**		**Men (N=33)**	
	Cut-off (% of respondents)	% of depicted relations all/direct	Cut-off (% of respondents)	% of depicted relations all/direct
A→C,V;	3 (10.7%)	38.5/29.5	3 (9.1%)	53.2/50.0
fC→C,V;	3 (10.7%)	54.1/64.3	3 (9.1%)	52.3/60.5
pC→pC, V;	3 (10.7%)	24.5/29.5	3 (9.1%)	29.9/30.8
iV→V;	2 (7.1%)	0/0	2 (6.1%)	43.5/35.3
tV→tV;	2 (7.1%)	52.2/47.6	2 (6.1%)	43.7/47.6
Average		Ø 33.9/34.2		Ø 44.5/44.8
% of all linkges		38.8/39.9		42.2/43.3

A=attributes; C=consequences; V= values; fC=functional consequences; pC= psychosocial consequences; iV= instrumental values; tV= terminal values;

Source: Own illustration.

As in the case of mycotoxins, the thin arrows indicate relations between concepts that are mentioned by less than 15% of the respondents, the medium arrows represent relations that are mentioned by eqal or more than 15%, but less than 35% of the respondents and the thick arrows indicate relations that are made by more than 35% of the respondents. Appendix F2 further depicts the related number of times a relation was mentioned.

Figure 12 and Figure 13 present the HVMs of pesticides for women and men. In these maps, the number of attributes, functional consequences, and instrumental values is similar, but men seem to link more different kinds of terminal values to pesticides (7 terminal values for women compared to 10 terminal values for men). Of the functional and psychosocial consequences, 14 of 19 consequences reach the value level in the women's HVM, compared to 16 of 22 consequences in the men's HVM.

The following summarizes the congruent parts of the two HVMs.

The HVMs share the following chains:

- intake in human body – health risk – health – wellbeing – self-direction – hedonism
- intake in human body – health risk – health – performance – hedonism
- intake in human body – health risk – health – long life – hedonism
- no information – uncertainty – freedom of choice – health
- environmental contamination – preservation nature

As in the case of mycotoxins, health concerns are dominant and 'health risk' together with 'health' are key concepts, with 6/5 incoming links and 12/9 outgoing links for women/men. For women and men, health concerns due to pesticides are linked to 'wellbeing' – 'self-direction', to 'performance' – 'hedonism' and to 'long life' – 'hedonism'.

For women and men, cognitions with regard to pesticides also seem to be linked to concepts other than health, such as 'environmental contamination – preservation of nature' and 'no information – uncertainty – freedom of choice'. Furthermore, for both women and men, other attributes in addition to 'harmful' are important: 'artificial' and 'plant protection' for women and 'artificial' and 'spreading in nature' for men. The terminal value 'hedonism', which summarizes concepts such as quality of life, happiness and satisfaction, is further important in the case of pesticides in both HVMs.

Figure 12: HVM for Pesticides (Women; N=28)

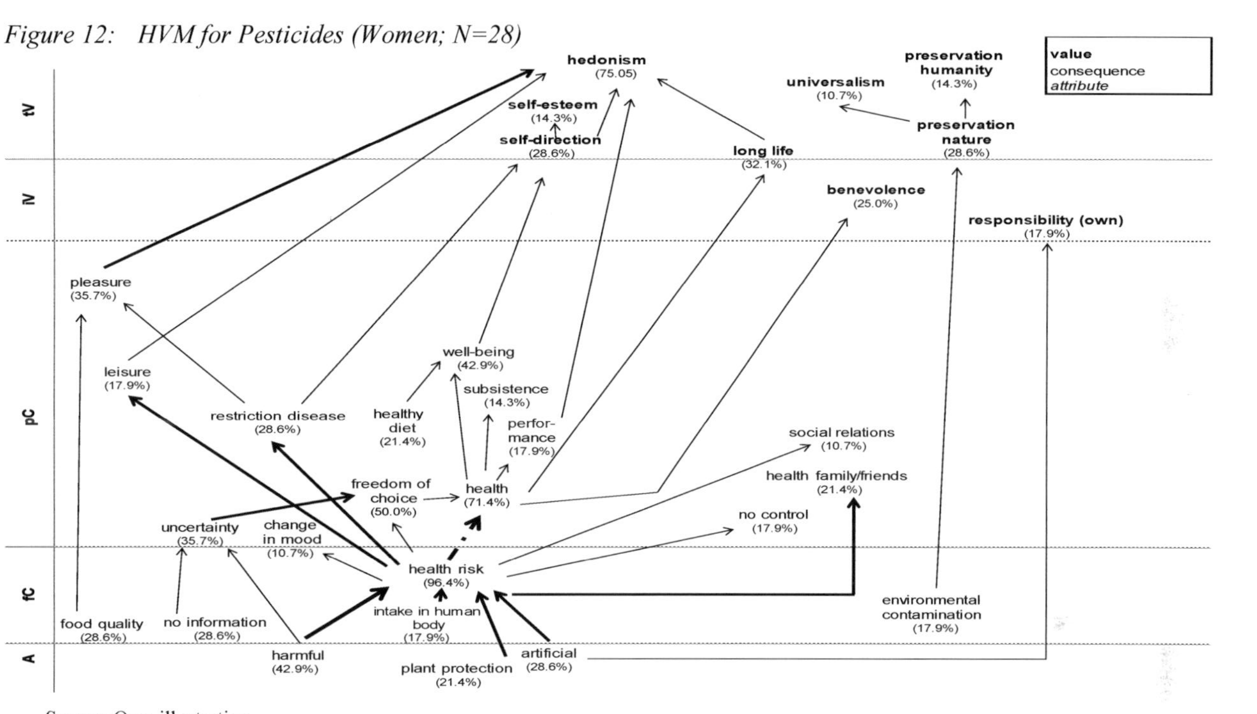

Source: Own illustration.

Figure 13: HVM for Pesticides (Men; N=33)

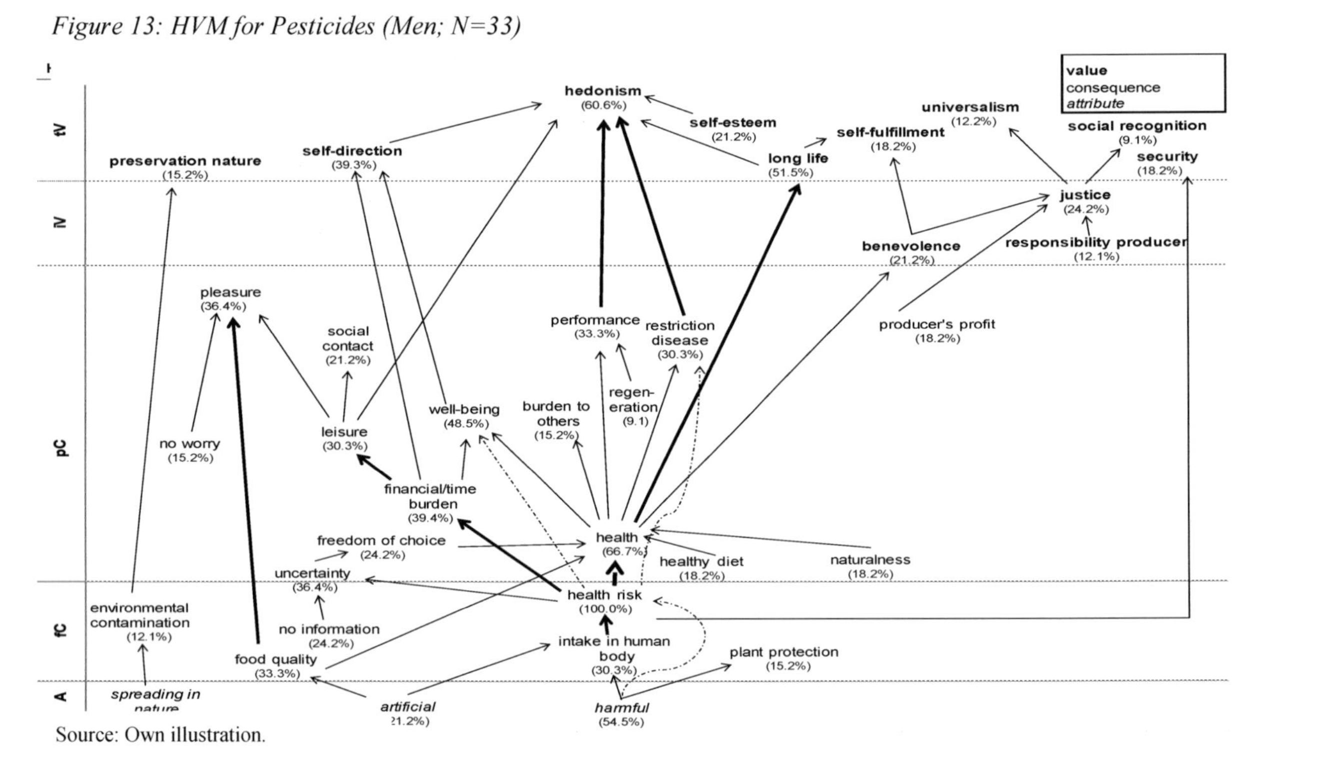

Source: Own illustration.

However, in the men's HVM, 'justice' is a second key value, with three incoming links and two outgoing links. For both women and men, not only 'hedonism' plays a role, but also more altruistic and biospheric values linked to the preservation of nature and/or humanity ('preservation nature' and 'preservation humanity') and the wellbeing of close friends or family ('benevolence').

The following summarizes the key differences between the HVMs of women and men:

In the women's HVM, the path from 'health risk' to 'health family/friends' is important, but it is not at all important in the men's HVM.

In the men's HVM, the chain 'health risk – financial/time burden – leisure' is important, whereas the concept 'financial/time burden' does not play a role in the HVM of women. 'Financial/time burden' and 'leisure' are further key concepts in the HVM of men but not of women, with three outgoing paths for both concepts. The threat to 'performance' is perceived by more men than women, but women perceive the threat to their ability to organize everyday life ('subsistence') more strongly than men. The relation between 'uncertainty' and 'freedom of choice' is stronger for women than for men, and 'freedom of choice' is also mentioned by more women than men. For men, the values 'security' and 'long life' are more strongly linked to pesticides than for women.

Irradiation

Table 19 presents the selected cut-off levels for irradiation and the related percentage of links depicted in the HVM. The cut-off values in each abstraction level in the two maps are the same. The cut-off values are three for relations from functional and psychosocial consequences, two for relations from attributes and terminal values, and one for relations from instrumental values. The women's HVM represents 40.2% of all linkages and 43.6% of all direct linkages. For the men's HVM, these are 41.6% and 47.7% respectively. As with the HVMs of mycotoxins and pesticides, the share of depicted relations departing from psychosocial consequences is quite low, with 26.7% for the women's HVM and 33.0% for the men's HVM. Moreover, in the women's and men's HVM, all relations (100%) are depicted that depart from instrumental values as there are only a few.

Table 19: Selection of Cut-Off Values and Related Information Content of HVM for Each Abstraction Level (Irradiation)

Irradiation	**Women (N=30)**		**Men (N=29)**	
	Cut-off (% of respon-dents)	% of depict-ed relations all/direct	Cut-off (% of respon-dents)	% of depict-ed relations all/direct
A→C,V;	2 (6.7%)	52.1/51.4	2 (6.9%)	49.6/53.3
fC→C,V;	3 (10.0%)	50.5/67.1	3 (10.3%)	43.9/61.6
pC→pC, V;	3 (10.0%)	26.7/27.5	3 (10.3%)	33.0/33.1
iV→V;	1 (3.3%)	100/100	1 (3.4%)	100/100
tV→tV;	2 (6.7%)	47.4/60.0	2 (6.9%)	46.7/41.7
Average		55.3/61.2		54.6/57.9
% of all linkges		40.2/43.6		41.6/47.7

A=attributes; C=consequences; V= values; fC=functional consequences; pC= psychosocial consequences; iV= instrumental values; tV= terminal values;

Source: Own illustration.

Figure 14 and Figure 15 present the HVMs for irradiation of women and men. As above, the arrow thickness (thin, medium and thick) indicates the importance of relations between concepts with relations mentioned by less than 15%, greater equal 15% and smaller 35% and greater equal 35% of the respondents. Appendix F3 depicts the number of times a relation is mentioned that is related to these three groups.

In these two maps, the number of attributes, functional consequences, and instrumental values is similar, with a few more different kinds of values by men (10 values by women compared to 12 values by men). Of the functional and psychosocial consequences, 11 of 16 consequences reach the value level in the women's HVM compared to 12 of 16 consequences in the men's HVM.

The following summarizes the congruent parts of the two HVMs. The HVMs share the following chains and the following elements are important elements in the HVMs of both subgroups:

- intake in human body – health risk – health – long life
- intake in human body – health risk – health – restriction disease

- no information – uncertainty – freedom of choice – self-direction
- no information – uncertainty – freedom of choice – health
- food quality – no information – health risk – restriction – disease

In the case of irradiation too, concerns about health are dominant in both HVMs. Health concerns are linked to physical restriction due to illness ('restriction disease'), and irradiation poses a threat to a long and healthy life ('long life') for women and men.

The 'no information – uncertainty – freedom of choice' chain is an important cognitive road, albeit more important in the HVM of men.

Next to the attribute 'harmful', both women and men link several kinds of attributes to irradiation, such as 'not beneficial', 'not visible', or 'radioactive/roentgen'. For women also 'artificial' is important with regard to irradiation.

The following summarizes the key differences between the HVMs of women and men:

For men but not for women, there exists an important chain from 'food quality' via 'pleasure' to 'hedonism'.

The two emotional concepts 'anxiety' and 'worry' are important with regard to the cognitions that women link to irradiation. Both emotional concepts seem to pose a threat to hedonistic aspects such as fun and the enjoyment of concrete things ('pleasure') and happiness or quality of life ('hedonism') in women's minds.

Furthermore, 'benevolence' constitutes a key value in the women's HVM, with three outgoing links and a higher frequency of women who mention it. Similarly, the value 'self-direction' is mentioned by a higher share of women than men.

Generally, the men's HVM has two strong health paths ('health risk – health – long life' and 'restriction disease – hedonism'), an important path between 'food quality' and 'pleasure', and a strong cognitive path: 'no information – uncertainty – freedom of choice'. In the women's HVM, only one health path is strong ('harmful – health – restriction disease').

Figure 14: HVM for Irradiation (Women; N=30)

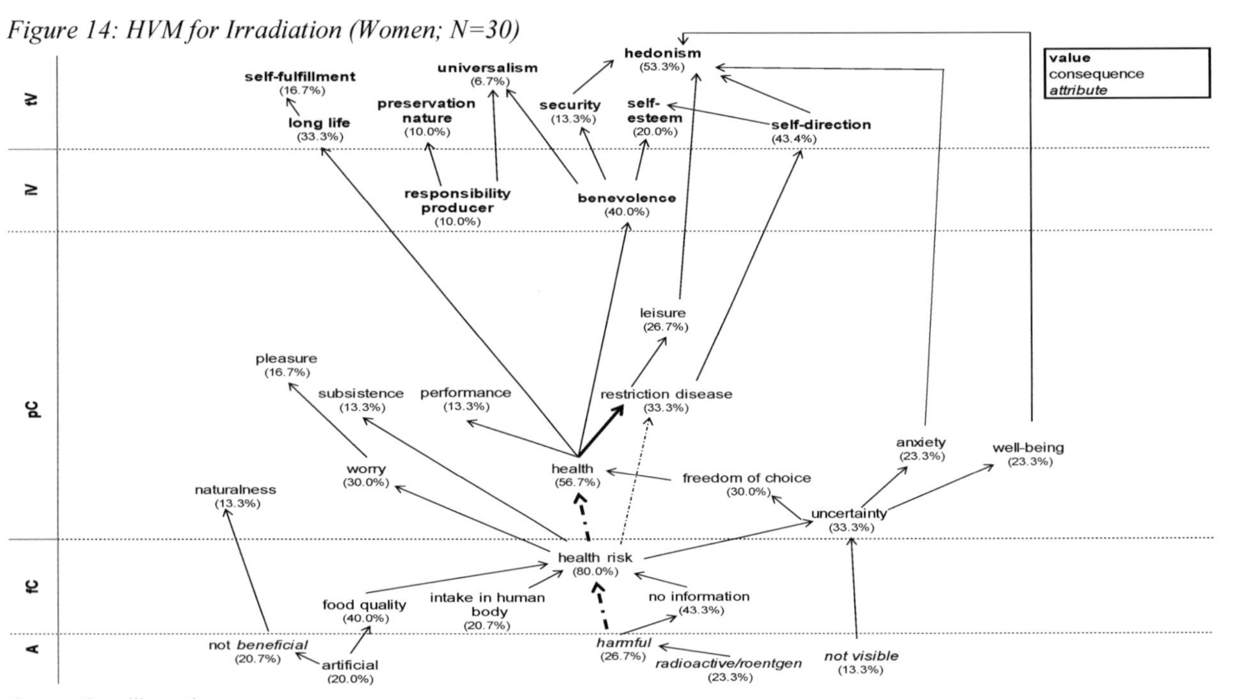

Source: Own illustration.

Figure 15: HVM for Irradiation (Men; N=29)

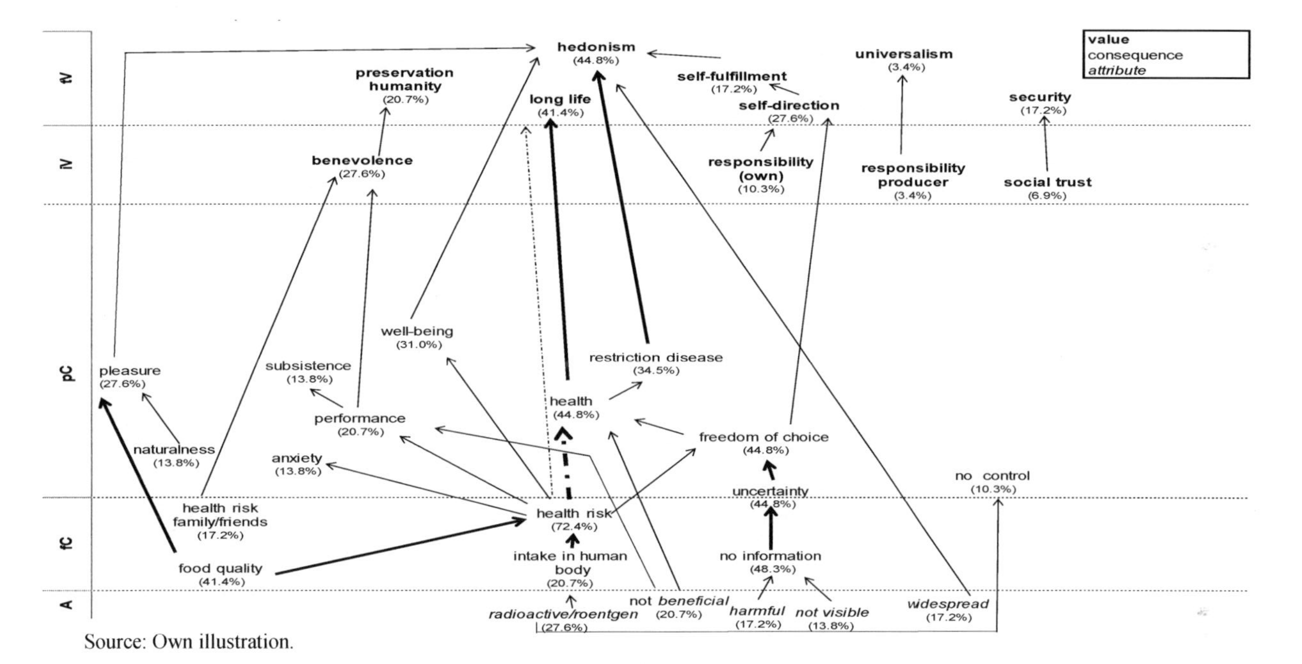

Source: Own illustration.

6.3.3.4 Summary

Across all food hazards the higher order concepts (psychosocial consequences and terminal values) are clearly dominant. Moreover, number of elicited concepts and ladders are especially high with regard to pesticides for women and men, which indicates a higher level of involvement for pesticides compared to mycotoxins and irradiation.

Across all three food hazards and both sexes, concepts related to health, personal wellbeing, and the wellbeing of close-ones are important concepts for women and men. With regard to pesticides and irradiation, perceptions of not being adequately informed and feelings of uncertainty are further important for both women and men. Furthermore, the concept'artificial' is mentioned in relation to pesticides by women and men, and by women also in relation to irradiation. For both women and men, concepts and paths related to environmental contamination and biospheric values are important with regard to pesticides.

However, beyond the concepts that are related to all food hazards and shared by both sexes, each specific food hazard is partly differently constructed for women and men.

Only for women, the ability to take informed decisions and have alternatives if necessary is important for all food hazards. Justice and security values are however only important for men with regard to mycotoxins and pesticides.

Women seem to be more strongly involved with regard to *mycotoxins* as expressed in a higher number of elicited concepts and ladders, longer ladders, a higher variability of concepts, and an overall higher level of abstraction of the concepts. This is mainly due to a higher variety of psychosocial consequences and a stronger importance of each of the psychosocial consequences. It is noticeable that the women's HVM shows strong interconnections between psychosocial consequences, but not that of men. For women too, mycotoxins are mainly constructed around restrictions and burdens in everyday life as a consequence of illness, threat to the ability to perform, to have good social relations, and to be able to take care of other people with whom they have close relationships. And (for women only), the emotions 'anxiety' and 'worry' are found to be important. Men's cognitive structures related to mycotoxins are much less complex, and images that are shared between women and men (such as the threat to the ability to perform, physical restrictions, and care of other people) are less important for men. More important, men's meanings related to mycotoxins are linked to mycotoxins' bad effect on food quality and therefore to being able to enjoy food, as well as the threat to self-fulfillment as a consequence of bad health. However, for more men than women, mycotoxins seem to be a threat to social and personal stability and harmony ('security'), justice and moral values concerning the equality of human beings, and the relationship between humans and nature.

With regard to *pesticides* compared to mycotoxins, the picture related to gender is reversed for some measures or concepts mentioned: Men's involvement seems to be stronger than women's. This is expressed in men's higher complexity of their cognitive structures in terms of number of concepts and ladders, ladder length and a higher level of abstraction. While similar kinds of psychosocial consequences are linked to pesticides for women and men, relatively more men mentioned concepts related to burdens in everyday life, threat to performance ability, and having good social relationships. Moreover, women more strongly than men link altruistic values (such as the perception of being responsible for protecting nature) to pesticides, while pesticides pose a threat to egoistic values for men (self-direction, self-esteem, self-fulfillment). In addition, concepts related to the social order and stability (justice and security) and the political concept of trust in governing institutions (social trust) are more strongly activated by pesticides in the minds of men.

With regard to *irradiation*, no clear picture emerges for levels of involvement, with men eliciting a higher number of concepts and longer ladders, but women a higher number of ladders and a larger number of abstract self-related aspects.

With regard to negative associations, women's cognitive structures are much more health-centered: all health-related concepts are more important in the women's HVM and only one health path constitutes an important path in that HVM. The threat to health also plays a role for men. However, other concepts (such as the feeling of not being adequately informed, uncertainty, and threat to freedom of choice, as well as the negative effect on food quality and the ability to enjoy food) also play an important role in the men's HVM. This does not mean that these concepts do not play a role in the women's HVM, but in women's minds they are in some way related to health concerns, while in men's minds, these concepts are largely independent of health. Addionally, in the women's HVM, negative emotions and self-centered values such as self-direction, self-esteem, and self-fulfillment do play a more important role than in the men's HVM. Similarly, concern for other, related people is more strongly activated in the HVM of women than in the HVM of men.

Positive ladders do only play a role with regard to irradiation. For many of the respondents, cognitions are split between positive and negative forms of irradiation. Positive associations mainly relate to natural and not harmful forms of irradiation such as sunlight. Some respondents also mention the possibility that irradiation eliminates mycotoxins and makes pesticides unnecessary.

Positive associations are much more important for male respondents as men elicit twice as many positive ladders than women, and the more abstract psycho-social consequences are only relevant for men.

6.4 Discussion

Functional consequences followed by attributes are most important among the first concepts that come to mind when respondents are confronted with food hazards. Fazio (1986) assumes a negative relation between the level of cognitive effort and the impact on consumer decision-making, and also Fishbein and Ajzen (1980) propose that the top of mind cognitions are the ones that are relevant for people's attitudes and behavior. The results of this thesis confirm that relationship in so far as the top of mind associations mirror the overall evaluations with regard to general affect and risk/benefit perceptions of women and men.

Whereas gender differences are small with regard to the judgment about mycotoxins and pesticides, the questionnaires revealed that women are somewhat more negative with regard to mycotoxins, and men with regard to pesticides. This picture also emerges with regard to cognitions related to the risk and benefit judgments, with more men tending to be less concerned about the harmful potential of mycotoxins, and more women tending to be less concerned about pesticides. Furthermore, women strongly believe that it is mycotoxins that nullify a product's benefit, whereas men think that it is pesticides that do this. However, with regard to the vividness of the most salient associations, the picture seems inconsistent with regard to pesticides and mycotoxins. Whereas men's 'top of mind' associations with mycotoxins are fairly unspecific negative affections, these are related to pesticides for women. This seems inconsistent against the background that during product rankings men would rather choose product A (mycotoxins) over product B (pesticides), and women preferred product B over product A. This might point to a stronger negative attitude towards pesticides than towards mycotoxins for men, and a stronger negative attitude towards mycotoxins than towards pesticides for women, which was confirmed in ratings of overall affect. However, a closer look at the data indicates that the rather unspecific negative salient emotions seem to replace more specific and concrete associations related to consequences. Thus, the most salient negative emotional statements seem to point to an overall negative evaluation of the product or hazard in question, but also indicate a lack of spontaneous concrete associations and knowledge, which seems to be the case for pesticides for women and for mycotoxins for men. Elicited affect-related statements allow a good prediction of respondents' overall evaluations. However, they do not seem to be a good measure for respondents' vividness of the first images, as at least these unspecific affect-related statements point rather to the lack of concrete spontaneous images.

As expected, irradiation is a relatively unknown food technology, with both women and men indicating their lack of knowledge. Accordingly, concepts are fairly heterogeneous, including positive aspects. However, more women than men are found to have negative associations, which are mirrored in women's higher risk and lower benefit ratings.

During the second interview day, the nuclear accident at Fukushima occurred[19]. Against this background, it seems surprising that only a minority of respondents mentioned this nuclear catastrophe (10% of women and 17.6% of men) or the attribute 'radioactive' (20% of women and 14.7% of men) when asked about their spontaneous thoughts about food irradiation. Moreover, according to the findings of the study by Visschers et al. (2007), people make sense of unknown things by relating them to known ones, and this relation is often drawn on the basis of semantic similarity. The working of a similarity heuristic from 'irradiation' to 'radiation' seems to be relevant only for a sub-sample of the respondents. This is not surprising as the German word for irradiation is also used in the context of cancer therapy and is thus much more often associated with health treatment than with nuclear radiation. The nuclear accident of Fukushima activated the concepts related to nuclear radiation in respondents' minds. Therefore, it is likely, that much more respondents linked food irradiation to nuclear radiation than it would have been the case before the accident.

In addition, this study can confirm the findings by Alhakami and Slovic (1994) that people's risk and benefit judgments are strongly interrelated, with a considerable number of respondents clearly formulating a negation of benefit in the presence of a potential harm. This study cannot confirm the general inverse relationship between risk and benefit perception in both directions, as participants' first thoughts when making risk judgments were elicited before the same was done for the assessment of benefits. Thus it is possible that if elicitation was reversed more benefits and fewer risks would have been elicited. The relationship between risk and benefit judgment is further mediated by an underlying overall affect towards the object in question, which is called 'affect heuristic' (Finucane et al., 2000a). Thus people's first affective evaluations do play an important role, and these tend to be negative (considering affect ratings and elic-

19 Data were collected between March 10th 2011 and March 29th 2011. The nuclear accident of Fukushima happened on March 11th.

ited affect) for all hazards for women, and for mycotoxins and pesticides for men.

The results of the laddering interviews show that, across all food hazards and both sexes the higher order concepts (psychosocial consequences and terminal values) are clearly dominant. At first glance, this seems surprising, as MEC studies in the food domain generally report a dominance of attribute and functional consequences (Costa, 2003). Food purchase decisions are characterized as low-involvement decisions that, once taken, have a strong habitual character (Costa et al., 2003a; Steenkamp, 1997). However, the focus on risk in this study seems to dramatically change consumers' perception of relevance and involvement, as suggested by Peter and Olson (2010).

Especially with regard to pesticides, the high number of concepts and ladders point to consumers' high level of involvement. This is not surprising as in risk perception studies that report the risk ranking of different hazards, pesticides are generally among the most dreaded and often even perceived as riskier than all other hazards (Byrne, Gempesaw and Toensmeyer, 1991; Ohtsubo and Yamada, 2007; Hohl and Gaskell, 2008; Federal Research Center for Nutrition and Food, 2008). For instance, in the study by Hohl and Gaskell (2008) in 25 European countries, consumers' main worry was about pesticides. This was also confirmed in a German study (Federal Research Center for Nutrition and Food, 2008), which showed that respondents ranked pesticides at the top of 14 interrogated food hazards, with 77.6% of the respondents assessing pesticides as the riskiest food hazard. Similarly, in another German study of the Federal Institute for Risk Assessment, pesticides were among the three most dreaded risks with 80% of the respondents judging pesticides as a high or very high risk (Dressel et al., 2010).

Overall, similarities between women and men concerning the meanings they attach to the food hazards are as important as the differences. Across all three food hazards and both sexes, concepts related to health and personal wellbeing are important concepts for women and men, and the large majority of cognitive paths are related to health. This concurs with the findings of the study by Miles and Frewer (2001), where health concerns were shared by all of the five investigated food hazards. Moreover, this mirrors findings in the literature that reported that in people's minds food and health are strongly connected and that health is a strong motive when purchasing food (Connors et al., 2001; Lookie et al., 2002; Lookie et al., 2004). Related to that, this study further shows that all three food hazards activate negative images regarding the consequences of illness such as restrictions in mobility. The results of this study further show that these health-related associations are linked to overall live goals such as happiness, satisfaction and quality of life. Next to personal health and wellbeing, women and men perceive the wellbeing of close friends and family members to be threatened by all three food hazards. Thus, next to egoistic values also socio-altruistic values seem to be activated by all three food hazards. Moreover, food quality is an important concept with regard to all three food hazards for both sexes. Women and men fear negative consequences for the products' healthiness, taste, appearance and freshness due to the food hazards/technologies. The perception of negative effect on the quality of food seems to be the underlying reason for respondents' low perceptions of benefits with regard to the products.

With regard to the technological food hazard of pesticide residues and the less-known food technology of irradiation, perceptions of not being adequately informed and feelings of uncertainty are further important for both women and men. It thus seems that lack of consumer confidence in the safety of food as reported in previous studies (Knox, 2000; Bergmann, 2000; Berg, 2004), and consumers' wishes for informed choice (Frewer et al., 2002), are also expressed here with regard to the man-made technological food risks. This is also evident in consumer responses to the consumer typology questionnaire of Berg (2004), where the majority of respondents can be classified as skeptical consumers. With regard to pesticides, cognitive paths that are related to environmental contamination and biospheric values such as the preservation of nature and humanity also play an important role for women and men. Thus, consumers' associations with pesticides go beyond concerns about the safety to humans.

In addition, the characteristic 'artificial' is mentioned as an important negative attribute by women for pesticides and irradiation and by men for pesticides. Among the few positive associations with regard to mycotoxins, 'not artificial' is elicited. This is not surprising if studies on consumers' motives behind their food choices are considered again. The preference for natural products is reported in several studies (Lookie et al. 2002; Rozin et al., 2004; Rozin, 2005). And according to the US study by Rozin et al. (2004), consumer preference for natural food is not only due to a perceived greater healthiness of natural foods, but exists independently of health as an aesthetic or moral correlate. 'Naturalness' is further regarded as opposed to several food technologies such as genetic engineering, the use of pesticides and irradiation (Lookie et al., 2004), and is considered as a main factor in consumer resistance to novel food technologies (Siegrist, 2007). In addition, 'naturalness' seems to be related to dichotomous conceptualizations such as 'nature, culture' and 'respect for nature, mastery of nature'. Thus, preference for natural products can also be regarded as a criticism of humans interfering with nature (Rozin et al., 2004).

Next to important similarities in the meanings women and men attach to food hazards, several differences emerge as well. These differences concern important concepts across two or all three hazards and also the construction of each food hazard.

Across all food hazards, it is important for women to be able to take informed decisions and have alternatives if necessary. This might be related to women's overall more 'virtuous' relationship towards food that was also found in the sample of this study regarding the food health reflexivity measure (Beardsworth et al., 2002; Berg, 2004).

On the other hand, the justice and security values are only important for men with regard to mycotoxins and pesticides. This concurs with the findings of the classical study by Gilligan (1982), who examined human judgments about hypothetical moral dilemmas such as risking breaking the law in order to help a sick relative. She found that most women and girls more strongly valued being able to help people they have close relationships with, while many men and boys discussed the issues in terms of rules and law. Similarly, the concepts social trust with regard to pesticides and food control with regard to irradiation are important cognitive concepts only for men, but not for women. It thus seems that for men, the food hazards activate political concepts concerning the organization of the state and society.

As already described a considerable number of concepts related to health-related consequences and quality of life or wellbeing of family members are shared between all three hazards and across sexes. However, beyond the concepts that are related to all food hazards, each specific food hazard is partly differently constructed for women and men.

In order to remind the main differences with regard to *mycotoxins*, women have more complex and vivid cognitive structures linked to concrete images of everyday life and fear of not being able to perform and live good personal relationships with other people. Men's cognitive structures are less complex. This may be due to less concrete images regarding threats to everyday life for men with regard to mycotoxins. For men, mycotoxins seem to rather question more general values such as the social and natural order and stability.

Regarding *pesticides* another picture emerges with regard to the gender gap: Men are more strongly involved compared to women. More men compared to women mentioned concepts related to burdens in everyday life, threat to performance ability, and having good social relationships. Moreover, while pesticides pose a threat to egoistic values for men, altruistic values, especially those related to the preservation of the nature are more important for women. As was the case for mycotoxins, moral understanding about social order and stability (justice and security) and the political concept of trust in governing institutions (social trust) are more strongly activated by pesticides in the minds of men.

Complexity seems to be linked to the extent that concrete images related to respondents' everyday life are activated. This is the case for women especially with regard to mycotoxins and for men especially with regard to pesticides.

Reasons for women's more concrete images with regard to *mycotoxins* might be that women are often still the ones who are responsible for food shopping and cooking (Lake et al., 2006) and thus being more often in contact with moulds. However, food shopping responsibilities do no differ that much between women and men in our sample.

The higher complexity of men's cognitive strucutures with regard to *pesticides* is surprising against the background that risks are perceived as higher by women than men also in two recent German studies (Dressel et al., 2010;. Federal Research Center for Nutrition and Food, 2008). However, in this study no gender gap exists for the risk ratings with regard to pesticides, which might be related to the small and therefore non-representative sample. On the other hand, risks due to pesticides residues in food are subject of public discussion since years in Germany and are regularly reported in the media (Dressel et al., 2010). Possibly, high public awareness has sensitized especially men to the risks of pesticides in food, whereas women are involved with regard to several food hazards due to a more skeptical and more reflexive approach to food in general. Moreover, in this study women are also strongly involved with regard to pesticides in food, but links to everyday consequences are less strong than for men. However, similar to the study by the Federal Institute for Risk Assessment (Dressel et al., 2010) that found women to be more concerned about the risks for environment, biospheric values are more important for women in this study, too.

As expected and already evident in the 'top of mind' associations, the largest differences in the meanings held by women and men exist for *irradiation*.

With regard to negative associations, women's cognitive structures are much more health-centered, while for men, other concepts (such as the feeling of not being adequately informed, as well as the negative effect on food quality) are also important. Linked to women's stronger focus on health concern seems to be the greater importance of negative emotions, the greater importance of self-centered values such as self-direction, self-esteem, and self-fulfillment, and also a stronger activation of concern for other, related people.

While positive ladders can be neglected in the case of mycotoxins and pesticides, they are important with regard to irradiation. Respondents' lack of knowledge about food irradiation leads to very heterogeneous evaluations. For many respondents, cognitions are split between positive and negative forms of irradiation and some respondents mention the possibility that irradiation eliminates mycotoxins and makes pesticides unnecessary. This is however probably an artifact of the design of this study rather than the expression of consumers' knowledge about the effect of food irradiation. Moreover, positive associations are much more important for male respondents. As already evident from the more positive 'top of mind' associations with regard to irradiation by men, it seems that while both sexes lack knowledge with regard to this food technology, men are more willing to also anticipate positive aspects, which might be linked to a gendered construction of science and technology (Faulkner, 2000). Furthermore, food plays a stronger role in women's health concepts. Whereas for men physical training seems to be most relevant for staying healthy, choice of food is dominant in women's mind (Berg, 2004; Fagerli and Wandel, 1999; Prahl and Setzwein, 1999). The results of this thesis confirm this, especially with regard to the salient concepts for irradiation. With regard to irradiation, health risks were only salient and central for women but not for men. As shown in previous research, people rely on several heuristics in order to be able to make judgments and take decisions, when people lack knowledge (Visschers et al., 2007; Tversky and Kahneman, 1974; see chapter 2.2.2.1), and thus irradiation as a food technology is likely to be linked to participants' health concepts as well as their meanings related to technology. Thus, in the case of an almost unknown food technology, the stronger link between health and food for women compared to men might explain women's salience of health and women's less multidimensional cognitive structures compared to men. In the same way, a gendered construction of technology (Faulkner, 2000; Henwood, Parkhill and Pidgeon, 2008) leading men to be rather positive about technology and women to be rather negative about it, might be the reason underlying men's much more positive images with regard to food irradiation. Contrary to previous studies (Fox and Firebaugh, 1992; Trankina, 1993; Bieberstein et al., 2011), however, no gender gap is found in this sample with regard to general attitude towards science and technology. However, the results relating to food irradiation clearly show men to anticipate more positive aspects of this food technology than women.

As seen above, 'naturalness' with regard to food seems to be an important concept for women and men. However, it is more strongly activated by food irradiation in the minds of women than in men. Thus, for women more than for men, naturalness seems to be a main underlying criterion for the positive versus negative overall evaluation of food irradiation. This is also reflected in a relatively stronger importance of the food choice motive 'natural' for women (Roininen, Lähteenmäki and Tuorilla, 1999; Lookie et al., 2004). Technology and thus technological hazards are viewed as man-made products (Cutter, Tiefenbacher and Solecki, 1992), and the preference for naturalness is an expression of opposition towards technology (Lookie et al., 2007). Thus, in the context of food, women more than men, seem to question technocentric worldviews that preach the domination of nature through technology. This does not automatically mean that women are more favorable than men towards ecocentric worldviews as detailed in chapter 3.3.4, but that these are more strongly activated by the relatively unknown technology of food irradiation.

Overall, it seems that self-centered values such as self-esteem, self-direction and self-fulfillment as well as the feeling of being responsible for the wellbeing of close-ones are directly related to concern about health. This concurs with previous studies, that found that health is multidimensional in terms of being related to ego-related goals and at the same time being linked to concerns about the wellbeing of close family and friends (socio-altruistic values) (Olson, Grunert and Sonne, 2010; Sørensen and Henchion, 2011). Sørensen and Henchion (2011) further found the link between health concerns and concerns and feelings of responsibility for the wellbeing of family members to be especially strong for participants in the family life stage. Theories about a gendered socialization to care for women would expect here a difference between the cognitive paths of women and men. However, the results of this thesis show that 'caring' for family members and close friends is activated for both women and men to the extent that health concerns and the effect of illness on everyday life play an important role in their cognitive maps. However, the later seems to be different for women and men with regard to the different food hazards. For women, this is especially true for mycotoxins and irradiation, and for men with regard to pesticides.

From a methodological point of view, this study shows how consumers' MECs can be investigated also in the context of more abstract issues such as in this case of food hazards. As with Bredahl (2001), the stimuli for the elicitation of the starting concepts were also products that were linked to the different food hazards and hypothetical purchase decisions, but the subsequent laddering interviews focused on the cognitions that were mentioned in relation to the food hazards only. Thus the rather abstract topic of food risks was more closely related to real purchase decisions, but final cognitive maps represent respondents' cognitions with regard to the hazards only.

Limitations of this thesis are clearly related to its 'sex-difference' approach, which is linked to the thesis' overall objective to understand differences between women's and men's perceptions of food risks. Future research that analyzes (food) risk meanings linked to gender identity could help to get a deeper understanding of the factors that determine the conceptualization of risks.

Moreover, as this thesis aimed at getting a closer picture of people's meanings they relate to food hazards, qualitative laddering interviews were conducted for collecting the data. As a consequence, the sample is small. Besides, as the specific interview method demands that people are somewhat interested in the topic in question, only people that are interested in food issues were selected as interviewees. Hence, the male sample is likely to be biased in terms of a relatively high share of men with interest in food issues compared to the overall male population. This might also be the underlying reason for the lack of the gender gap in general attitude towards science and technology, and the evaluation of mycotoxins and pesticides in the questionnaires. Therefore, future research based on quantitative approaches, that allow a representative sample, would be useful to verify the results. Based on the here elicited concepts, hard laddering methods could be used. This would also allow to control for other sociodemographic variables such as age and income or to create HVMs for subgroups relating to levels of risk perception.

7 Summary

Consumers' perceptions and judgments of risks is an important field of study in consumer research (Mitchell, 1999), and people's risk perceptions of food products and technologies are important determinants of food choice, food preparation behavior, and acceptance of food technologies (Frewer and Miles, 2001; Knox, 2000). Interest in the study of food risk perception is also due to widespread concern about the safety of food (Hohl and Gaskell, 2008).

Whereas concern about food risks is widespread, consumers are found to differ in terms of levels of worry and in regard to what kinds of hazards they are worried about. The most prominent finding in the risk perception literature is related to gender. Many studies report men to be less worried about environmental and technological risks than women, which is also the case with regard to food hazards. However, gender theorists often criticize researchers for taking the gender gap in risk perceptions for granted, for overlooking similarities, for exaggerating differences, and for the lack of systematic investigations with regard to the underlying reasons (Lorber, 1991; Gustafson, 1998).

This thesis therefore fills this research gap by providing a systematic investigation of the perceptions of food hazards of women and men. In order to reach this goal, the first target is to examine whether a consistent gender gap in existing food risk perception studies exists and if so, how it is dependent on the type of food hazard. Second, meanings that women and men attach to various food risks are the focus of this thesis. In this regard, based on the means-end chain (MEC) theory, the images, associations, and feelings that women and men attach to the investigated food risks, as well as the underlying values that are perceived to be threatened, are examined in detail according to a possible gendered construction. A further contribution to the existent literature is the thesis' methodological approach, as the MEC theory, mainly applied to understand consumers' product perceptions, is adopted to study the more abstract issue such as the perception of food hazards.

The thesis starts with a comprehensive overview of theoretical approaches to risk perception and empirical work that has been done in the field of risk perception. While different approaches exist to risk and risk perception that are introduced, risk perception research is interested in how people judge risks and tries to find out why people differ in their assessments of risks (Slovic, 1987). 'Hazard' and 'risk' are two different concepts, where 'hazard' relates to the source of an adverse effect and 'risk' to the possibility and probability of an adverse effect (Kaplan and Garrick, 1981). As in the risk perception literature, these concepts are usually used interchangeably, as is also the case in the present thesis. In this thesis, however, the meaning of risks relates in general to the source of an adverse effect (hazard).

Cognitive processes and affective processes as well as the interplay between the two processes guide all human decision-making and behavior and therefore also people's assessments of hazards. A general introduction into the working of both processes and especially the interplay between them is given in order to outline the most basic mechanisms underlying risk assessment.

Next, the cognitive and affective processes important for the evaluation of risks are described. The early psychological studies on risk perception focused on the cognitive factors. Tversky and Kahneman's (1974) research about intuitive judgment of probability revealed that people use heuristic strategies in order to reduce the mental complexity of judging probabilities that, while often useful, also lead to biases. One example is the representativeness heuristic where people infer their judgments about a new event/issue by comparing it with an event/issue they perceive to be similar. This has not only been found for the judgment about probabilities, but also for assessments of perceived risk levels (Visschers et al., 2007). The psychometric paradigm as the most influential cognitive approach is further presented. For the psychometric paradigm, risk perception is the subjectively defined severity of a risk and its characteristics and research in this school of thought investigates the impact of risk characteristics on levels of perceived risk. The 'affect heuristic' (Peters and Slovic, 1996) and the 'risk as feeling hypothesis' (Loewenstein et al., 2001) are further introduced as important models for the effect of affect and emotion on risk perception. According to the 'affect heuristic', people's associations linked to a hazard or technology are tagged with affect, and people's overall feelings decide whether risk perception outweigh benefit benefits and vice versa (Peters and Slovic, 1996). In addition, the 'risk as feeling hypothesis' postulates that both emotions and cognitions have a direct and sometimes even divergent impact on people's judgments. The effect of emotions is hereby strongly dependent on the vividness of mental images people have in mind (Loewenstein et al., 2001).

Subsequently, approaches coming from different scientific disciplines that are relevant for understanding differences in risk assessments are introduced and conclusions are drawn for their ability to research differences in risk perception.

Whereas the psychometric approach focuses on explaining differences in risk perception by applying approaches of cognitive psychology, it neglects the social context. The Cultural Theory approach (Douglas 1978; Douglas and Wildavsky, 1982) focuses on the influence of culture and is able to explain inter-group differences, but it fails to take into account individual responses to risk (Jackson, Allum and Gaskell, 2006). During recent years, the strengths of both schools of thoughts have been combined, and a socio-psychological (Jackson, Allum and Gaskell, 2006) as well as a socio-cultural approach (Tulloch and Lupton, 2003) to the research into risk perception has been evolved. Socio-psychological approaches suppose that a consistent system of attitudes and motives as well as people's social affiliations determine people's risk perception. Socio-cultural approaches consider the role of personal values, worldviews, and the role of religiosity or spiritual beliefs as important predictors in risk perception (Banse and Bechmann, 1998). Related to this, empirical results with regard to effect of socio-demographic factors such as gender and age, socio-structural factors such as income and education, socio-psychological factors such as world views and values, as well as socio-political factors such as social trust or general scientific attitudes are presented.

Following this comprehensive overview of theoretical as well as empirical work in the field of risk perception, chapter 3 focuses on gender and risk perception. The concepts 'sex' and 'gender' are briefly introduced and the role that sex and gender plays in consumer research in general and subsequently in risk research is discussed from a gender theory perspective. It is concluded that an androcentric perspective (Briston and Fischer, 1993) is even prevalent in recent risk research, since differences between women and men are always framed in terms of women showing deviant risk assessments. Furthermore, the 'sameness taboo' presupposing that women and men have to be distinguishable is likely to lead to an exaggeration of the gender gap in risk perception research too.

Chapter 3.2 starts by presenting studies that investigated the impact of sex on levels of risk perception with regard to environmental, technological and lifestyle risks, and presents results of studies investigating risky behavior. Whereas with regard to risks due to nuclear power and waste, as well as industrial and chemical risks, men are mostly found to be less concerned, results with regard to gene technology and general environmental concern are mixed. The most thorough review of empirical work on gender and risk perception has been performed by Davidson and Freudenburg (1996), who found that the gender gap in risk perception is only consistent and statistically significant in cases where specific risks are addressed or when hazards (even though quite general such as air pollution) are framed as locally effective environmental and health risks. The results of most food risk perception studies also point to a considerable effect of sex on risk perception, with men often being less concerned than women, but only a systematic investigation on food risk perception and gender can examine whether this is the case for all kinds of food hazards and take magnitude and significant levels into account. The last part of this chapter presents in detail the theoretical and empirical work that has been made in order to understand the underlying reasons for the often reported gender differences in risk perception in general. Among others, hypotheses related to gender role theories, gender identity, and socio-political approaches focusing on gender power relations are discussed, and the explanatory value of these hypotheses in empirical work is outlined.

In order to meet the first goal of this thesis, a systematic literature review of quantitative studies investigating the effect of sex on levels of food risk perception or acceptance of food technologies was performed. We examined whether there is a consistent gap between the perceptions of women and men and in which direction, taking the magnitude of the differences into account. In addition, we investigated whether gender differences differ dependent on the type of food hazards. Based on an already exhaustive literature base, studies were searched by means of the snowballing technique, by considering the reference sections of existing articles, by reading through relevant journals and homepages of institutions, and by ranning searches in electronic databases. Literature search was performed between March and August 2010 including studies that were published between 1978 and 2010. From the overall data base of 196 studies that investigated risk perception, 132 studies had to be excluded as they either did not investigate food hazards or did not report any results with regard to gender. 64 studies were included for the systematic review. Studies were categorized according to type of food hazard, and according to magnitude and direction of the gender-related results. As with the literature review on technological and environmental risks and gender by Davidson and Freudenburg (1996), the findings indicate that in the case of food hazards too, a consistent gender gap exists, with men being mostly less concerned. In addition, except for nanotechnology, in 70 to 100% of the results related to technology-based food hazards such as pesticides, food additives or gene technology, women perceived risks as higher than men, whereas with regard to life-style risks such as an unhealthy diet or natural food hazards such as food bacteria, results with regard to women's and men's perceptions are more balanced. This finding is discussed against the background of a gendered construction of technology, as well as different conceptualizations of food for women and men. Previous findings on gender and technology found men to be more positive about technology and engineering (Fox and Firebaugh, 1992) which is due to a masculine connotation of technology and engineering (Faulkner, 2000; Henwood, Parkhill and Pidgeon, 2008). As a consequence, women more strongly than men question the utility of technology (Fox and Firebaugh, 1992), which is also likely to play a role for food technology. Furthermore, greater preference for the naturalness of food on behalf of women, which is perceived as being opposed to technology (Lookie et al., 2004), might be a further reason for this finding.

Somewhat more balanced are the results with regard to risk due to an unhealthy diet such as fatty eating, but still the majority of the results indicate men to be less worried about that. Here, the often reported stronger focus on health with regard to food by women (Fagerli and Wandel, 1999; Lookie et al., 2002; Setzwein, 2004), as well as a close link between attractiveness and weight especially for young women (Beardsworth, Bryman and Keil, 2002; Chaiken and Pliner, 1987), are likely to play a role here.

Finally, the findings indicate that the gender differences in the assessments of food risks and technologies are clearly consistent, but also small.

However, understanding the reasons behind the gender gap is the aim of empirical investigation that examined women's and men's meanings that they attach to various food risks. The methodological background of these empirical investigations builds the MEC theory, which is presented in detail. The MEC theory models how knowledge is organized in human memory and presupposes hierarchically organized knowledge structures. It focuses on the relationship between an object in question and the person by allowing the exploration of the conscious and unconscious rationales of people's evaluations of objects, in this case hazards. The MEC theory is described alongside an alternative model – the network model – and the application of the MEC model is justified beyond the background that, in addition to associations and images, consumers' motivational basis in terms of underlying values is also of interest. Before the commonly used MEC models by Gutman and Reynolds (1979), Gutman (1982) and Olson and Reynolds (1983) are introduced, a historical overview is given of the precursor models of the current MEC approach, which also includes work on human values by Rokeach (1973) and Schwartz (1994). According to the current model, consumers evaluate certain product attributes according to their consequences, which in turn help to achieve life goals and values (Gutman, 1992). Additionally, a distinction is drawn between concrete and abstract attributes, functional and psychosocial consequences, and between instrumental and terminal values. Walker and Olson (1991) further point to the situational dependence of the knowledge that is activated. According to them, the ends of an MEC (the psychosocial consequences, instrumental values and terminal values) constitute a person's self-relevant knowledge, and that different aspects of a person's self-schema are activated in different situations. Related to that, consumer involvement regarding an issue or situation depends on how strongly associations with that situation or issue are connected to central aspects of the person's self (Celsi and Olson, 1988; Fotopoulos, Krystallis and Ness, 2003). With regard to the product characteristics, perceived risks of products are supposed to greatly increase consumers' involvement, according to Peter and Olson (2010).

Based on the findings of the systematic review supposing a 'natural, technological' distinction, three types of food hazards were chosen: Mycotoxins as a natural food hazard, pesticides as a technological food hazard, and irradiation as a technological but fairly unknown food technology. A twofold approach was chosen for investigating the meaning women and men attach to the three selected food hazards. First, women's and men's first associations that were activated when they were confronted with a stimulus were investigated. These salient concepts are supposed to be especially important for guiding behavior (Fishbein and Ajzen, 1980). Linked to this, the emotional intensity of consumers' first associations in mind were also of interest. The second part focused on the more underlying cognitive structures of women and men, the consequences and values that are activated and perceived to be threatened by the three food hazards, and levels of complexity of women's and men's cognitive structures.

34 women and 35 men were recruited and invited to participate in a study in Munich, Germany in March 2011. In order to reveal consumers' salient associations, data was collected by means of the free elicitation technique. In addition, the soft-laddering interview technique was used to elicit people's detailed MECs with regard to the three food hazards. With the use of entry and exit questionnaires, respondents were asked additional questions concerning their sociodemographic background, risk and benefit assessments, and several food and technology related questions.

With regard to the salient concepts, results across all elicitation tasks (general, risk and benefit-related) show that health concerns and complete rejection are most important for all food hazards for women and for mycotoxins and pesticides for men, but health concern is somewhat less important for pesticides than for mycotoxins. Considering irradiation, the perception of not being adequately informed is further important for both sexes. Whereas women only mentioned negative aspects of irradiation among the top four concepts, men mentioned positive and negative concepts. Most important differences between women and men concern the associations linked to the risk assessment of food irradiation: only women have a clear negative position and have a few concepts such as health concerns and lack of information in mind, whereas men's thoughts are quite sparse. Across all products and both sexes, but somewhat less for pesticides, benefit and risk perception seem to be interlinked for a considerable number of respondents, which confirms findings by Alhakami and Slovic (1994). In the perception of women, mycotoxins and irradiation nullify the possible benefits of the herbs, whereas for men this is the case with pesticides.

The results further show that the most salient concepts in people's minds mirror the overall evaluations according to the questionnaire with regard to general affect and risk/benefit perceptions of women and men, and thus confirm the suggestions by Fishbein and Ajzen (1980). However, a less consistent picture emerges with regard to the vividness of the 'top of mind' associations: Product rankings point to stronger negative attitude towards pesticides than to mycotoxins for men, and a stronger negative attitude towards mycotoxins than to pesticides for women. However, in men's 'top of mind' associations unspecific negative affections are dominant for pesticides, whereas this is the case in women's 'top of mind' associations with mycotoxins. A closer look at the data reveals that specific and concrete associations related to consequences are replaced by fairly unspecific negative salient emotions. Thus, the most salient negative emotional statements indicate a lack of spontaneous concrete associations and knowledge, which seems to be the case for pesticides for women and for mycotoxins for men. The results of this thesis suggest that elicited spontaneous affect is a good predictor of respondents overall judgments. However, they also point to the lack of concrete spontaneous images and cannot be used as a measure for respondents' vividness of the first images.

Results of the soft-laddering interviews indicate that across all three food hazards concepts related to health, personal wellbeing and the wellbeing of close people are important concepts for women and men. This concurs with the findings by Miles and Frewer (2001), and mirrors findings in previous literature that has shown that health is an important motive of food choice (Connors et al., 2001; Lookie et al., 2002; 2004). With regard to pesticide residues and irradiation, perceptions of not being adequately informed and feelings of uncertainty are further important for both women and men. It thus seems that lack of consumer confidence in the safety of food as reported in previous studies (Knox, 2000; Bergmann, 2000; Berg, 2004) and consumers' wish for informed choice (Frewer et al., 2002) is also expressed here with regard to the technological food risks. In addition, the characteristic 'artificial' was mentioned as an important negative attribute by women for pesticides and irradiation and by men for pesticides, which is also evident in people's general preference for natural products (Lookie et al. 2002; Rozin et al., 2004; Rozin, 2005); naturalness is often seen as an opposite of technology (Lookie et al., 2004). In addition, with regard to pesticides, cognitive paths that are related to environmental contamination and biospheric values such as the preservation of nature and humanity also play an important role for both women and men. Thus, consumers associations with pesticides go beyond concerns about the safety to humans.

In addition to the concepts that refer to all three food hazards, each specific food hazard is partly differently constructed for women and men.

Regarding mycotoxins, women have more complex and vivid cognitive structures linked to concrete images of everyday life. Men's cognitive structures are much less complex and have less concrete images with regard to threats to everyday life. On the contrary, for men more than for women, mycotoxins seem to question more general and overall values such as the social order and stability.

In the case of pesticides, the picture related to sex is reversed: Men's involvement seems to be stronger, and more men mentioned concepts related to burdens in everyday life, threat to performance ability, and having good social relationships. In addition, pesticides pose a threat to egoistic values for men, whereas altruistic values (such as the perception of being responsible for protecting nature) are more important for women with regard to pesticides. Pesticides more strongly activate values related to social order and stability in the minds of men.

The greatest differences between the cognitions of women and men exist for food irradiation. With regard to the negative associations, women's cognitive structures are much more health-centered. For women and men, health concerns and other concerns such as the feeling of not being adequately informed do play a role, but in women's mind all concepts are in some way linked to the health concerns, while in the minds of men these concepts are largely independent of health.

Whereas with regard to mycotoxins and pesticides, positive ladders can be neglected, they are important with regard to irradiation and are much more important for male respondents.

As already evident from the more positive 'top of mind' associations with regard to irradiation by men, it seems that while both sexes lack knowledge with regard to this food technology, men are more willing to anticipate positive aspects too, which is likely to be linked to a gendered construction of science and technology (Faulkner, 2000; Henwood, Parkhill and Pidgeon, 2008). Furthermore, food plays a relatively stronger role in women's health concepts (Berg, 2004; Fagerli and Wandel, 1999; Prahl and Setzwein, 1999) that are activated by food irradiation.

Similarly, for women, naturalness seems to be a main underlying criterion for the positive versus negative overall evaluation of food irradiation. The preference for 'naturalness', which is conceptualized as being opposed to technological (Lookie et al., 2004), shows that, in the context of food, women more than men seem to question technocentric worldviews that preach the domination of nature through technology. This does not automatically mean that women are more favorable than men towards ecocentric worldviews as detailed in chapter

3.3.4, but that these are more strongly activated by food irradiation in the minds of women.

Theories about a gendered socialization to care for women would expect differences between the cognitive paths of women and men. However, the results show that 'caring' for family members and close friends is activated for both women and men to the extent that health concerns and the effect of illness on everyday life play an important role in their cognitive maps. However, the latter seems to be different for women and men with regard to the different food hazards. For women, this is especially true for mycotoxins and irradiation, and for men with regard to pesticides.

Across all food hazards, it is important for women to be able to take informed decisions and have alternatives if necessary, which confirms findings about women's overall more 'virtuous' relationship towards food. This was also found in the sample of this study regarding the food health reflexivity measure (Beardsworth et al., 2002; Berg, 2004). On the other hand, the justice and security values are only important for men with regard to mycotoxins and pesticides. This concurs with the findings of the classical study by Gilligan (1982) according to which male respondents discussed the issues in terms of rules and law. It thus seems that for men, food hazards activate political concepts concerning the organization of the state and society.

The design of this study shows how consumers' MECs can be investigated also in the context of more abstract issues such as in this case of food hazards: Starting point of the data collection was a hypothetical product choice situation and food hazards were linked to specific products, which allowed to elicit concrete associations. As only associations that were related to the hazards were further investigated in the indepth interviews, resulting cognitive maps were related to the hazards only.

Overall, this thesis contributes to research about risk perception by providing detailed information about the meanings people attach to food risks. This is crucial for understanding consumers' judgments of food risks and technology, for the design of effective risk communication, and above all for taking the 'consumer voice' in decisions about food safety management into account. More specifically, the thesis' results also add to literature that is interested in the relationship between consumers' risk and benefit assessments and how consumers make assessments about technologies about which they lack knowledge.

Most important, the thesis adds to the research aiming at understanding gender differences in risk assessment. Review of previous literature reveals that the gap between women's and men's risk evaluations is especially consistent for technological hazards and in general rather small. In contrast to what the gender gap in quantitative risk assessment studies would point to, women and men seem to share a considerable number of meanings related to all food hazards. And these similarities are as important as the revealed differences. Interestingly, women and men have the same concepts in mind but they are activated by different kinds of food hazards, as was the case here for mycotoxins and pesticides. That means that underlying cognitive structures with regard to food risks are similar between women and men, but that specific types of food hazards are somewhat differently constructed for women and men. Results of this thesis further conflict with theories based on assumptions of general differences between women and men, such as women's stronger socialization to care. Caregiving associations were activated for both sexes to the extent that health concerns were activated by the food hazards. However, the cognitive structures revealed point to different conceptualizations by women and men of food and even more of technology.

8 Zusammenfassung

Die Sorge um die Sicherheit von Lebensmitteln ist ein weit verbreitetes Phänomen (Hohl und Gaskell, 2008). Allerdings unterscheiden sich Menschen im Grad ihrer Besorgnis. Vielfach zitiert sind insbesondere Geschlechterunterschiede in der Bewertung von Risiken, wobei Männer im Vergleich zu Frauen viele Risiken häufig als weniger besorgniserregend einstufen, was auch für viele Studien zur Bewertung von Lebensmittelrisiken zutrifft.

Von Seiten der Geschlechterforschung wird wiederholt die Kritik geäußert, dass Geschlechterunterschiede auf Kosten von Gemeinsamkeiten häufig übertrieben dargestellt werden und dass systematische Untersuchungen über die zugrunde liegenden Ursachen fehlen.

Diese Kritik wird in der vorliegenden Arbeit aufgegriffen, indem die Bewertung und Wahrnehmung von Frauen und Männern in Bezug auf Lebensmittelrisiken systematisch untersucht werden.

Um dies zu erreichen, werden zunächst die bisherigen Studien, die die Bewertung von Lebensmittelrisiken untersuchen, mittels eines systematischen Literaturüberblicks dahingehend untersucht, ob ein konsistenter (signifikanter wie auch genügend großer) Unterschied in der Bewertung von Frauen und Männern besteht und ob etwaige Geschlechterunterschiede von der Art des Risikos abhängen.

Hauptziel ist es herauszufinden, welche Bedeutung verschiedene Lebensmittelrisiken für Frauen und Männer besitzen. Basierend auf der Theorie der Means-End-Chains werden die Assoziationen, Bilder und Gefühle, wie auch die als bedroht wahrgenommen Werte bezüglich verschiedener Lebensmittelrisiken auf eine mögliche ‚geschlechtliche Konstruktion' analysiert.

Die Means-End-Chains-Theorie wurde bisher vor allem zur Untersuchung der Konsumentenwahrnehmung für konkrete Produkte herangezogen. Die Anwendung der Theorie auf ein kognitiv abstraktes Thema stellt eine Erweiterung der bestehenden Literatur dar.

Die Arbeit beginnt mit einer detaillierten Übersicht über die bestehenden theoretischen Ansätze in der Risikowahrnehmungsforschung, wie beispielsweise dem Psychometrischen Paradigma oder den Ansätzen der Cultural Theory. Sie erläutert die Forschung zu kognitiven und affektiven Faktoren, welche die Bewertung von Risiken beeinflussen, und liefert einen umfassenden Überblick über empirische Arbeiten zu den Einflussfaktoren der Risikobewertung.

Im anschließenden Kapitel liegt der Fokus auf dem Zusammenhang zwischen Geschlecht und Risikobewertung. Eine kritische Auseinandersetzung mit der Rolle des Geschlechts in der Risikoforschung zeigt, dass die Risikoforschung ähnlich wie die Konsumforschung androzentrische Merkmale besitzt und dem sogenannten ‚Gleichheitstabu' unterliegt, das besagt, dass Frauen und Männer sich unterscheiden müssen. Des Weiteren wird ein Überblick über die Ergebnisse zum Einfluss von Geschlecht auf die Bewertung von Technikrisiken, Umweltrisiken, sogenannte Lebensstilrisiken und Lebensmittelrisiken gegeben. Forschung wird vorgestellt, die versucht, Geschlechterunterschiede in der Bewertung von Risiken zu erklären, wie beispielsweise Hypothesen, die auf Geschlechterrollen- oder Identitätstheorien basieren.

Im Systematischen Literaturüberblick wurden 132 Ergebnisse aus 64 verschiedenen Studien berücksichtigt. Die Ergebnisse des Systematischen Literaturüberblicks zeigen, dass auch bei Lebensmittelrisiken konsistente Geschlechterunterschiede bestehen, die durchwegs allerdings eher klein ausfallen, hingegen bei den technikbasierten Risiken wie Pestiziden, Gentechnik und Lebensmittelzusatzstoffen besonders ausgeprägt sind. Diese Ergebnisse deuten auf eine ‚geschlechtliche Konstruktion' von Technik hin (Faulkner, 2000; Henwood, Parkhill und Pidgeon, 2008) und zeigen, dass Frauen stärker als Männer auch im Lebensmittelbereich den Nutzen von Technologien hinterfragen (Fox und Firebaugh, 1992).

Basierend auf diesen Ergebnissen wurden in der hier vorliegenden Arbeit die Lebensmittelrisiken unterschieden in natürliche Risiken wie Schimmelpilzgifte, in technik-basierte Risiken, denen die Pestizide zugeordnet werden, und in Risiken, die auf unbekannten Lebensmitteltechnologien basieren, wie der Bestrahlung. Die kognitiven Strukturen von Frauen und Männern wurden hinsichtlich dieser drei Risikoarten untersucht. 34 Frauen und 35 Männer wurden in einem speziellen Verfahrens des Tiefeninterviews zu den drei Lebensmittelrisiken/-technologien befragt. Die empirische Untersuchung der kognitiven Strukturen gliedert sich in zwei Teile: zunächst wurden diejenigen Assoziationen erhoben, die als erste auftauchen, wenn TeilnehmerInnen mit einem Stimulus, in diesem Fall ein Lebensmittelrisiko, konfrontiert werden. Diese ersten Assoziationen gelten als besonders verhaltensrelevant (Fishbein und Ajzen, 1980) und somit auch hinsichtlich der Bewertung von Risiken. Im zweiten Teil lag der Fokus auf den tiefer liegenden Kognitionen, beispielsweise die als bedroht wahrgenommen Werte.

Die Ergebnisse bezüglich der ersten Konzepte zeigen, dass die Sorge um die Gesundheit und eine spontane Ablehnung der Produkte aufgrund der Risiken bei Frauen und Männern dominant sind, was auch die Bewertungen in den Fragebögen widerspiegeln. Zudem scheinen die Bewertung von Nutzen und Risiken in den Konzepten von KonsumentInnen insofern verknüpft zu sein, als diese häufig jeglichen Nutzen negieren, wenn gleichzeitig Risiken bestehen. Dies ist für Pestizide und Bestrahlung besonders stark bei den Frauen ausgeprägt. Deutliche Unterschiede zwischen den Geschlechtern bestehen in erster Linie hinsichtlich der Bestrahlung, mit der Frauen ausschließlich negative Konzepte verknüpfen, während Männer auch positive Assoziationen damit verbinden.

Ergebnisse der Tiefeninterviews zeigen, dass viele der kognitiven Strukturen, die durch die drei Lebensmittelrisiken aktiviert werden, zwischen Frauen und Männern gleich sind. So verknüpfen beide Geschlechter die Sorge um die Gesundheit, Wohlbefinden und das Wohlergehen von nahestehenden Personen mit allen drei Lebensmittelrisiken. Für die technikbasierten Risiken Pestizide und Bestrahlung sind zudem noch der Wunsch nach mehr Information und Gefühle von Unsicherheit von Bedeutung. Im Zusammenhang mit Pestiziden wird häufig die Sorge über die Verschmutzung der Umwelt genannt und der damit verbundene Wunsch der Erhaltung von Natur und Mensch.

Neben den Gemeinsamkeiten bezüglich jedes einzelnen Lebensmittelrisikos werden jedoch auch Unterschiede in der Kognition deutlich. Während die Art der Konzepte, die durch die drei untersuchten Risiken aktiviert werden, für Männer und Frauen ähnlich sind, verknüpfen Männer viele dieser Konzepte beispielsweise eher mit Pestiziden, Frauen die gleichen Konzepte jedoch mit Schimmelpilzgiften. So sind beispielsweise die Sorgen um Leistungsfähigkeit für Frauen stark mit Schimmelpilzgiften verbunden, während dies für Männer stark mit Pestiziden verbunden ist. So bestehen auch keine grundsätzlichen Unterschiede in der Stärke der Aktivierung von Kognitionen bezüglich Betreuung und Versorgung, wie dies Theorien zu Geschlechterrollen vermuten lassen. Kognitionen bezüglich Betreuung und Fürsorge werden bei beiden Geschlechtern in dem Maße aktiviert, in dem gesundheitsbezogene Sorgen wichtig sind.

Die größten Unterschiede zwischen Frauen und Männern bestehen bezüglich der Bestrahlung. Während für Schimmelpilzgifte und Pestizide nur negative Assoziationen von Relevanz sind, werden in Bezug auf Bestrahlung auch einige positive Assoziationen genannt - in erster Linie von Männern. Während die Ergebnisse zeigen, dass beide Geschlechter geringes Wissen bezüglich Lebensmittelbestrahlung besitzen, sind Männer im Vergleich zu Frauen eher bereit, auch positive Aspekte mit der Bestrahlung zu antizipieren.

Ähnlich verhält es sich mit dem Wunsch nach ‚Natürlichkeit', der verstärkt von Frauen als das zugrundeliegende Kriterium für die Entscheidung zu einer positiven oder negativen Bewertung der Bestrahlung angesehen wurde. ‚Natürlichkeit' wird häufig als Gegensatz zu Technik konzeptualisiert (Lookie et al., 2004). Der Wunsch nach ‚Natürlichkeit' weist somit auf eine pessimistischere Einstellung von Seiten der Frauen gegenüber Lebensmitteltechnologien aus.

References

Adeola, F.O. (2004). Environmentalism and risk perception: Empirical Analysis of black and white differentials and convergence. Society and Natural Resources, 17(19): 1-29.

Adeola, F.O. (2007). Nativity and environmental risk perception: An empirical study of native-born and foreign-born residents of the USA. Human Ecology Review, 14 (1): 13-25.

Alhakami, A. S., Slovic, P. (1994). A psychological study of the inverse relationship between perceived risk and perceived benefit. *Risk Analysis*, 14 (6): 1085-1096.

Anderson, J.R. (1983). Retrieval of information from long-term memory. *Science*, 220: 25-30.

Anderson, J.R. (2007). Kognitive Psychologie. *Springer*, Berlin, Germany. 6th edition.

Armaş, Iuliana. (2006): Earthquake Risk Perception in Bucharest, Romania. *Risk Analysis,* 26 (5): 1223–1234.

Asselbergs, W.J.M. (1993). Betekenis structuur analyse – Wat, waroom en hoe? In: Nederlandse Vereniging van Marktonderzoekers (eds.): Recente ontwikkelingen in het marktonderzoek-jaarboek 92-93 van de. De Vrieseborch, Haarlem: 99-115.

Atkinson, R.C., Shiffrin, R.M. (1968). Human memory: A proposed system and its control processes. In: Spence, K.W., Spence, J.T. (eds.): The psychology of learning and motivation (Volume 2), *Academic Press*, New York, USA: 89-195.

Audenaert, A., Steenkamp, J.-B. (1997). Means-end chain theory and laddering in agriculture marketing research. In: Wierenga, B., van Tilbury, A., Grunert, K., Steenkamp, J.-B. (eds.): Agricultural marketing and consumer behavior in a changing world. *Kluwer Academic*, Boston, USA: 217-230.

Bänsch, A. (2002). Käuferverhalten. Oldenbourg, München, Wien, Germany, 9th edition.

Bajtelsmit, V.L., Bernasek, A., Jianakoplos, N.A. (1999). Gender differences in defined contribution pension decisions. *Financial Services Review,* 8: 1-10.

Banse, G., Bechmann, G. (1998). Interdisziplinäre Risikoforschung. Eine Bibliographie. *Westdeutscher Verlag*, Wiesbaden, Germany.

Barke, R., Jenkins-Smith, H., Slovic, P. (1997). Risk perceptions of men and women scientists. *Social Science Quartlery,* 78 (1): 167-176.

Barrena, R., Sánchez, M. (2010). Differences in consumer abstraction levels as a function of risk perception. *Journal of Agricultural Economics,* 61 (1): 34-59.

Barry, A., Osborne, T., Rose, N. (1996). Foucault and political reason. *UCL Press*, London, England.

Bastide, S., Moatti, J-P., Pages, J-P., Fagnani, F. (1989). Risk perception and the social acceptability of technologies: the French case, *Risk Analysis,* 9(2): 215–23.
Baumer, T.L. (1978). Research on fear of crime in the United States. *Victimology*, 3: 254-264.
Beardsworth, A., Bryman, A., Keil, T., Goode, J., Haslam, C., Lancashire, E. (2002). Women, men and food: the significance of gender for nutritional attitudes and choices. *British Food Journal,* 104 (7): 470-491.
Bech-Larsen, T. (1996). Danish consumers' attitudes to the functional and environmental characteristics of food packaging. MAPP Working paper, No.32, Aarhus School of Business, Aarhus, Denmark. Retrieved [11\02\2011], from http://pure.au.dk/portal/files/32300145/wp32.pdf
Bech-Larsen, T., Nielsen, N.A. (1999). A comparison of five elicitationtechniques for elicitation of attributes of low involvement products. *Journal of Economic Psychology,* 20: 315-341.
Beck, U. (1986). Risikogesellschaft: Auf dem Weg in eine andere Moderne. Suhrkamp, Frankfurt am Main, Germany.
Beck, U. (1992). Risk Society: Towards a New Modernity. *Sage*, New Delhi, London.
Berg, L. (2004). Trust in food in the age of mad cow disease: a comparativestudy of consumers' evaluation of food safety in Belgium, Britain and Norway. *Appetite* 42 (1): 21-32.
Bergmann, K. (2000). Der verunsicherte Verbraucher. Neue Ansätze zur unternehmerischen Informationsstrategie in der Lebensbranche. Schriftenreihe herausgegeben von der Dr. Reiner Wild-Stiftung. *Springer*, Berlin, Germany.
Bettman, J.R., Payne, J.W., Staelin, R. (1987). Cognitive considerations in designing effective labels for presenting risk information. In: Viscusi, K., Magat, W. (eds.): Learning about risk: Evidence on the economic responses to risk information. *Harvard University Press*, Cambridge, MA, USA: 1-28.
Bieberstein, A., Vandermore, F., Roosen, J., Blanchemanche, S., Marette, S. (2011). Revisiting social trust with regard to gendered perception of new food technologies: The case of nanofood. In: B. Curtis (ed.): Psychology of Trust, *Nova Science Publishers*, USA, chapter 8.
Bloch, P.H., Richins, M. (1983). A theoretical model for the study of product importance perceptions. *Journal of Marketing,* 47(3): 69-81.
Blocker, T.J., Eckberg, D., L. (1989). Environemtnal issues as women's issues: General concerns and local hazards. *Social Science Quarterly*, 70: 586-593.
Böcker, A. (2003). Geschlechterdifferenzen in der Risikowahrnehmung bei Lebensmitteln genauer betrachtet: Erfahrung macht den Unterschied. *Hauswirtschaft und Wissenschaft*, 2: 65-75.
Böcker, A., Hartl, J., Kliebisch, C., Engelken, J. (2005). Extern segmentierte Laddering Daten: Wann sind Segmentvergleiche zulässig und wann Unterschiede zwischen Segmenten signifikant? Ein Vorschlag für einen Homogenitätstest. Agrarökonomische Diskussionbeiträge. Working paper, No.75, Gießen, Germany. Retrieved [10\13\2011], from
http://www.geb.uni-giessen.de/geb/volltexte/2005/2115/pdf/Agraroekonomie-2005-75.pdf

Böcker, A., Hartl, J., Nocella, G. (2008). How different are GM food accepters and rejecters really? A means-end chains application to yoghurt in Germany. *Food Quality and Preference*, 19: 383-394.

Bøholm, A. (1998). Comparative studies of risk perception: a review of twenty years of research. *Journal of Risk Research,* 1(2): 135-163.

Bord, R.J., O'Connor, R.E. (1992). Determinants of risk perceptions of a hazardous waste site. *Risk Analysis*, 12(3): 411-416.

Bord, R.J., O'Connor, R.E. (1997). The gender gap in environmental attitudes: The case of perceived vulnerability of risk. *Social Science Quarterly*, 78(4): 830-840.

Botschen, G., Thelen, E.M. (1998). Hard versus soft laddering: Implications for appropriate use. In: Balderjahn, I., Menniken, C., Vernette, E. (eds.): New developments and approaches in consumer behavior research. *Schäfer-Poeschel Verlag*, Stuttgart, Germany: 321-339.

Botschen, G., Thelen, E.M., Pieters, R. (1999). Using means-end structures for benefit segmentation. An application to services. *European Journal of Marketing,* 33 (1/2): 38-58.

Bredahl, L. (1999). Consumers' cognition with regard to genetically modifiedfoods – results of a qualitative study in four countries. *Appetite,* 33: 343-360.

Bredahl, L. (2001). Determinants of consumer attitudes and purchase intentions with regard to genetically modified foods. Results of a cross-national survey. *Journal of Consumer Policy,* 24: 23-61.

Breivik, E., Supphellen, M. (2003). Elicitation of product attributes in an evaluation context: A comparison of three elicitation techniques. *Journal of Economic Psychology,* 24: 77-98.

Brenot, J., Bonnefous, S., Mays, C. (1996). Cultural Theory and risk perception: Validity and utility explored in the French context. *Radiation Protection Dosimetry,* 68 (3/4): 239-243.

Briston, J. M., Fischer, E. (1993). Feminist thought: Implications for consumer research. *The Journal of Consumer research*, 19(4): 518-536.

Brody, B.N.R. (1986). Tolerance for environmental helth risks: the influence of knowledge, benefits, voluntariness, and environmental attitudes. *Risk Analysis,* 6: 425-435.

Brosius, H.-B., Koschel, F., Haas, A. (2009). Methoden der empirischen Kommunikationsforschung. Eine Einführung. *VS Verlag für Sozialwissenschaften*, Wiesbaden, Germany, 5th edition.

Brossard, D., Scheufele, D.A., Kim, E., Lewenstein, B.V. (2009). Religiosity as a perceptual filter: examining process of opinion formation about nanotechnology. *Public Understanding of Science,* 18(5): 546-558.

Browne, M.J., Hoyt, R.E. (2000). The demand for flood insurance: Empirical evidence. *Journal of Risk and Uncertainty,* 20: 271-289.

Brunsø, K., Scholderer, J, Grunert, G. (2004). Closing the gap between values and behavior – a means-end theory of lifestyle. *Journal of Business Research,* 57(6):665-670.

Buchler, S., Smith, K., Lawrence, G. (2010). Food risks, old and new. Demographic characterisitcs and perspectives of food additives, regulation and contamination in Australia. *Journal of Sociology,* 46(4): 353-374.

Byrne, Patrick J.: Gempesaw, Conrado M.: Toensmeyer, Ulrich C. (1991). An evaluation of consumer pesticide residue concerns and risk information sources. *Southern Journal of Agricultural Economics*: 167–174.

Byrnes, J.P., Miller, D.C., Schafer, W.D. (1999). Gender differences in risk taking: A meta-analysis. *Psychological Bulletin,* 125: 367-383.

Campbell, H., Fitzgerald, R. (2001). Follow the fear: A multi-sited approach to GM. *Rural Society,* 11(3): 211-224.

Cantor, N., Mischel, W. (1979). Prototypes in person perception. In: Berkowitz, L. (ed.): Advances in Experimental Social Psychology (Volume 12), *Academic Press*, New York, USA 3-52.

Carrol, D., Baker, J. and Preston, M. (1979). Individual differences in visual imagery and the voluntary control of heart rate. *British Journal of Psychology,* 70: 39-49.

Celsi, R.L., Olson, J.C. (1988). The role of involvement in attention and comprehension processes. *Journal of Consumer Research,* 15(2): 210-224.

Chaiken, S. (1980). Heuristic versus systematic information processing andthe use of source versus message cues in persuasion context. *Journal of Personaility & Social Psychology*, 39: 752-756.

Chaiken, S., Trope, Y. (eds.) (1999). Dual process theories in social psychology. *Guilford Press*, New York, USA.

Chaiken, S., Pliner, P. (1987). Women, but not men, are what they eat. The effect of meal size and gender on perceived femininity and masculinity. *Personality and Social Psychology Bulletin,* 13(2): 166-176.

Christoph, I.B, Bruhn, M., Roosen, J. (2008). Knowledge, attitudes towards and acceptability of genetic modification in Germany. *Appetite,* 51: 58-68.

Claeys, C., Swinnen, A.,Vanden Abeele, P. (1995). Consumers' means-end chains for "think" and "feel" products. *International Journal of Research in Marketing,* 12(3): 193–208.

Clore, G.L., Gasper, K. (2000). Feelings is believing: Some affective influences on belief. In: Frijda, N.H., Manstead, A.S.R., Bem, S. (eds.): Emotions and Beliefs. How feelings influence thoughts. *Cambridge University Press*, Cambridge, UK: 10-37.

Clore, G.L., Schwarz, N., Conway, M. (1994). Affective causes and consequences of social information processing. In: Wyer, R.S., Scrull, Jr. T.K. (eds.): Handbook of social cognition. Volume 1: Basic processes. *Lawrence Erlbaum Associates*, New Jersey, USA: 323-411.

Cobb, M. and Macoubrie, J. (2004). Public Perceptions about Nanotechnology: Risk, Benefits and Trust. *Journal of Nanoparticle Research,* 6: 395–405.

Cohen, J. (1960). A coefficient of agreement of nominal scales. *Educational and Psychological Measurement,* 20: 37-46.

Cohn, L.D., Macfarlane, S., Yanez, C., Imai, W.K. (1995). Risk-percpetion: Differences between adolescents and adults. *Health Psychology,* 14(3): 217-222.

Cole, M.J., Zhang X., Liu J., Liu C., Nicholas J., Belkin N.J., Bierig, R., Gwizdka J. (2010). Are Self-Assessments Reliable Indicators of Topic Knowledge? *Proceedings of the American Society for Information Science and Technology,* 47(1):1-10.

Combs, B. Slovic, P. (1979). Newspaper coverage of causes of death. *Journalism Quarterly,* 56: 837-843.

Connell, R.W. (1995). Masculinities. Polity Press, Cambridge, UK.

Connors, M., Bisgoni, C.A., Sobal, J., Devine, C.M. (2001). Managing values in personal food systems. *Appetite*, 36: 189-200.

Costa, A.I.A. (2003). New insights into consumer-oriented food-product design. Ph.D. thesis, Wageningen. Netherlands. Retrieved [10\05\2011], from http://edepot.wur.nl/121401

Costa, A.I.A., Dekker, M., Jongen, W.M.F. (2004). An overview of means-end theory: potential application in consumer-oriented food product design. *Trends in Food Science and Technology,* 15: 403-415.

Costa-Font, M., Gil, J.M., Traill, W.B. (2008). Consumer acceptance, valuation of and attitudes towards genetically modified food: Review and implications for food policy. *Food Policy,* 33: 99-111.

Costa, A.I.A., Schoolmeester, D., Dekker, M., Jongen, W.M.F. (2003). Exploring the use of consumer collages in product design. *Trends in Food Science and Technology*, 14: 17-31.

Cottle, T.J., Klineberg, S.L. (1974). The present of things future, Free Press-MacMillian, New York.

Cowley, E., Mitchell, A.A. (2003). The moderating effect of product knowledge on the learning and organization of product information. *Journal of Consumer Research*, 30: 443-454.

Coxon, A.P.M., Davies, P.M. (1982). The user's guide to multidimensional scaling. *Heinemann*, London, England.

Cross, F.B. (1998). Facts and values in rsik assessment. *Reliability and Engineering and System Safety,* 59: 27-40.

Cunningham, S.M. (1967). The major dimensions of perceived risk. In: Cox, D.F. (ed.): Risk taking and information handling in consumer behavior. Graduate School of Buisness Administration, *Harvard University Press*, Boston, MA, USA: 82-108.

Cutter, S. (1981). Community concern for pollution: social and environmental infleunces. *Journal of Environmental Psychology,* 13: 105-124.

Cutter, S., Tiefenbacher, J., Solecki, W.D. (1992). En-gendered fears: femininity and technological risk perception. *Organization and Environment*, 6: 5-22.

Cvetkovich, G. (1999). The attribution of social trust. In: Cvetkovich, G., Löfstedt, R. (eds.): Social Trust and the management of risk, *Earthscan*, London, England: 53-61.

Dacin, P.A., Mitchell, A.A. (1986). The measurement of declarativeknowledge. *Advances in Consumer Research,* 13: 454-459.

Dake, K. (1990). Technology on trial: Orienting dispositions towardenvironmental and health hazards. Unpublished Ph.D. thesis. University of California, Berkely, USA.

Dake, K. (1991). Orienting dispositions in the perception of risk: An analysis of contemporary worldviews and cultural biases. *Journal of Cross-Cultural Psychology,* 22(1): 61-82.

Damasio, A.R. (1994). Descartes' error: Emotion, reason, and the human brain.*Putnam*, New York, USA.

Davidson, D.J., Freudenburg, W.R. (1996). Gender and environmental riskconcerns. A review and analysis of available research. *Environment and Behavior,* 28(3): 302-339.
De Jonge J.H., Frewer, L., Van Trijp, R., Renes R. J., De Witt, W., Timmers, J. (2004): Monitoring consumer confidence in food safety: an exploratory study. British Food Journal, 106(10/11): 837-849.
De Jonge, J.H.; Van Trijp, R., Renes R: J., Frewer, L. (2007): Understanding Consumer Confidence in the Safety of Food: Its Two Dimensional Structure and Determinants. *Risk Analysis,* 27(3): 729-740.
De Silva, M.J., McKenzie, K., Harpham, T., Huttly, S.R.A. (2005). Social capital and mental illness: a systematic review. *Journal of Epidemilogical Community Health,* 59: 619-627.
Devlin, D., Birtwistle, G. (2003). Food retail positioning strategy: A means-end chain analysis. *British Food Journal,* 105(9): 653-670.
Dickson-Spillmann, M. Siegrist, M., Keller, C. (2011). Attitude towardschemicals are associated with preference for natural food. *Food Quality and Preference,* 22(1):149-156.
Dietz, T., Stern, P.C., Guagnano G.A. (1998). Social structural and social sociological bases of environmental concern. *Environment and Behaviour,* 30: 450-471.
Dosman, D.M., Adamowicz, W.L., Hrudey, S.E. 2001. Socioeconomic determinants of health- and food safety-related risk perceptions. *Risk Analysis,* 21(2): 307-317.
Douglas, M. (1978). Cultural Bias. Occasional Paper No.35. Royal Anthropological Institute, London.
Douglas, M. (1990). Risk as a forensic resource. *Daedalus,* 119(4): 1-16.
Douglas, M., Wildavsky, A. (1982). Risk and culture: an essay on the selection of technical and environmental dangers. *University of California Press,* Berkely, USA.
Dressel, K., Böschen, S., Hopp, M., Schneider, M., Viehöver, W., Wastian, M. (2010). Planzenschutzmittel – Rückstände in Lebensmitteln. Die Wahrnehmung der Deutschen Bevölkerung – Ein Ergebnisbericht. In: Epp., A., Michalski, B., Banasiak, U., Böl, G.-F. BfR-Wissenschaft (Bundesinstitut für Risikobewertung), 07/2010, Berlin, Germany. Retrieved [01/06/2012], from
http://www.bfr.bund.de/cm/350/pflanzenschutzmittel_rueckstaende_in_lebensmitteln.pdf
Drottz-Sjöberg, B.M., Sjöberg, L. (1991). Attitudes and conceptions of adolescents with regard to nuclear power and radioactive wastes. *Journal of Applied Social Psychology,* 21: 2007-2035.
Dunlap, R.E., Beus, C.E. (1992). Understand public concerns about pesticides: An empirical examination. *The Journal of Consumer Affairs,* 26(2): 418-438.
Dunlap, R.E., Van Liere, K. D. (1978). The new environmental paradigm: A proposed measuring instrument and preliminary results. *Journal of Environmental Education,* 9: 10-19.
Dunlap, R.E., Van Liere, K.D., Mertig, A.G., Jones, R.E. (2000). Measuring endorsement of the new ecological paradigm: A revised NEP scale. *Journal of Social Issues,* 56(3): 425-442.

Eagly, A.H. (1987). Sex differences in social behavior: A social roleinterpretation. *Erlbaum Associaties*, Hilsdale, New Jersey, USA.

Earle, T.C., Cvetcovich, G.T. (1995). Social trust. Toward a cosmopolitan society. *Praeger Publishers*,Westport, CT, London, England.

Eiser, J.R., Miles, S., Frewer, L.J. (2002). Trust, perceived risk and attitudes towards food technologies. *Journal of Applied Social Psychology*, 33(1): 2423-2433.

Eisler, A.D., Eisler, H., Yoshida, M. (2003). Perception of human ecology:cross-cultural and gender comparisons. *Journal of Environmental Psychology,* 23: 89-101.

Epstein, S. (1994). Integration of the cognitive and psychodynamic unconscious. *American Psychologist*, 49: 709-724.

European Commission (eds): (1999). Eurobarometer 52.1. The Europeans and Biotechnology. Retrieved [01/16/09], from http://ec.europa.eu/research/eurobarometer-1999.pdf

European Commission (eds): (2006). Europeans and Biotechnology in 2005: Patterns and trends. Eurobarometer 64.3. Retrieved [01/16/09], from http://www.ask-force.org/web/Eurobaro/Eurobaro-2005-ebs_244b_en.pdf

Evans, D.G.R., Maher, E.R., Macleaod, R., Davies, D.R., Crauford, D. (1997). Uptake of genetic testing for cancer predisposition. *Journal of Medical Genetics,* 34: 746–8.

Fagerli, R.A., Wandel, M. (1999). Gender differences in opinions and practises with regard to a “healthy diet”. *Appetite* 32: 171-90.

Faulkner, W. (2000). The power and the pleasure? A research agenda for “making gender stick” to engineers. *Science, Technology and Human Values,* 25: 87-119.

Farmer F. (1967). Reactor safety and siting: a proposed risk criterion, *Nuclear Safety,* 539–548.

Fazio, R.H. (1986). How do attitudes guide behaviour. In: Sorrentino, R.M., Higgins, E.T. (eds.): The handbook of motivation and cognition. Foundations of social behavior. *Guilford Press*, New York, USA: 204-243.

Feather, N.T. (1975). Values in education and society. *Free Press*, New York, USA.

Federal Research Centre for Nutrition and Food (2008). National Nutrition Survey II. Retrieved [10/02/2011] from www.was-esse-ich.de

Finucane, M.L., Alhakami, A., Slovic, P., Johnson, S.M. (2000a). The affect heuristic in judgements of risks and benefits. *Journal of Behavioral Decision-Making,* 13:1-17.

Finucane, Melissa L., Holup, J.L. (2005). Psychosocial and cultural factorsaffecting the perceived risk of genetically modified food: an overview of the literature. *Social Science & Medicine*, 60: 1603–1612.

Finucane, M.L., Slovic, P., Mertz, C.K., Flynn, J., Satterfield, T.A. (2000b). Gender, race and perceived risk: the ‘white male’ effect. *Health, Risk & Society,* 2(2): 159-172.

Fischer, G.W., Morgan, M.G., Fischhoff, B., Naire, I., Lave, L.B. (1991). What risks are people concerned about? *Risk Analysis,* 11(2): 303-314.

Fishbein, M., Ajzen, I. (1980). Understanding attitudes and predicting social behavior. *Englewood Clies,* New Jersey: Prentice Hall, USA.

Fischhoff, B.; Slovic, P.; Lichtenstein, S.; Red, S.; Combs, B. (1978): How safe is safe enough? A psychometric study of attitudes towards technological risks and benefits. *Policy Sciences,* 9: 127–152.

Fischler, C. (1988). Anthropology of food. *Social Science Information,* 27(2): 275-292.

Flynn, J., Burns, W., Mertz, C.K., Slovic, P. (1992). Trust as a determinant ofopposition to a high-level radioactive waste respository: analysis of a structural model. *Risk Analysis,* 12: 417-429.

Flynn, J., Slovic, P., Mertz, C. K. (1994). Gender, race, and perception of environmental health risks. *Risk Analysis,* 14(6): 1101-1107.

Fotopoulos, C., Krystallis, A., Ness, M. (2003). Wine produced by organic grapes in Greece: using means-end chains analysis to reveal organic buyers'purchasing motives in comparison tot he non-buyers. *Food Quality and Preference*, 14(7): 549-566.

Fox-Keller, E. (1985). Reflections on gender and socience, *Yale University Press*, New Haven, CT, USA.

Fox, M.F., Firebaugh, G. (1992). Confidence in Science: The Gender Gap, *Social Science Quarterly,* 73:101–13.

Freudenburg, W.R. (1993). Risk and recreancy: Weber, the division of labor, and the rationality of risk percpetions. *Social Forces,* 71: 909-932.

Frewer, L., Howard, C., Shepherd, R. (1998). The importance of initial attitudes on responses to communication about genetic engineering in food production. Agriculture and Human Values, 15: 15-30.

Frewer, L.J. (1999). Risk perception, social trust and public participation into strategic decision-making – Implications for emerging technologies. *Ambio,* 28: 569- 574.

Frewer, L.J. (2000). Risk perception and risk communication about food safety issues. *Nutrition Bulletin*, 25: 31-33.

Frewer, L.J., Howard, C., Shepherd, R. (1996). The influence of realisitc product exposure on attitudes towards genetic engineering of food. *Food Quality and Preference,* 7: 61-67.

Frewer, L.J., Miles, S. (2001). Risk perception, communication and trust. How might consumer confidence in the food supply be maintained? In: Frewer, L.J., Risvik, E., Schifferstein, H. (eds.): Food, people and society: a European Perspective of consumers' food choices. *Springer*, Berlin, Germany: 401-413.

Frewer, L. F., Miles, S., Brennan, M., Kuznesof, S., Ness., M., Ritson, C. (2002). Public preference for informed choice under conditions of risk uncertainty. *Public Understanding of Science*, 11: 363-372.

Frewer, L.J., Scholderer, J., Bredahl, L. (2003). Communicating about the risks and benefits of genertically modified foods: the mediating role of trust. *Risk Analysis,* 23(6): 1117-1133.

Früh, W. (2007). Inhaltsanalyse – Theorie und Praxis. *UVKVerlagsgesellschaft*. Konstanz, Germany. 6th edition.

Gannon, L.R. (1999). Women and aging. Transcending the myths. *Routledge*, London, UK.

Gaskell, G., Allum, N., Wagner, W., Kronberger, N., Torgeresen, H., Hampel, J., Bardes, J. (2004). GM foods and the misperception of risk perception. *Risk Analysis,* 24(1): 185-194.

Geis, A. (1992). Computerunterstützte Inhaltsanalyse - Hilfe oder Hinterhalt? In: Züll, C., Mohler, P.P (eds.): Textanalyse. Anwendungen der computergestützten Inhaltsanalyse. *Westdeutscher Verlag*, Opladen, Wiesbaden, Germany: 7–32.

Gengler, C.E., Mulvey, M.S., Oglethorpe, J.E. (1999). A means-end analysis of mother's infant feeding choices. *Journal of Public Policy & Marketing,* 18(2): 172-188.
Gengler, C.E., Reynolds, T.J. (1993). Laddermap. A Software Tool for Analyzing Laddering Data, Version 5.4, computer software, Means-End Software, Camden, New Jersey, USA.
Gengler, C.E., Reynolds, T.J. (1995). Consumer understanding and advertising strategy: Analysis and strategic translation of laddering data. *Journal of Advertising Research,* 35: 19–33.
Gengler, C.E., Reynolds, T.J. (2001). Consumer understanding and advertising strategy: Analysis and strategic translation of laddering data. In: Reynolds, T.J., Olson, J.C. (eds.): Understanding consumer decision making. The means-end approach to marketing and advertising strategy. *Lawrence Erlbaum Associates*, Mahwah, New Jersey, USA: 119-144.
George, M.R. (1999). National Institute of mental health, Research described in : Do male and female brains repond differently to severe emotional stress?: In a flurry of new research, scientists are finding tantalizing clues. Newsweek, Special Edition: What every women needs to know: 68-71.
Gildemeister, R., Wetterer, A., (1991). Wie Geschlechter gemacht werden. Die soziale Konstruktion der Zweigeschlechtlichkeit und ihre Reifizierung in der Frauenforschung. In: Knapp, A.-G., Wetterer, A. (eds.): Traditionen und Brüche. Entwicklung feministischer Theorie. *Kore Verlag*, Freiburg, Germany: 201-254.
Gilman, C.P. (1911). The Man-Made World; or, Our Androcentric Culture. *Echo Library,* Teddington.
Gilligan, C. (1982). In a different voice: Psychological theory and women's development. *Harvard University Press*, Cambridge, MA, USA.
Goszzczynska, M., Tysaka, T., Slovic, P. (1991). Risk perception in Poland: acomparison with three other countries. *Journal of Behavioral Decision Making,* 4: 179-193.
Govindasamy, R., Italia, J., Adelaja, A. (1998). Predicting consumer risk perceptions towards pesticide residue: a logistic analysis. *Applied Economics Letters,* 5: 793-796.
Grayson, K., Rust, R. (2001). Interrater reliability. *Journal of Consumer Psychology,* 10 (1&2): 71-73.
Grebitus, C. (2008). Food quality from the consumer's perspective – an empirical analysis of perceived pork quality. *Cuvilier Verlag*, Göttingen, Germany.
Greenberg, M.R., Schneider, D.F. (1995). Gender differences in risk perception: Effects differ in stressed vs. non-stressed environments. *Risk Analysis,* 15(4): 503-511.
Gregory, R. Flynn, J., Slovic, P. (2001). Technological stigma. In: Flynn, J., Slovic, P., Kunreuther, H. (eds.): Risk, media and stigma. Understanding public challenges to modern science and technology. *Earthscan Publications Ltd.*, London, England: 3-8.
Grobe, D., Douthitt, R., Zepeda, L. (1999). A model of consumers' risk perception toward recombinant bovine growth hormone (rbGH): the impact of risk characteristics. *Risk Analysis,* 19: 661-673.
Grunert, K.G. (1990). Kognitive Strukturen in der Konsumforschung – Entwicklung und Erprobung eines Verfahrens zur offenen Erhebung assoziativer Netzwerke. *Physica-Verlag*, Heidelberg, Germany.

Grunert, K.G., Grunert, S.C. (1995). Measuring subjective meaning structures by the laddering method: Theoretical considerations and methodological problems. *International Journal of Research in Marketing*, 12: 209-225.

Grunert, S.C., Juhl, H.J. (1995). Values, environmental attitudes, and buying of organic foods. *Journal of Economic Psychology*, 16: 39–62.

Grunert, K.G., Grunert, S.C., Sørensen, E. (1995). Means-End Chains and laddering: An inventory of problems and an agenda for research. MAPP Working paper, No.34, Aarhus School of Business, Aarhus, Denmark.Retrieved [10\13\2011], from http://pure.au.dk/portal/files/32299631/wp34.pdf

Gupta, N., Fischer, R.H., Frewer, L.J. (2011). Social-psychological determinants of public acceptance of technologies – A review. *Public Understanding of Science*, DOI: 10.1177/0963662510392485.

Gustafson, P. E. (1998). Gender and risk perception: Theoretical and methodological perspectives. *Risk Analysis,* 18(6): 805-811.

Gutman, J. (1982). A Means-end chain model based on consumer categorization processes. *Journal of Marketing,* 46 (2): 60-72.

Gutman, J., Reynolds, T.J. (1979). An investigation of the levels of cognitive abstraction utilized by consumers in product differentiation. In: Eighmey, J. (eds.): Attitude research under the sun. *American Marketing Association*, Chicago, 128B150.

Gutteling, J.M., Wiegman, O. (1993). Gender-specific reactions to environmental hazards in the Netherlands. *Sex Roles*, 28(7&8): 433-447.

Hallman, W.K., Hebden, W.C., Aquino, H.L., Cuite, C.L. and Lang, J.T.. (2003). Public Perceptions of Genetically Modified Foods: A National Study of American Knowledge and Opinion. Food Policy Institute, Cook College, Rutgers - The State University of New Jersey., New Brunswick, New Jersey.

Hamilton, L. C. 1985: Concern about toxic wastes: three demographic predictors. *Sociological Perspectives,* 28(4): 463-486.

Hansen, J., Holm, L., Frewer, L., Robinson, P., Sandøe, P. (2003). Beyond the knowledge deficit: recent research into lay and expert attitudes to food risks. *Appetite,* 41: 111-121.

Harris, C.R., Jenkins, M., Glaser, D. (2006). Gender differences in risk assessment: Why do women take fewer risks than men? *Judgment and Decision Making,* 1(1): 48-63.

Harshman, R.A. and Paivio, A. (1987). Paradoxical sex differences in self-reported imagery. *Canadian Journal of Psychology,* 41: 303-316.

Harvey, J., Erdos, G., & Callingor, S. (2001). The relationship between attitudes, demographic factors and perceived consumption of meat and other proteins in relation to the BSE crisis: A regional study in the United Kingdom. *Health, Risk and Society,* 3: 181–197.

Haukenes, A. (2004). Perceived health risk and perceptions of expert consensus in modern food society. *Journal of risk Research,* 7(7&8): 759-774.

Henchion, M., Sørensen, D. (2011). Understanding consumers' cognitivestructures with regard to high pressure processing: A means-end chain application to the chilled ready mealy category. *Food Quality and Preference,* 22: 271-280.

Hendick, L., Vlek, C. and Oppewal, H. (1989). Relative importance of scenario and information and frequency information in the judgement of risk. *Acta Psycholgica,* 72: 41-63.

Henwood, K.I., Parkhill, K.A., Pidgeon, N.F. (2008). Science, technology and risk perception. From gender differences to the effects made by gender. *Equal Opportunities International,* 27(8): 662-676.

Hermann, A. (1996). Nachfrageorientierte Produktgestaltung. Ein Ansatz auf Basis der „Means-End"-Theorie. *Gabler-Verlag Woodside*, Wiebaden, Germany.

Hermand, D., Mullet, E., Rompteaux, L. (1999). Socital risk perception among children, adolescents, adults and elderly people. *Journal of Adult Development,* 6(2): 137-143.

Hersch, J. (1996). Smoking, seat belts, and other risky consumer decision: differences by gender and race. *Managerial and Decision Economic,* 17 (5): 471-481.

Hinkle, D. (1965). The change of personal constructs from the viewpoint of theory of construct implications. Unpublished doctoral dissertation, Ohio state University, Columbus, Ohio, USA.

Hoban, T., Woodrum, W., Czaja, R. (1992). Public opposition to genetic engineering. *Rural Sociology,* 57: 476-493.

Hohl, K., Gaskell, G. (2008). European public perceptions of food risk: cross-national and methodological camparisons. *Risk Analysis,* 28(2): 311-324.

Hollander, J.A., Howard, J.A. (2000). Social psychological theories on social inequalities. *Social Psychology Quarterly*, 63: 338-351.

Hossain, F., Onyango, B., Schilling, B., Hallman, W., Adelaja, A. (2003).Product attributes, consumer benefits and public approval of genetically modified foods. *International Journal of Consumer Studies,* 27: 353-365.

Howard, J.A. (1977). Consumer behavior: Application of theory. *McGraw-Hill,* NewYork, USA.

Howard, J.A., Hollander, J.A. (1996). Gendered situations, gendered selves. A gender lens on social psychology. *Sage*, Newbury Park, CA, USA.

Hwang, Y.-J., Roe, B., Teisl, M. (2005). An empirical analysis of United states Consumers' conerns about eight food production and processing technologies. *AgBioForum,* 8(1): 40-49.

Jackson, J., Allum, N., Gaskell, G. (2006). Bridging Levels of Analysis in Risk Perception Research: The Case of the Fear of Crime. In: Forum: *Qualitative Social Research,* 7 (1/20): 1–19.

Jacobsen, L., Karlsson, J.C. (1996). Vardasuppfattningar inom riskområdet. Enander and Jacobsen, L. (eds.): Risk och hot i den svenska vardagen: *Allt från Tjernobyl till skuren sås.,* 9-15.

Japp, K.P. (1997). Die Beobachtung von Nichtwissen. *Soziale Systeme*, 3(2): 289-312.

Japp, K.P. (2000). Risiko. *Transcript Verlag*, Bielefeld, Germany.

Japp, K.P., Kusche, I. (2008). Systems theory and risk. In: Zinn, J.O. (eds.): Social theories of risk and uncertainty. An introduction. *Blackwell Publishing*: 76-105.

Jenkins-Smith, H.C. (1993). Nuclear imagery and regional stigma: testing hypotheses of image acquisition and valuation regarding Nevada. University of New Mexico, Institute for Public Policy, Albuquerque, New Mexico.

Jianakoplos, N.A., Bernasek, A. (1998). Are women more risk averse? *Economic Inquiry,* 36(4): 620-630.

Johnson, B.B., Covello, V.T. (1987). Introduction: The Social and Cultural Construction of Risk: Issues, Methods, and Case Studies. In: Johnson, B.B., Covello, V.D. (eds.): The Social and Cultural Construction of Risk: Essays on risk selection and perception. *Springer*, Dortrecht, The Netherlands.

Jonas, M.S., Beckmann, S.C. (1998). Functional foods: consumer perceptions in Denmark and England. MAPP Working paper, No.55, Aarhus School of Business, Aarhus, Denmark.

Jungermann, H., Slovic, P. (1993). Die Psychologie der Kognition und Evaluation von Risiko. In: Bechmann, G. (ed.): Risiko und Gesellschaft - Grundlagen und Ergebnisse interdisziplinärer Risikoforschung. *Westdeutscher Verlag*, Opladen, Germany:167–208.

Kaciak, E., Cullen, E.W. (2005). Consumer purchase motives and product perceptions: A "hard" laddering study of smoking habits of poles. *International Business and Economic Research Journal,* 4(5): 69-86.

Kahan, D.M., Braman, D., Gastil, J., Slovic, P., Mertz, C.K. (2005). Gender, race and risk perception: the influence of cultural status anxiety. Public Law & Legal theory Research Paper Series, Research Paper, No.86. Yale Law School. Cambridge, USA. Retrieved [01\05\2012], from http://www.stat.columbia.edu/~gelman/stuff_for_blog/SSRN-id723762.pdf

Kahan, D.M., Braman, D., Gastil, J., Slovic, P., Mertz, C.K. (2007). Culture and identity-protective cognition: Explaining the white male effect in risk perception. *Journal of Empirical Legal Studies,* 4(3): 465-505.

Kahan, D.M. (2009a). Cultural cognition as a conception of the Cultural Theory of risk. Cultural Cognition Project Working paper, No.73. Retrieved [03/06/2011], from http://ssrn.com/abstract=1123807

Kahan, D., Braman, D., Slovic, P., Gastil, J., Cohen, G. (2009b). Cultural cognition of the risks and benefits of nanotechnology. *Nature Nanotechnology,* 4: 87-90.

Kahle, L.R:, Beatty; S.E. and Homer, P. (1986). Alternative measurement approaches to consumer values: the list of values (LOV) and values and life style (VALS), *Journal of Consumer Research,* 13: 405-409.

Kahneman, D., Tversky, A. (1972). A judgment of representativeness. *Cognitive Psychology,* 3(3): 430-454.

Kanwar, R., Olson J.C., Sims, L.S. (1980). Toward conceptualizing and measuring cognitive structures. *Advances in Consumer Research,* 7: 122–127.

Kapferer, J.N., Laurent, G. (1985). Consumers' involvement profile: New empirical results. *Advances in Consumer Research,* 12: 290-295.

Kaplan, S., Garrick, B.J. (1981). On The Quantitiative Definition of Risk. *Risk Analysis,* 1(1): 11–27.

Kasperson, R., Berk, G., Pijawka, D., Sharaf, A., Wood, J. (1980). Public opposition to nuclear energy: Retrospects and prospects. In: Unseld, C.T., Morrison, D.E., Sills, D.L., Wolf, C.P. (eds.): Sociopolitical effects of energy use and policy. Supporting paper, No.5, National Academy of the Sciences. Washington, D.C.: 259-292.

Keller, K.L. (1993). Memory retrieval factors and advertising effectiveness. In: Mitchell, A.A. (ed.): Advertising, exposure, memory and choice. *Lawrence Erlbaum Associates*, Hillsdale, New Jersey, USA: 11-48.

Keller, C., Siegrist, M., Gutscher, H. (2006). The role of the affect and availability heuristic in risk communication. *Risk Analysis,* 26(3): 631-639.

Kelly, G.A. (1955). The psychology of personal constructs. *Norton*, New York, USA.

Kessler, S. J., McKenna, W. (1978). Gender: An Ethnomethodoloigal Approach. *University of Chicago Press*, New York, USA.

Kihlstrom, J.F., Cantor, N. (1984). Mental representations of the self. In: Berkowitz L. (eds.): Advances in experimental social psychology. Vol.17, *Academic Press*, New York, USA.

Kirk S.F.L., Greenwood, D., Cade, J.E., Pearman, A.D. (2002). Public perception of a range of potential food risks in the United Kingdom. *Appetite*, 38: 189-197.

Kleinhesselink, R. and Rosa, E.A. (1994). Nuclear trees in a forest of hazards: a comparison of risk perceptions between Americans and Japanese university students. In: Lowinger, T.C., Hinman, G.W. (eds.): Nuclear Power at the Crossroads: Challenges and Prospects for the Twenty-First Century. International Research Center for Energy and Economic Development.

Kliebisch, C. (2002). Kommunikationskonzepte für das Gemeinschaftsmarketing von Lebensmitteln. Eine empirische Studie unter Berücksichtigung der Means-End-Chain-Theorie. Logos, Berlin, Germany.

Knight, F. (1921). Risk, uncertainty and profit. *Houghton Mifflin Co.*, Boston, MA, USA.

Knight, A., Warland, R. (2004). The relationship between sociodemographics and concern about food safety issues. *Journal of Consumer Affairs,* 38(1): 107–120.

Knox, B. (2000): Consumer perception and understanding of risk from food. *British Medical Bulletin,* 56(1): 97–109.

Köhler, F. (2005). Wohlbefinden landwirtschaftlicher Nutztiere: Nutztierwissenschaftliche Erkenntnisse und gesellschaftliche Einstellungen. Dissertation, Christian-Albrechts-Universität zu Kiel, Kiel, Germany. Retrieved [10\13\2011], from http://deposit.ddb.de/cgi-bin/dokserv?idn=978442911&dok_var=d1&dok_ext=pdf&filename=978442911.pdf

Köhler, F., Junker, K. (2000). Motivational bases of consumer concerns about animal welfare - the German laddering interviews report. EU FAIR - CT 98 – 3678, Germany - 3 rd. Report.

Kogan, N., Wallach, M.A. (1964). Risk-taking: A study in cogntion and personality. *Holt, Rhinehart &Winstin*, New York, USA.

Kraus, N., Malmfors, T., Slovic, P. (1992). Intuitive toxicology: Expert and lay judgments of chemical risks. *Risk Analysis,* 12(2): 215-232.

Krewski, D., Lemyre, L., Tuerner, M.C., Lee, J.E.C., Dallaire, C., Bouchard, L., Brand, K., Mercier, P. (2006). Public Perception of Population Health Risks in Canada: Health Hazards and Sources of Information. *Human and Ecological Risk Assessment,* 12: 626–644.

Kroeber-Riel, W. (1979). Activation Research: Psychobiological Approaches in consumer research. *Journal of Consumer Research,* 3: 240-250.

Kroeber-Riel, W., Weinberg, P., Gröppel-Klein, A. (2009). Konsumentenverhalten. *Verlag Franz Vahlen*, München, Germany: 9th revised edition.

Krugman, H. (1966). The measurement of advertising involvement. *Public Opinion Quarterly*, 30: 583-596.

Kunreuther, H., Desvousges, W., Slovic, P. (1988). Nevada's predicament: Public perceptions of risks from the proposed nuclear waste repository. *Environment,* 30: 16-20.

Kuß, A., Tomczak, T. (2007). Käuferverhalten. *Lucius & Lucius*. Stuttgart, Germany, 4th edition.

Lähteenmäki, L., Grunert, K., Ueland, Ø., Aström, A., Arvola, A., Bech-Larsen, T. (2002). Acceptability of genetically modified cheese presented as real product alternative. *Food Quality and Preference,* 13: 523-533.

Lake, A.A., Hyland R.M., Mathers, J.C., Rugg-Gunn, A.J., Wood, C.E.,Adamson A.J. 2006. Food shopping and preparation among the 30-somethings: whose job is it? (The ASH30 study) *British Food Journal,* 108(6): 475-468.

Larson, T.J., Montén, R. (1986). Upplevda risker för sjukdom och olycksfall 1986: Attidyder hos förvärvarbetade svenskar med kroppsarbete. IPSO Factum 6, The Institue for Human Safety and Accident Research, Stockholm.

Lastocicka, J.L., Gardner, D.M. (1978). Low involvement versus high involvement cognitive structures. *Advances in Consumer Research,* 5: 87-92.

Lastovicka, J.L. (1995). Laddermap: Version 4.0 by Chuck Gengler. *Journal of Marketing Research,* 32(4): 494-497.

LeDoux, J. (1996). The emotional brain. Simon and Schuster. New York, USA.

Leikas, S., Lindeman, M., Roininen, K., Lähteenmäki, L. (2007). Food risk perceptions, gender, and individual differences in avoidance and approach motivation, intuitive and analytic thinking styles, and anxiety. *Appetite,* 48: 232–240.

Lemyre, L., Lee, E.C., Mercier, P., Bouchard, L., Krewski, D. (2006). The structure of Canadians' health risk percpetions: Environmental, therapeutic and social health risks. *Health, Risk & Society,* 8(2): 185-195.

Leppard, P., Russell, D.N., Cox, D.N. (2004). Improving means-end-chains studies by using a ranking method to construct hierarchical value maps. *Food Quality and Preference,* 15: 489-497.

Lerner, J.S., Gonzales, R.M., Small, D.A., Fischhoff, B. (2003). Effects of fear and anger on perceived risks of terrorism: A national field experiment. *Psychologicla Science,* 14: 144-150.

Lerner, J.S., Keltner, D. (2000). Beyond valence: toward a model of emotion-specific influences in judgement and choice. *Cognition and Emotion,* 14: 473-493.

LeRoy, S.F., Singell, L.D. Jr. (1987). Knight on Risk and Uncertainty. *Journal of Political Economy*, 95(2), 394-406.

Lichtenstein, S., Slovic, P., Fischhoff, B., Layman, M., Combs, B. (1978). Judged frequency of lethal events. *Journal of Experimental Psychology and Human Learning Memory,* 4: 551-578.

Lin, C.T.J. (1995). Demographic and socioeconomic influences on the importance of food safety in food shopping. *Agricultural and Resource Economics Review*: 190-198.

Lin, C. (2002). Attribute-consequence-value linkages: a new technique for understanding customer's product knowledge. *Journal of Targeting, Measurement and Analysis for Marketing,* 10: 339-352.
Lines, R., Breivik, E., Supphellen, M. (1995). Elicitation of attributes: Acomparison of preference model structures derived from two elicitation techniques. In: Proceedings of the 24th European Marketing Academy Conference, *Essec*, France: 641-656.
Loewenstein, G.F., Weber, E.U., Hsee, C.K., Welch, N. (2001). Risk as feelings. *Psychological Bulletin,* 127: 267-286.
Lookie, S., Lyons, K., Lawrence, G., Grice, J. (2004). Choosing organics: a path analysis of factors underlying the selection of organic food among Australian consumers. *Appetite*, 43: 135-146.
Lookie, S., Lyons, K., Lawrence, G., Mummery, K. (2002). Eating 'green': Motivations behind organic food. *Sociologica Ruralis*, 42(1): 23-39.
Lorber, J. (1991). Dismantling Noah's Ark. In: Lorber J., Farrell S.A. (eds.): The social construction of gender. *Sage*, Newbury Park, CA, USA.
Luhmann, N. (1989). Trust: A mechanism for the reduction of social complexity. In: Luhmann, N (ed.): Trust and power. *Wiley*, New York, USA: 4-103.
Luhmann, N (1993). Risk: A sociological theory; *Walter de Gruyter*, New York, USA.
Lupton, D. (1999). Risk. *Routledge*, New York, USA.
MacGregor, D., Slovic, P., Mason, R., Detweiler, J., Binne, S., Dodd, B. (1994). Perceived risk of radioactive waste transport through Oregon: Results of a statewide survey. *Risk Analysis,* 14: 5-14.
Macoubrie, J. (2006). Nanotechnology: Public concerns, reasoning and trust in government. *Public Understanding of Science,* 15: 221-241.
Marks, L.J., Olson, J.C. (1981). Toward a cognitive structure of conceptualization of product familiarity. *Advances in Consumer Research,* 8: 145-150.
Markus, H., Nurius, P. (1986). Possible selves. *American Psychologist,* 41(9): 954-969.
Marris, C., Langford, I.H., O'Riordan, T. (1998). A Quantitative test of the Cultural Theory of risk perceptions: Comparison with the psychometric paradigm. *Risk Analysis,* 18(5), 635-647.
Mayring, P. (2010). Qualitative Inhaltsanalyse. Grundlagen und Techniken. *Beltz*, Weinheim und Basel: Switzerland: 11th edition.
Marshall, B.K. (2004). Gender, race, and perceived environmental risk: the 'white male' effect in Cancer Alley, LA. *Sociological Spectrum,* 24: 453-478.
Maslow, A.H. (1954). Motivation and Personality. *Harper*, New York, USA.
Miles, S., Brennan, M., Kuznesof, S., Ness, M., Ritson, C. (2004). Public worry about specific food safety issues. *British Food Journal,* 106(1): 9-22.
Miles S., Frewer, L.J. (2001). Investigating specific concerns about different food hazards. *Food Quality and Preference,* 12: 47-61.
Mitchell, V.W. (1999). Consumer perceived risk: conceptualisations and models. *European Journal of Marketing,* 33(1&2): 163-195.
Mitchell, A. (1979). Involvement: A potentially important mediator of consumer behavior. In: Wilkie, W.L., Arbor, A. (eds.): *Advances in Consumer Research*, Vol.6, Association for Consumer Research, Michigan, USA: 35-30.

Mitchell, V.W. (1999). Consumer perceived risk: conceptualisations and models. *European Journal of Marketing,* 33: (1&2): 163-195.
Moerbeck, H., Casimir, G. (2005). Gender differences in consumers' acceptance of genetically modified food. *International Journal of Consumer Studies,* 29: 308-318
Mohr, P., Harrison, A., Wilson, C., Badhurst, K.I., Syrette, S. (2007). Attitudes, values, and socio-demographic characteristics that predict acceptance of genetic engineering and applications of new technology in Australia. *Biotechnology Journal,* 2: 1169-1178.
Moon, W., Balasubramanian, S.K. (2004). Public attitudes toward agrobiotechnology: the mediating role of risk percpetions on the impact of trust, awareness, and outrage. *Review of Agricultural Economics,* 26: 186-208.
Mulvey, M.S., Olson, J.C., Celsi, R.L., Walker, B.A. (1994). Exploring the relationships between means-end knowledge and involvement. *Advances in Consumer Research,* 2: 51-57.
Mulrow, C.D. (1994). Systematic Reviews: Rationale for systematic reviews. BMY, 309: 597-599.
Nayga, R.M. (1996). Sociodemographic Influences on Consumer Concern for Food Safety: The Case of Irradiation, Antibiotics, Hormones, and Pesticides. *Review of Agricultural Economics,* Vol.18, 3: 467-475.
Nielsen, N.A., Bech-Larsen, T., Grunert, K.G. (1998). Consumer purchase motives and product perceptions: A laddering study on vegetable oil in three countries. *Food Quality and Preference,* 9(6): 455-466.
Nordenstedt, H., Ivanisevic, J. (2010). Values in risk perception – studying the relationship between values and risk perception in three countries. *Journal of Disaster Risk Studies,* 3(1): 335-345.
Nyland, L.G. (1993). Risk perception in Brazil and Sweden, Stockholm: Center for Risk Research.
Ohtsubo, H., Yamada, Y. (2007). Japanese public perceptions of food-related hazards. *Journal of Risk Research,* 10(6): 805-819.
Olson, J.C. (1995). Introduction. Special issue on means-end chain analysis. *International Journal of Research in Marketing,* 12:189-191.
Olson, R.A., Cox, C.M. (2001). The influence of gender on the perception and response to investment risk: the case of professional investors. *Journal of Psychology & Financial Markets,* 2: 29-36.
Olson, N.F., Grunert, K.G., Sonne, A.-M. (2010). Consumer acceptance of high-pressure processing and pulsed-electric field: A review. *Trends in Food Science and Technology,* 21: 464-472.
Olson, J.C., Reynolds, T.J. (1983). Understanding consumers cognitivestructures: Implications for advertising strategy. In: Percy, L., Woodside, A. (eds.): Advertising and consumer psychology. Vol.1. *Lexington Books* 77B90, Massachusetts, USA: 77-80.
Olson, J.C., Reynolds, T.J. (2001). The means-end approach to understanding consumer decision making. In: Reynolds, T.J., Olson, J.C. (eds.): Understanding consumer decision making. The means-end approach to marketing and advertising strategy. *Lawrence Erlbaum Associates*, Mahwah, New Jersey, USA: 3-20.

Oltedal, S., Bjørg-Elin M., Hroar K., Torbjørn R. (2004). Explaining risk perception: evaluation of cultural theory: Rotunde (85), Trondheim, Norway.

Ott, S.L., Maligaya, A. (1989). An analysis of consumer attitudes Toward pesticide use and the potential market for pesticide residue-free fresh produce." Paper Presented at the Southern Agricultural Economics Association Annual Meetings, Nashville, TN, 5–8 February.

Palmer, C.G.S. (1996). Risk perception: An empirical study of the relationship between world views and the risk construct. *Risk Analysis,* 16(5): 717-723.

Palmer, C.G.S. (2003). Risk perception: antoher look at the 'white male' effect. *Health, Risk & Society,* 5(1): 71-83.

Perrault, W.D. Jr., Leigh, L.E. (1989). Reliability of nominal data based on qualitative judgments. *Journal of Marketing Research,* 26: 135-148.

Peter, J.P., Olson, J.C. (2010). Consumer Behavior and Marketing strategy. *McGraw-Hill,* Chicago, USA, 9th edition.

Peters, E., Burraston, B., Mertz, C.K. (2004). An emotion-based model of risk perception and stigma sudceptibility: Cognitive appraisals of emotion, affective reactivity, worldviews, and risk perceptions in the generaton of technological stigma. *Risk Analysis,* 24: 1349-1367.

Peters, R.G., Covello, V.T., McCallum, D.B. (1997). The determinants of trust and credibility in environmental risk communication: an empirical study. *Risk Analysis,* 17(1): 43-54.

Peters, E., Slovic, P. (1996). The role of affect and worldviews as orienting dispositions in the perception and acceptance of nuclear power. *Journal of Applied Social Psychology,* 26(16): 1427-1453.

Petty, R.E., Cacioppo, J.T. (1984). Sources factors and the elaboration likelihood model of persuasation. *Advances in Consumer Research,* 11: 667-672.

Petty, R.E., Cacioppo, J.T., Schumann, D. (1983). Central and peripheral routes to advertising effectiveness: The moderating role of involvement. *Journal of Consumer Research,* 10: 135-146.

Pidd, M. (2005). Perversity in public service performance measurement. *International Journal of Productivity and Performance Management*, 54 (5/6): 482-493.

Pidegon N., Roger E.K., Slovic P. (Ed.): The Social Amplification of Risk. Cambridge: *Cambridge University Press,* 47–79.

Pieters, R., Baumgartner, H., Allen, D. (1995). A means-end approach to consumer goal structures. *International Journal of Research in Marketing,* 12: 227-244.

Pilisuk, M., Acredolo, C. (1988). Fear of technological hazards: One concern or many? *Social Behavior,* 3: 17-24.

Plapp, T. (2004). Wahrnehmung von Risiken aus Naturkatastrophen. Eine empirische Untersuchung in sechs gefährdeten Gebieten Süd- und Westdeutschlands. Karlsruher Reihe II, Risikoforschung und Versicherungsmanagement. Karlsruhe, Germany.

Poortinga, W., Pidgeon, N.E. (2004). Trust, the asymmetry principle, and the role of prior beliefs. *Risk Analysis,* 24(6): 1475-1486.

Poortinga, W., Pidgeon, N.F. (2005). Trust in risk regulation: Cause or consequence of the acceptability of GM food? *Risk Analysis,* 25(1): 199-209.

Prahl, H.W., Setzwein, M. (1999). Soziologie der Ernährung. *Leske und Budrich*. Opladen, Germany.

Quillian, M.R. (1968). Semantic memory. In: Minsky, M. (eds.): Semantic information processing. *MIT Press*, Cambridge, England: 227-270.

Qin, W., Brown, J.L. (2007). Public reactions to information about genetically engineered foods: effects of information formats and male/female differences. *Public Understanding of Science,* 16: 471-488.

Rayner, S. (1992). Cultural theory and risk analysis. In: Krimsky, S., Golding, D. (eds.): Social theories of risk. *Praeger Publishers*, New York: 83-115.

Rayner, S., Cantor, R. (1987). How fair is safe enough? The cultural approach to societal technology choice. *Risk Analysis,* 7(1): 3-9.

Renn, O., Zwick, M.M. (1997). Risiko- und Technikakzeptanz. *Springer*, Germany.

Reynolds, T.J, Dethloff, C., Westberg, S.J. (2001). Advancements in laddering. In: Reynolds, T.J., Olson, J.C. (eds.): Understanding consumer decision making. The means-end approach to marketing and advertising strategy. *Lawrence Erlbaum Associates*, Mahwah, New Jersey, USA: 91–118.

Reynolds, T.J., Gutman, J. (1988). Laddering theory, method, analysis, and interpretation. *Journal of Advertising Research*, 28: 11-31.

Reynolds, T.J., Gutman, J. (2001). Laddering theory, method, analysis, and interpretation. In: Reynolds, T.J.,Olson, J.C. (eds.): Understanding consumer decision making. The means-end approach to marketing and advertising strategy. *Lawrence Erlbaum Associates*, Mahwah, New Jersey, USA: 25–62.

Reynolds, T.J., Gutman, J., Fiedler, J.A (1985). Understanding cognitive structures: the relationship of levels of psychological distance and preference. In: Alwith, L.F., Mitchell, A.A. (eds.): Psychological processes and advertising effects. *LEA*, New Jersey, USA: 262-271.

Reynolds, T., Whitlark, D. (1995). Applying laddering data tocommunications strategy and advertising practice. *Journal of Advertising Research,* 35: 9-16.

Richins, M.L. (1997). Measuring emotions in the consumption experience. *The Journal of Consumer Research,* 24(2): 127-146.

Riger, S., Gordon, M.T., LeBailly, R. (1978). Women's fear of crime: From blaming to restricting the victim. *Victimology*, 3: 274-284.

Roininen, K., Lähteenmäki, L., Tuorila, H. (1999). Quantification of consumer attitude to health and hedonic characteristics of food. *Appetite*, 33: 71-88.

Rohrmann, B. (1994). Risk perception of different societal groups: Australian findings and cross-national comparisons. *Australian Journal of Psychology,* 46: 150-163.

Rohrmann, B., Renn, O. (2000). Cross-cultural risk perception. A survey of empirical studies. *Kluwer Academic*, Dordrecht, The Netherlands.

Rokeach, M.J. (1973). The nature of human values. *The Free Press*, NewYork, USA.

Roosen, J., Thiele, S., Hansen, K. (2005). Food risk perceptions by different consumer groups in Germany. *Acta Agriculture Scand Section* C 2: 13-26.

Rosa, E.A. (2003). The logical structure of the social amplification of risk framework (SARF): Metatheoretical foundation and policy implications. In: Pidegeon, N., Kaspersen, R.E., Slovic, P. (eds.): The social amplification of risk. *Cambridge University Press*, Cambridge, UK.

Rosenberg, M.J. (1956). Cognitive structure and attitudinal affect. *Journal of Abnormal and Social Psychology,* 53: 367-372.
Rottenstreich, Y., Hsee, C.K. (2001). Money, kisses, and electric shockes: On the affective psychology of risk. *Psychological Science,* 12: 185-190.
Rothschild, M.L. (1975). Involvement as a determinant of decision making styles. In: Mazze, E.M. (eds.): Combined Proceedings, *American Marketing Association*, Chicago, USA: 216-220.
Rozin, P. (2005). The meaning of natural. Psychological Science, 16: 652-658.
Rozin, P., Spranca, M., Krieger, Z., Neuhaus, R., Surillo, D., Swerdlin, A., Wood, K. (2004). Preference for natural: instrumental and ideational/moral motivations, and contrast between foods and medicines. *Appetite*, 43(2): 147-154.
Rozin, P. (1976). Food, self and identity. The anthropology of *food. Social Science Information*, 27(2): 275-292.
Russell, C.G., Busson, A., Flight, I., Bryan, J., van Pabst van Lawick, J.A. (2004a). A comparison of three laddering techniques applied to an example of a complex food choice. *Food Quality and Preference,* 15: 569-583.
Russell, C.G., Flight, I., Leppard, P.,van Pabst van Lawick, J.A., Syrette, J.A., Cox, D.N. (2004b). A comparison of paper-and-pencil and computerized methods of "hard" laddering. *Food Quality and Preference,* 15: 279-291.
Satterfield, T.A., Mertz, C.K., Slovic, P. (2004). Discriminiation, vulnerability and justice in the face of risk. *Risk Analysis,* 24(1): 115-129.
Savage, I. (1993). Demographic influences on risk perceptions. *Risk Analysis,* 13(4):413-420.
Schan, A.K., Holzer, E. (1990). Studies of individual environmental concern. *Environment and Behavior*, 22: 767-786.
Scheufele, D., Corley, E., Shih, T., Dalrymple, K., Ho, S. (2009). Religious beliefs and public attitudes toward nanotechnology in Europe and the United States. *Nature Nanotechnology,* 4(2): 91-94.
Scheufele, D., Lewenstein, B. (2005). The public and nanotechnology: how citizens make sense of emerging technologies. *Journal of Nanoparticle Research,* 7: 659-667.
Schneider, W., Shiffrin, R.M. (1977). Controlled and automatic human information processing. In: Detection, search and attention. *Psychological Review,* 84: 1-66.
Schubert, R., Brown, M., Gysler, M., Brachinger, H.W. (1999). Financial decision-making: are women really more risk-averse? *The American Economic Review*, 89(2): 381-385.
Schütz, H., Wiedemann, P.M., Gray, P.C.R. (2000). Risk perception beyond the psychometric paradigma. Arbeiten zur Risikokommunikation, Heft 78. Programmgruppe Mensch, Umwelt, Technik (MUT), Forschungszentrum Jülich GmbH.
Schütz, H., Wiedemann, P., Hennings, W., Mertens, J., Clauberg, M. (2003). Vergleichende Risikobewertung Konzepte, Probleme und Anwendungsmöglichkeiten. Abschlussbericht zum BfS-Projekt StSch 4217 "Risikobewertung und -management: Ausarbeitung von Konzepten eines integrierten und vergleichenden Risikoansatzes". Programmgruppe Mensch, Umwelt, Technik (MUT), Forschungszentrum Jülich GmbH.

Schwartz, S.H. (1992). Universal in the content and structure of values: theoretical advances and empirical tests in 20 countries. *Advances in Experiemntal Social Psychology*, 25: 1-65.
Schwartz, S.H. (1994). Are there universal aspects in the structure and content of human values? *Journal of Social Issues*, 50: 19-45.
Schwartz, S.H., Bilsky, W.(1987). Towards a universal structure of human values. *Journal of Personality and Social Psychology*, 53: 550-562.
Seel, B. (2004). Ernährung im Haushaltszusammenhang – Befunde und ökonomische Erklärungsansätze zu geschlechtsdifferentem Verhalten. In: Rückert-John, J. (ed.): Hohenheimer Beiträge zu Gender und Ernährung, 1: 8-49.
Setbon, M., Raude, J., Fischler, C., Flahault, A. (2005). Risk perception of the „Mad Cow Disease"in France: Determinants and consequences. *Risk Analysis,* 25(4):813-821.
Setzwein, M. (2004). Ernährung als Thema der Geschlechterforschung. In: Rückert-John, J. (ed.) Hohenheimer Beiträge zu Gender und Ernährung 1: 50-72.
Siegrist, M. (1998).Belief in gene technology: The influence of environmental attitudes and gender. *Personality and Individual Differences,* 24(6): 861-866.
Siegrist, M. (1999). A causal model explaining the perception and acceptance of gene technology. *Journal of Applied Social Psychology,* 29: 2093-2106.
Siegrist, M. (2000). The influence of trust and perceptions of risks and benefits on the acceptance of gene technology. *Risk Analysis,* 20(2): 195-203.
Siegrist, M. (2002). The influence of trust and perceptions of risks and benefits on the acceptance of gene technology. *Risk Analysis,* 20,(2), 195-204.
Siegrist, M. (2003). Perception of gene technology, and food risks: results of a survey in Switzerland. *Journal of Risk Research,* 6(1): 45-60.
Siegrist, M. (2007). Consumers attitudes to food innovation and technology. In: Frewer, L., van Trijp (eds.): Understanding consumers of food products. *Woodhead Publishing*, Cambridge, England: 236-253.
Siegrist, M., Cvetkovich, G. (2000). Perception of hazards: the role of social trust and knowledge. *Risk Analysis,* 20(5): 713-718.
Siegrist, M., Cvetkovich, G., Roth, C. (2000). Salient value similarity, social trust, and risk/benefit perpcetion. *Risk Analysis,* 20(2): 353-362.
Siegrist, M., Keller, C., Kastenholz, H., Frey, S., Wiek, A. (2007). Laypeople's and experts' perception of nanotechnology hazards. *Risk Analysis,* 27(1): 59-69.
Sjöberg, L. (1997). Explaining risk perception: An empirical and quantitative evaluation of Cultural Theory. *Risk Decision and Policy*: 113.
Sjöberg, L. (1998).World views, political attitudes and risk perception. *Risk: Health, Safety and Environment*, 9: 137-152.
Sjöberg, L. (2000a). Consequences matter, "risk" is marginal. *Journal of Risk Research,* 3(3): 287-295.
Sjöberg, L. (2000b). Factors in risk perception. *Risk Analysis,* 20(1): 1-11.
Sjöberg, L. (2006). Will the real meaning of affect please stand up? *Journal of Risk Research,* 9(2): 101-108.
Sjöberg, L. (2007). Emotions and risk perception. *Risk management,* 9(4): 223-237.

Sjöberg, L., Kolarova, D., Rucai, A.A., Bernström, M-L., Flygelholm H. (1996). Risk Perception and Media Reports in Bulgaria and Romania, Stockholm: Center for Risk Research.

Sjöberg, L., Moen, B.E., Rundmo, T. (2004). Explaining risk perception. An evaluation of the psychometric paradigm in risk perception research: Rotunde (84), Trondheim, Norway.

Sjöberg, L., Wahlberg, A. (2002). Risk Perception and New Age Beliefs. *Risk Analysis,* 22(4): 751-764.

Slimak, M.W., Dietz, T. (2006). Personal values, beliefs, and ecological risk perception. *Risk Analysis,* 26(6): 1689-1705.

Sloman, S.A. (1996). The empirical case for two systems of reasoning. *Psychological Bulletin,* 119 (1): 3-22.

Slovic, P. (1987). The perception of risk. *Science*, 236: 280-285.

Slovic, P. (1992). Perception of Risk: Reflections on the Psychometric Paradigm. In: S. Krimsky, Golding, D. (eds.): Social Theories of Risk. *Praeger*, London: 117–152.

Slovic, P. (1993). Perceived risk, trust, and democracy. *Risk Analysis,* 13(3): 675-682.

Slovic, P. (1999). Trust, emotion, sex, politics, and science: surveying the risk-assessment battlefield. *Risk Analysis,* 19(4): 689-700.

Slovic, P., Finucane, M., Peters, E., MacGregor, D.G. (2002). The affect heuristic. In: Gilovich, T., Dale, G., Kahnemann, D. (eds.): Heuristics and biases: the psychology of intuitive judgment. *Cambridge University Press*, New York, USA: 397-420.

Slovic, P., Finucane, M., Peters, E., MacGregor, D.G. (2004). Risk as analysis and risk as feelings: Some thoughts about affect, reason, risk, and rationality. *Risk Analysis,* 24(2): 311-322.

Slovic, P., Fischhoff, B., Lichtenstein, S. (1982). Facts versus fears: Understanding perceived risk. In: Kahneman, D., Slovic, P., Tversky, A. (eds.): Judgment under uncertainty: Heuristics and biases. *Cambridge University Press*, Cambridge, USA: 463-492.

Slovic, P., Flynn, J.H., Layman, M. (1991). Perceived risk, trust, and the politics of nuclear waste. *Science,* 254: 1603-1607.

Slovic, P., Lichtenstein, S., Fischhoff, B. (1979). Which risks are acceptable? *Environment,* 21(4): 17–20.

Slovic, P., Malmfors, T., Mertz, C.K., Neil, N., Purchase, I.F. (1997). Evaluating chemical risks: results of a survey of the British Toxicology Society. *Human & Experiemental Toxicology*, 16(6): 289-304.

Slovic, P., Malmfors, T., Mertz, C.K., Neil, N., Purchase, I.F.H. (1997). Evaluating chemical risks: results of a survey of the British Toxicology Society. *Human & Experimental Toxiciology,* 16: 289-304.

Slovic, P., Monahan, J., Macgregor, D.G. (2000). Violence risk assessment and risk communication: The effects of using actual cases, providing instruction, and employing probability versus frequency formats. *Law and Human Behavior,* 24: 271-296.

Slovic, P., Peters, E. (2006). Risk perception and affect. *Current Directions in Psychological Science*, 15 (6): 322-325.

Smith, C.A., Ellsworth, P.C. (1985). Patterns of cognitive appraisal in emotion. *Journal of Personaility and Social Psychology*, 48: 813-838.
Solomon, R.M., Bamossy, G., Askegaard, S., Hogg, M.K. (2010). Consumer behaviour. A European perspective. *Pearson Education*, Harlow, England.
Sørensen, E., Grunert, K.G., Nielsen, N.A. (1996). The impact of product experience, product involvement and verbal processing style on consumers' cognitive structures with regard to fresh fish. MAPP Working paper, No.42, Aarhus School of Business. Retrieved [10\03\2011], from http://pure.au.dk/portal/files/118/wp42.pdf
Sørensen, D., Henchion, M. (2011). Understanding consumers' cognitive structures with regard to high pressure processing: A means-end chain application to the chilled ready meals category. *Food Quality and Preference*, 22: 271-280.
Sparks, P., Shepperd, R., Frewer, L. (1995). Assessing and structuring attitudes towards the use of gene technology in food production: the role of perceived ethical obligation. *Journal of Basic and Applied Social Psychology,* 16: 267-285.
Squire, L.R. (1987). Memory and brain. *Oxford University Press*, New York, USA.
Starr, C. (1969). Social benefits versus technological risks. *Science,* 165(3899): 1232-1238.
Starr, G., Langley, A., Taylor, A. (2000). Environmental health risk perception in Australia. A research report to the commonwealth department of Health and Aged Care. Centre for Population Studies in Epidemiology, South Australian Department of Human Services.
Stallen, P.J.M., Tomas,A. (1988). Rublic concern about industrial hazards. *Risk Analysis,* 8(2): 237-245.
Stedman, R.C. (2004). Risk and climate change: Perceptions of key policy actors in Canada. *Risk Analysis,* 24(5): 1395-1406.
Steg, L., Sievers, I. (2000). Cultural Theory and individual perceptions of environmental risks. *Environment and Behavior,* 23: 250-269.
Steger, M.A.E., Witte, S.L. (1989). Gender differences in environmental orientations: A comparison of publics and activists in Canada and the U.S.. *Western Political Quarterly*, 42: 627-649.
Stern, P.C., Dietz, T., Kalof, L. (1993). Value orientations, gender, and environmental concern. *Environment and Behavior,* 25(3): 322-348.
Stern, P.C.; Dietz, T., Kalof, L., Guagnano, G.A. (1995). Values, Beliefs, and Proenvironmental Action: Attitude Formation Toward Emergent Attitude Objects. *Journal of Applied Social Psychology,* 25(18): 1611–1636.
Storbeck, J., Robinson, M.D., McCourt, M.E. (2006). Semantic processing precedes affect retrieval: the neurological case for cognitive primacy in visual processing. *Review of General Psychology,* 10 (1): 41-55.
Steenkamp, J.-B. E.M. (1997). Dynamics in consumer behavior with respect to agricultural and food products. In: Wierenga, B. (eds.): Agricultural marketing and consumer behavior in a changing world, *Kluwer Academic*, Boston, MA: 143-188.
Steenkamp, J.-B.E.M., van Trijp, H.C.M. (1997). Attribute elicitation in marketing research: a comparison of three procedures. *Marketing Letters,* 8 (2): 153-165.

Steinbrugge, K.V., McClure , F.E., Snow, A.J. (1969). Studies in seismicity and earthquake damage statistics. Washington D.C.: U.S. Department of Housing and Urban Development.

Tanner, M., Young, M.A. (1985). Modeling agreement among raters. *Journalof the American Statistical Association,* 80(389): 175-180.

Thompson, P. B., Dean, W. (1996). Competing conceptions of risk. *Risk: Health Safety Environment,* 7:361-384.

Thompson, M., Ellis, R., Wildavsky, A. (1990). Cultural Theory. Boulder Colo.: *Westview Press.*: Westport, Conn., USA.

Tibben, A., Frets, P.G., van de Kamp, J.J.P., Niermeijer, M.F., Vegter-van der Vlis, M., Roos, R.A.C., Vanommen,G.J.B., Uivenvoorden, H.J. and Verhage, F. (1993). Presymptomatic DNA testing for Huntington Disease:Pretest Attitudes and Expectations of Applicants and their Partners in the Dutch Program. *American Journal of Medical Genetics* 48: 10–16.

Townsend, E., Clarke, D.D., Travis, B. (2004). Effects of context and feelings on perception of genetically modified food. *Risk Analysis,* 24(5): 1369-1383.

Trankina, M. (1993). Gender differences in attitudes toward science.*Psychological Reports,* 73: 123–130.

Tulloch, J., Lupton, D. (2003). Risk and everyday life. *Sage*, London, England.

Tulloch, K. (2008). Culture and risk. In: Zinn, J.O. (eds.): Social theories of risk and uncertainty. An introduction. *Blackwell Publishing*: 138-167.

Tversky, A.; Kahneman, D. (1972). Subjective probability: Judgement of representativeness. Cogntive Psychology, 3(3): 430-454.

Tversky, A.; Kahneman, D. (1973). Availability: A heuristic for judging frequency and probability. *Cognitive Psychology,* 5(2): 207–232.

Tversky, A., Kahneman, D. (1974). Judgement under uncertainty: Heuristics and biases. *Science,* 185: 1124-31.

Tversky, A., Kahneman, D. (1983). Extensional versus intuitive reasoning: The conjuction fallacy in probability judgments. *Psychological Review,* 90: 293-315.

Ter Hofstede, F., Audenaert, A., Steenkamp, J.B.E.M., Wedel, M. (1998).An investigation into the association pattern technique as a quantitative approach to measuring means-end chains. *International Journal of Research in Marketing,* 15(1): 37-50.

Tolman, E.C. (1932). Purposive behavior in animals and men. *Century*, New York, USA.

Trommsdorff, V., Teichert, T. (2011). Konsumentenverhalten. Kohlhammer, Stuttgart, Germany, 8th edition.

Tuncalp, S., Sheth, J.N. (1975). Prediction of attitudes: A comparative study of Rosenberg, Fishbein and Sheth models. Advances in Consumer Research, 2: 389-404.

Ulbig, E., Hertel, R.F., Böl, G.F. (eds.) (2010). Kommunikation von Risiko und Gefährdungspotenzial aus Sicht verschiedener Stakeholder. Abschlussbericht. Bundesinstitut für Risikobewertung. Berlin, Germany.

Urban, D., Hoban, T.J. (1997). Cognitive determinants of risk perception associated with biotechnology. *Scientimetrics,* 40: 299-331.

Valette-Florence, P., Rapacchi, B. (1991). Improvements in means-end chain analysis: using graph theory and correspondence analysis. *Journal of Advertising Research,* 31: 30-45.

Vandermoere, F., Blanchemanche, S., Bieberstein, A., Marette, S., Roosen, J. (2009). The public understanding of nanotechnology in the food domain: the hidden role of views on science, technology, and nature. *Public Understanding of Science,* 20(2): 195-206.

Vandermoere, F., Blanchemanche, S., Bieberstein, A., Marette, S., Roosen, J. (2010). The morality of attitudes toward nanotechnology: About God, techno-scientific progress, and interfering with nature. *Journal of Nanoparticle Research,* 12(2): 373-381.

Vannoppen, J., Van Huylenbroek, G., Verbeke, W., Viaene, J. (1999).Consumers values with regard to buying food from short mark channels. In: Sylvander, B., Barjolle, D., Arfini, F. (eds.): The socio-economics of origin labelled products in agri-food supply chains: spatial, institutional and co-ordination aspects. Proceedings of the 67th EAAE seminar, *INRA Editions*, 28-30 October, Le Mans, France: 223-236.

Vaughan, E., Nordenstam, B. (1991). The perception of environmental risks among ethnically diverse groups. *Journal of Cross-Cultural Psychology*, 22: 29-60.

Veludo-de-Oliveira, M.T., Akemi, I.A., Cortez, C.M. (2006). Discussing laddering application by the means-end chain theory. The Qualitative Report 11 (4): 626-642. Retrieved [10\03\2011], from http://www.nova.edu/ssss/QR/QR11-4/veludo-de-oliveira.pdf

Viklund, M. (2003). Trust and risk perception in Western Europe: A cross-national study. *Risk Analysis,* 23(4): 727-738.

Vinson, D.E., Scott, J.E., Lamont, L.M. (1977). The role of personal values in marketing and consumer behavior. *Journal of Marketing,* 41: 44-50.

Viscusi, W.K. (1991): Age Variations in Risk Perceptions and Smoking Decisions. *The Review of Economics and Statistics,* 73(4), 577–588.

Visschers, H.M., Meertens R.M., Passchier W.F., deVries N.K. (2007). How does the general public evaluate risk information? The impact of associations with other risks. *Risk Analysis,* 27(3), 715-727.

Vriens, M., Ter Hofstede, F. (2000). Linking attributes, benefits, and consumer values. A powerful approach to market segmentation, brand positioning and advertising strategy. *Journal of Marketing Research,* 12(3): 4-10.

Walker, B.A., Olson, J.C. (1991). Means-end chains: Connecting products with self. *Journal of Business Research,* 22: 111-118.

Weitkunat, R., Pottgiesser, C., Meyer, N., Crispin, A., Fisher, R., Schotten, K., Kerr, J.U., Berla, K. (2003). Perceived risk of bovine spongiform encephalopathy and dietary behaviour. *Journal of Health Psychology,* 8(3), 373–381.

West, C., Fenstermaker, S. (1995). Doing difference. *Gender and Society,* 9(8): 37.

West, C., Zimmerman, D.H. (1987). Doing Gender. *Gender and Society,* 1(2): 125-151.

West, C., Zimmerman, D.H. (1991). Doing Gender. In: Lorber J. and Farrell S. A. (eds.): The social construction of gender. *Sage*, Newbury Park, CA: 13-37.

Wester-Herber, M., Warg, L.E. (2002). Gender and regional differences in risk perception: results from implementing the Seveso II Directive in Sweden. *Journal of Risk Research,* 5(21): 69-81.

Wharton, A.S. (2005). The sociology of gender. An introduction to theory and research. *Blackwell Publishing,* Malden, MA, USA.

Wiedemann, P.M., Balderjahn, I. (1999). Risikobewertung im kognitiven Kontext. Arbeiten zur Risiko-Kommunikation, 3, Programmgruppe Mensch, Umwelt, Technik (MUT), Forschungszentrum Jülich GmbH. Retrieved [10\13\2011], from http://www2.fz-juelich.de/inb/inb-mut/publikationen/hefte/heft_73.pdf

Wiedemann, P.M., Eitzinger, C. (2006). Risikowahrnehmung und Gender. Arbeiten zur Risikokommunikation, Heft 93. Forschungszentrum Jülich, Progra gruppe Mensch, Umwelt, Technik (MUT), Jülich, Germany. Retrieved [01/05/2012], from http://www2.fz-juelich.de/inb/inb-mut/publikationen/hefte/heft_93.pdf

Wildavsky, A. (1987). Choosing preferences by constructing institutions: Acultural theory of preference formation. *American Political Science Review*, 81(1): 3-21.

Wildavsky, A., Dake, K. (1990). Theories of risk perception: Who fears what and why?. *Daedalus,* 19(4): 41-60.

Wilkie, W.L., Farris, P.W. (1976). Consumer information processing: Perspectives and implications for advertising. Marketing Science Institute, Report Number 76-113, Cambridge, Massachusetts, USA.

Worsley, A., Lea, E. (2008). Consumer concern about food and health. *British Food Journal*, 110 (11): 1106-1118.

Worsley, A., Scott, V. (2000). Consumers' concerns' about food and health in Australia and New Zealand. *Asia Pacific Journal of Clinical Nutrition,* 9(1): 24-32.

Young, S., Feigin, B. (1975). Using the benefit chain for improved strategy formulation. *Journal of Marketing,* July: 72-74.

Zajonc, R.B. (1980). Feelings and thinking: Preferences need no inferences. *American Psychologist,* 35(2): 151-175.

Zanoli, R., Naspetti, S. (2002). Consumer motivations in the purchase of organic food. A means-end approach. *British Food Journal,* 104(8): 643-653.

Zelezny, L., Poh-Pheng, C., Aldrich, C. (2000). Elaborating on gender differences in environmentalism. *Journal of Social Issues,* 56: 443-457.

Zinn, J.O. (2004). Literature review: Economics and risk. Social contexts and responses to risk network (SCARR), ESRC Working paper, 2, Retrieved [09/03/2010] from www.kent.ac.uk/scarr/papers/Economics%20Lit%20Review%20WP2%20.04Zinn.pdf

Zinn, J.O. (2006a). Risk, affect and emotion. Forum: Qualitative Social Research, 7:1 (29), Retrieved [13/03/08], from http://www.qualitative-research.net/fqs-texte/1-06/06-1-29-e.html

Zinn, J.O. (2006b). Recent developments in sociology of risk and uncertainty. Forum: Qualitative Social Research, 7: 1 (30), Retrieved [11/12/11], from http://www.qualitative-research.net/fqs-texte/1-06/06-1-30-e.pdf

Zinn, J.O. (2008a). Introduction: the contribution of sociology to the discourse on risk and uncertainty. In: Zinn, J.O. (eds.): Social theories of risk and uncertainty. An introduction. *Blackwell Publishing:* 1-17.

Zinn, J.O. (2008b). Risk society and reflexive modernization. In: Zinn, J.O. (eds.): Social theories of risk and uncertainty. An introduction. *Blackwell Publishing:* 18-51.

Zwart, H. (2000). A short history of food ethics. *Journal of Agicultural and Environmental Ethics,* 12: 113-126.

Appendix

Appendix A1: **Overview Study Classification for the Systematic Literature Review**[1]

Sytematic Review							
Type of Risk	**Authors**	**Journal & publication date**	**Date of data collection**	**Country**	**Dependent variable**	**Scale**	**Group**
Pesticides							
pesticides use in agricul-ture	Dunlap, Beus	Journal of Consumer Af-fairs, 1992	1990	USA	worry about safety	1 to 5	2
pesticides	Govindasamy, Italia	Applied Economics Letters, 1998	1990	USA	likelihood of being highly risk adverse	1=highly risk adverse; 0=otherwise	2
pesticides	Byre, Gem-pesaw, Toensmeyer	Southern Journal of Agricul-tural Economics, 1991	1990	USA	probability of being uncon-cerned	1 to 7	2

pesticides	Nayga	Journal of Agricultural and Applied Economics, 1996	1991	USA	likelihood to purchase	0/1	2
pesticides in food	Flynn, Slovic, Mertz	Risk Analysis, 1994	1992/1993	USA	risk perception	1 to 4	2
pesticides in food	Schütz, Wie-demann	Risk Analysis, 1998	1993/1994	Germany	risk perception	1 to 7	2a
pesticides in food	Dosman, Adamowicz, Hrudey	Risk Analysis, 2001	1994/1995	Canada	health risk perception in 1994	0 to 3	2
pesticides in food	Dosman, Adamowicz, Hrudey	Risk Analysis, 2001	1994/1995	Canada	health risk perception in 1995	1 to 3	2
pesticides in food	Finucane et al.	Health Risk & Society, 2000	1997	USA	risk percpetion	1 to 4	2
pesticides	Satterfield, Mertz, Slovic	Risk Analysis, 2004	1997/1998	USA	risk perception	1 to 4	2
pesticides residues	Williams, Hammitt	Risk Analysis, 2001	1998	USA	risk to safety	1 to 5	3
pesticides in food	Knight, War-land	Rueal Sociology, 2005	1999	USA	conccern about food risk	1 to 4	2
pesticide in food	Krewski et al.	Human and Ecological Risk Assessment, 2006	2004	Canada	risk perception	1 to 4	2

pesticides/ insectici-des	Federal Re-search Center for Nutrition and Food	www.was-esse-ich.de	2005/2006	Germany	risk perception	1 to 2;1=risk to safety; 2= no risk to safety	3
pesticides	Riechard, Peterson	Journal of Environmental Education, 1998	n.i.	USA	risk perception	1 to 6	2
pesticides	Eiser, Coulson, Eiser	Journal of Risk Research, 1998	n.i.	UK	combined attitude factor	1 to 5 (1=strongly agree; 5=strongly disagree)	3
pesticides in food	Pilisuk, Parks, Hawkes	The Social Science Journal, 1987	n.i.	USA	very concerned to completely unconcerned	1 to 4	2a
Genetic modifica-tion in food							

genetically engineered strawberries	Schütz, Wiedemann	Risk Analysis, 1998	1993/1994	Germany	risk perception	1 to 7	2a
gen food	Kirk, Greenwood, Cade, Pearman	Appetite, 2002	1998/1999	UK	worry about potential risk	1 to 5	2
gen food	Huang, Qui, Bai, Pray	Appetite, 2006	2002/2003	Urban China	attitude towards specific GM foods		3
gentechnoloy for food production	Marlier	Eurobarometer 39.1, 1993	1993	Europe	risk to human health and environment	+2 (definitly agree)to '-2 (definitily disagree)	3
gentechnology for food production	Sparks, Shepherd, Frewer	Agricultural and Human Values, 1994	1994	UK	magnitude of risks	1 to 7	3

recombinant bovine growth hormone (rgBH)	Grobe, Douthitt, Zepeda	Risk Analysis, 1999	1995	USA	concern about consuming milk from rbGH treated herds	0 to 3	2
gen food	Moerbeek, Casimir	International Journal of Consumer Studies, 2005	1996	Europe, Eurobarometer 1996	acceptance of GM food		2
Genetically engineered crops	Finucane et al.	Health Risk & Society, 2000	1997	USA	risk perception	1 to 4	2
GM food	Siegrist	Journal of Risk Research, 2003	1997	Switzerland	importance that food is not genetically modified	1 to 5	2a
GM food	Cook, Kerr, Morre	Journal of Economic Psychology, 2002	1999	Newsealand	attitutde towards purchasing GM food	1 to 5	2a

gen food	Böcker	Hauswirtschaft und Wissenschaft, 2003	2000	Germany	worry about food risks	1 to 5	3
gentech-nology for meat produc-tion	Magnusson, Hursti	Appetite, 2002	2000	Sweden	risk perception	1 to 6	2
gen food	Moerbeek, Casimir	International Journal of Consumer Studies, 2005	2002	Europe, Euro barome-ter 2002	acceptance of GM food		2
gen food	Raude, Fisch-ler, Setbon, Flahault	Journal of Risk Research, 2005	2002	France	worry about risks	1 to 21	2
meat from animals feed with GM food	Onyango, Nayga, Schil-ling	AgBioForum, 2004	2003	USA	willingness to consume	0 to 1	2
GM food	Onyango et al.	Paper at Northeast Agricultural and Resource Economics Association/ Canadian Agricultural Eco-nomics Society Meeting	2003	South Corea	acceptance of GM food		3

gen food	Poortinga	Journal of Risk Reseaerch, 2005	2003	Great Britain	gen food acceptability	1 to 5 (1=very unaccepta-ble; 5= very acceptable) & 1 to 5 (1=risks>benefits; 5=benefits>risks)	2
gen food	Krewski et al.	Human and Ecological Risk Assessment, 2006	2004	Canada	risk perception	1 to 4	2
genetically modified salmon	Qin, Brown	Public Understanding of Science, 2007	2004	USA	attitude towards genetically engineered salmon	-3 to +3 (from strongly disapprove to strongly approve)	2
fibre-enriched potatoes that might	Christoph, Bruhn, Roosen	Appetite, 2006	2005	Germany	acceptance of GM food	yes or no	3

prevent colon cancer (GM)							
GM food	Leikas, Lindeman, Roininen, Lähteenmäki	Appetite, 2007	2005	Finnland	scariness of the risk	1 to 7	2a
gen food	Costa-Font, Mossialos	Food Quality and Prederence, 2007	2007	UK	risk percpetion	1 to 4 (1=strongly agree that it is risky; 4= strongly disagree that it is risky)	2
GM rice	Steur, Gellynck, Storozhenko, Liqun, Lambert, Van Der Straeten, Viaene	Appetite, 2009	2008	Shanxi Province, China	safety of GM rice	1 to 5	2
opposition towards GM food	Federal Research Center for Nutrition and Food,	www.was-esse-ich.de	2008	Germany	risk perception	yes or no	3

	2008						
gen food	Subrahman-yan, Cheng	Jounral of Consumer Affa-irs, 2000	n.i.	Singapor	combined factor: atti-tudes and worries about genetically modified foods	1 to 6 (1=strongly disagree; 6= strongly agree)	2a
GM food	Saher, Linde-mann, Hursti	Appetite, 2006	n.i.	Finnland	attitude towards GM food	1 to 9	2
GM food	Lusk, Coble	American Journal of Agricultural Economics, 2005	n.i.	USA	acceptance to eat GM food	1 to 9	3a
Nano-technolo-gy							
nano outside packaging	Siegrist, Stampfli, Kastenholz, Keller	Appetite, 2007	2007	Switzer-land	risk perception	1 to 5	3a

nano inside food	Siegrist, Stampfli, Kastenholz, Keller	Appetite, 2007	2007	Switzer-land	risk perception	1 to 5	3a
nano packaging	Zimmer, Her-tel, Böl	BfR Wissenschaft, 2008	2007	Germany	acceptance of nanotechnolo-gy products	1 to 4 (1= completely approve; 4= completely disapprove)	2
nano food	Zimmer, Her-tel, Böl	BfR Wissenschaft, 2008	2007	Germany	acceptance of nanotechnolo-gy products	1 to 4 (1= completely approve; 4= completely disapprove)	2
nano packaging	Vandermoere et al., 2009	Public Understanding of Science, 2009	2008	France	likelihood of being supportive of product	0/1	2
nano food	Vandermoere et al., 2010	Public Understanding of Science, 2010	2009	France	likelihood of being supportive of product	0/1	3
nano outside	Siegrist, Stampfli,	Appetite, 2008	n.i.	Switzer-land	benefit percep-tion	1 to 5	2

packaging	Kastenholz, Keller						
nano inside food	Siegrist, Stampfli, Kastenholz, Keller	Appetite, 2008	n.i.	Switzer-land	benefit percep-tion	1 to 5	2
Irradiati-on							
food irradiation	Nayga	Journal of Agricultural and Applied Economics, 1994	1991	USA	likelihood to purchase the product	0/1	2
food irradiation	Worsley, Scott	Asia Pacific Journal of Clinical Nutrition, 2000	1991	Australia	concern about food risk	n.i.	2
food irradiation	Flynn, Slovic, Mertz	Risk Analysis, 1994	1992/1993	USA	risk perception	1 to 4	2
food irradiation	He, Fletcher, Rimal	Journal of Food Distribution Research, 2005	1997/1998	USA	desirability of beef irradiation	1 to 5	4
Bacteria and							

mycoto-xins							
bacterial food contami-nation	Worsley, Scott	Asia Pacific Journal of Clinical Nutrition, 2000	1991	Australia	concern about food risk	n.i.	3
bacteria in food	Flynn, Slovic, Mertz	Risk Analysis, 1994	1992/1993	USA	risk perception	1 to 4	2
bacteria in food	McIntosh, Acuff, Chis-tensen	The Social Science Journal, 1994	1994	USA	awareness of danger	1 to 2 2=yes, 1=no	2
bacteria in food	Dosman, Adamowicz, Hrudey	Risk Analysis, 2001	1994	Canada	health risk perception	0 to 3	2
bacteria in food	Dosman, Adamowicz, Hrudey	Risk Analysis, 2001	1995	Canada	health risk perception	1 to 3	2
food poisson-ing	Redmond, Griffith	Appetite, 2004	1997	UK	perception of personal risk	1 to 10	4
bacteria, mycoto-xins	Williams, Hammitt	Risk Analysis, 2001	1998	USA	risk to safety	1 to 5	1

Salmonella	Knight, Warland	Rural Sociology, 2005	1999	USA	conccern about food risk	1 to 4	2
salmonella	Kirk, Greenwood, Cade, Pearman	Appetite, 2002	1998/1999	UK	worry about potential risk	1 to 5	3
listeria	Böcker	Hauswirtschaft und Wissenschaft, 2003	2000	Germany	worry about food risks	1 to 5	2
salmonella	Böcker	Hauswirtschaft und Wissenschaft, 2003	2000	Germany	worry about food risks	1 to 5	3
EHEC bacteria	Leikas, Lindeman, Roininen, Lähteenmäki	Appetite, 2007	2005	Finnland	scariness of the risk	1 to 7	2a
spoilt food	Federal Research Center for Nutrition and Food	www.was-esse-ich.de	2005/2006	Germany	risk perception	1 to 2;1=risk to safety; 2= no risk to safety	3
natural toxins	Federal Research Center for Nutrition	www.was-esse-ich.de	2005/2006	Germany	risk perception	2 to 2; 1=risk to safety; 2= no risk to	3

	and Food					safety	
mycoto-xins	Federal Re-search Center for Nutrition and Food	www.was-esse-ich.de	2005/2006	Germany	risk perception	3 to 2;1=risk to safety; 2= no risk to safety	3
bacterial food contami-nation	Buchler, Smith, Law-rence	Journal of Sociology, 2010	n.i.	Australia	risk percpetion	1 to 7	3
Food additives/ Contaminants							
artificial sweete-ners	Schütz, Wie-demann	Risk Analysis, 1998	1993/1994	Germany	risk perception	1 to 7	2a
food additives	Worsley, Scott	Asia Pacific Journal of Clinical Nutrition, 2000	1991	Newse-aland, Australia	concern about food risk	n.i.	2
food additives	Dosman, Adamowicz, Hrudey	Risk Analysis, 2001	1994	Canada	health risk perception	0 to 3	2
food additives	Dosman, Adamowicz,	Risk Analysis, 2001	1995	Canada	health risk perception	0 to 3	2

	Hrudey						
dioxin	Leikas, Lin-deman, Roini-nen, Lähteen-mäki	Appetite, 2007	2005	Finnland	scariness of the risk	1 to 7	2
vegetable sterols	Leikas, Lin-deman, Roini-nen, Lähteen-mäki	Appetite, 2007	2005	Finnland	scariness of the risk	1to 7	2
food colouring	Eiser, Coulson, Eiser	Journal of Risk Research, 1998	n.i.	UK	combined attitude factor	1 to 5 (1=strongly agree; 5=strongly disagree)	3
food additives and - preserva-tives	Riechard, Peterson	Journal of Environmental Education, 1998	n.i.	USA	risk percpetion	1 to 6	2

preserva-tives in food products	Pilisuk, Parks, Hawkes	The Social Science Journal, 1987	n.i.	USA	very concerned to completely unconcerned	1 to 4	2a
food additives	Buchler, Smith, Law-rence	Journal of Sociology, 2010	n.i.	Australia	concern about food risk	1 to 7	2
contami-nated drinking water	Pilisuk, Parks, Hawkes	The Social Science Journal, 1987	n.i.	USA	concern about food risk	1 to 4 con-cerned to completely unconcerned	2a
Hormo-nes/ antibio-tics							
hormones	Nayga	Journal of Agricultural and Applied Economics, 1994	1991	USA	likelihood to purchase	n.i.	2
antiobio-tics	Nayga	Journal of Agricultural and Applied Economics, 1994	1991	USA	likelihood to purchase	n.i.	2
hormones/ antibiotics	Finucane et al.	Health Risk & Society, 2000	1997	USA	risk percpetion	1 to 4	2

growth hormones	Kirk, Greenwood, Cade, Pearman	Appetite, 2002	1998/99	UK	worry about potential risk	1 to 5	2
BSE							
BSE	Harvey, Erdos, Callinger	Health, Risk and Society, 2001	1996-1999 (three periods)	England	attitude and reaction to BSE crisis	1 to 6	2
BSE	Finucane et al.	Health Risk & Society, 2000	1997	USA	risk percpetion	1 to 4	3
BSE	Kirk, Greenwood, Cade, Pearman	Appetite, 2002	1998/99	UK	worry about potential risk	1 to 5	2
BSE	Böcker	Hauswirtschaft und Wissenschaft, 2003	2000	Germany	worry about food risks	1 to 5	3a
BSE	Weikunat et al.	Journal of Health Psychology, 2003	2001	Germany	perceived threat from BSE	1 to 5	2
BSE	Setbon et al.	Risk Analysis, 2005	2001/2002	France	worry about the mad cow disease	1 to 4	2

BSE	Leikas, Lindeman, Roininen, Lähteenmäki	Appetite, 2007	2005	Finnland	scariness of the risk	1 to 7	2a
Unhealthy diet							
fatty food	Worsley, Scott	Asia Pacific Journal of Clinical Nutrition, 2000	1991	Newsealand, Australia	concern about food risk	n.i.	2
cardiovascular diseases due to diet	Worsley, Scott	Asia Pacific Journal of Clinical Nutrition, 2000	1991	Newsealand, Australia	concern about food risk	n.i.	2
alcohol consumption	Flynn, Slovic, Mertz	Risk Analysis, 1994	1992/1993	USA	risk perception	1 to 4	2
fatty meat	Goldberg, Strycker	Personality and Individual Differences, 2002	1993	USA	avoidance of fatty meat	1 to 5	2
eating fatty foods	Finucane et al.	Health Risk & Society, 2000	1997	USA	risk percpetion	1 to 4	2
saturated fats	Kirk, Greenwood, Cade,	Appetite, 2002	1998/1999	UK	worry about potential risk	1 to 5	2

	Pearman						
fatty food	Knight, Warland	Journal of Consumer Affairs, 2004	1999	USA	concern about food risk	1 to 4	2
natritional balance of diet	Miles, Brennan, Kuznesof, Ness, Ritson, Frewer	British Food Journal , 2004	2000	UK	worry about the safety of food	1 to 5	2
cardio-vascular dieseases due to diet	Leikas, Lindeman, Roininen, Lähteenmäki	Appetite, 2007	2005	Finnland	scariness of the risk	1 to 7	3
lack of ascorbin acid	Federal Research Center for Nutrition and Food	www.was-esse-ich.de	2005/2006	Germany	risk perception	1 to 2;1=risk to safety; 2= no risk to safety	3
lack of food variety and excessive	Federal Research Center for Nutrition and Food	www.was-esse-ich.de	2005/2006	Germany	risk perception	1 to 2;1=risk to safety; 2= no risk to safety	3

eating							
cho-lersterol	Federal Research Center for Nutrition and Food	www.was-esse-ich.de	2005/2006	Germany	risk perception	1 to 2;1=risk to safety; 2= no risk to safety	3
alcohol	Federal Research Center for Nutrition and Food	www.was-esse-ich.de	2005/2006	Germany	risk perception	1 to 2;1=risk to safety; 2= no risk to safety	3
obesity	Rozin, Fischler, Imada, Sarubin, Wresniewski	Appetite, 1999	n.i.	USA, Belgium, Japan, France	woory about weight		2
Food safety in general or combined factors							
technical food risks	Roosen, Thiele, Hansen	Acta Scandinavia, 2005	1992-2003	Germany	likelihood of being concerned about technical food risks	0/1	3

natural food risks	Roosen, Thie-le, Hansen	Acta Scandinavia, 2005	1992-2002	Germany	likelihood of being concerned about natural food risks	0/1	2
natural food risks (several com-bined)	Siegrist	Journal of Risk Research, 2003	1997	Switzer-land	risk perception	1 to 4	2
techno-logical food risks (several com-bined)	Siegrist	Journal of Risk Research, 2003	1997	Switzer-land	risk perception	1 to 4	2
con-fidence in food	Berg	Appetite, 2004	1999	Belgium, Great Britain, Norway	confindence in food	1 to 5	3

techno-logical food risks (com-bined factors)	Miles, Bren-nan, Kuznesof, Ness, Ritson, Frewer	British Food Journal, 2004	2000	UK	worry about the safety of food	1 to 5	2
natural food risks (com-bined factors)	Miles, Bren-nan, Kuznesof, Ness, Ritson, Frewer	British Food Journal, 2004	2000	UK	worry about the safety of food	1 to 5	2
food safety	de Jonge, Frewer, Trijp, Renes, de Wit, Timmers	British Food Journal, 2004	2002	Dane-mark	worry about the safety of food products	1 to 5	2a
techno-logical food risks (GM, hormones and irra-diation)	Hwang, Roe, Teisl	AgBioforum, 2005	2002	USA	concern about food technolo-gies	1 to 5	2
techno-logical food risks (artifical	Hwang, Roe, Teisl	AgBioforum, 2005	2002	USA	concern about food technolo-gies	1 to 5	3

colours, pasteurization, preservatives combined)							
technological food risks (pesticides and antibiotics combined)	Hwang, Roe, Teisl	AgBioforum, 2006	2002	USA	concern about food technologies	1 to 5	4
food safety	Baker	International Food and Agribusiness Management Review, 2003	2003	USA	reduction of consumption	n.i.	2
confidence in food	De Jonge, Van Trip, Renes, Frewer	Risk Analysis, 2007	2004	Belgium	pessimsm and opptimism about safety of	n.i.	3

safety					food		
mix of 14 different food risks consid-ered as mean risk perception	Hohl, Gaskell	Risk Analysis, 2008	2005	Europe	risk perception	1 to 4	2
food safety	De Jonge, Trijp, God-dard, Frewer	Food Quality and Prefe-rence, 2008	2005/2006	Nether-lands, Canada	level of worry about the safety of food	1 to 3	3

[1]Group 1= women perceive risks as much higher compared to men; Group 2= women perceive risks as higher compared to men; Group 2a= women perceive risks as higher compared to men, according to significance level, but no effect size indicated; Group 3= no gender differences or very small; Group 3a=gender differences, but not significant; Group 4=men perceive risks as higher compared to women; Group 4a= men perceive risks as higher compared to women, according to significance level, but no effect size indicated; Group 5= men perceive risks as much higher compared to women;

Appendix B 1: List of Instrumental and Terminal Values According to Rokeach

Instrumental Values	Terminal Values
Ambitious	A comfortable life
Broadminded	An exciting life
Capable	A sense of accomplishment
Cheerful	A world of peace
Clean	A world of beauty
Courageous	Equality
Forgiving	Family security
Helpful	Freedom
Honest	Happiness
Imaginative	Inner harmony
Independent	Mature love
Intellectual	National Security
Logical	Pleasure
Loving	Salvation
Obedient	Self respect
Polite	Social recognition
Responsible	True friendship
Self-controlled	Wisdom

Source: Rokeach (1973): 28

Appendix C: Interview Guide, Questionnaires, Consent

Appendix C 1: Interview Guide

A short version of the interview guide is presented below, followed by a detailed version in German.

- **A) General explanations and consent**
- **B) Introduction**
- **C) Entry questionnaire**
- **D) Product evaluations and attribute elicitation**
- **E) Sorting of elicited attributes**
- **F) Laddering interviews**
- **G) Exit questionnaire**
- **H) Disbursement of incentive**

A) Allgemeine Erklärungen & Einwilligung

B) Einführung

1. Bemühe Dich eine angenehme Interviewatmosphäre herzustellen. Stelle der/dem Befragten das Interview vor. Das Interview beginnt mit einem Fragebogen, dann kommt das eigentliche Interview und endet wieder mit einem kurzen Fragebogen.

Warne vor der eigenwilligen Form des Interviews.

Erkläre, dass die Art des Interviews an einem Beispiel geübt wird.

2. Beispiel: *Bitte stellen Sie sich vor, Sie wollen ein Auto kaufen. Was wäre Ihnen dabei wichtig. Auf was würden Sie achten?*

Nennungen:

Warum ist Ihnen „xy“ wichtig? Warum noch?

Warum ist das wichtig? Etc.

Ich interessiere mich dafür, was Sie über verschiedene Lebensmittel denken. Es gibt keine richtigen oder falschen Antworten; uns interessiert nur, was Sie über die Produkte denken.

C) Eingangsfragebogen (I)

Gewürzkräuter

*Im Folgenden sind verschiedene Gewürze (italienische Kräuter) abgebildet. Bitte stellen Sie sich vor, Sie sind bei **Ihrem Lebensmitteleinkauf im Supermarkt** und wollen **italienische Gewürzkräuter (getrocknet, im Glas)** kaufen. Sie haben folgende Gewürzkräuter zur Auswahl: (Produkte auf Kärtchen)*

***Bitte ordnen Sie diese nach Ihrer Kaufwahrscheinlichkeit.** Stellen Sie das Produkt, das Sie am wahrscheinlichsten kaufen würden auf Platz 1, das Produkt, das Sie dann kaufen würden, wenn Ihr bevorzugtes Produkt nicht verfügbar ist, auf Platz 2 usw.*

***Bitte beachten** Sie dabei, dass die Gewürze in **Geschmack, Preis und Gewicht identisch** sind.* Sie unterscheiden sich lediglich in den neben den Produkten stehenden Kriterien. (Darauf hinweisen, dass diese Informationen nicht auf den Produkten stehen, sondern die Teilnehmer/innen das aus anderer Quelle wissen).

Teilnehmer/in legt Karten auf Seite im Eingangsfragebogen

Interviewerin schreibt Produktbuchstaben neben das Ranking!

D) Produktbewertung & Elizitierung der Eigenschaften

➔ Weiter mit Eingangsfragebogen (Assoziationen, Risiko- und Nutzenbewertung je Produkt)

Wenn alle Fragen zu Assoziationen, Risiko- und Nutzenbewertung ausgefüllt sind (**von allen Gewürzen**!), werden Merkmale/Attribute erhoben (außer für Gewürz D-das ist das Referenzprodukt, das wir nur für das Ranking und die Nutzen/Risikobewertung benötigen)

! Fragebogen nicht zurückblättern lassen!

Gewürz A

Interviewerin notiert Nennungen von Fragebogen auf **Blatt I Gewürz A**

Interviewerin stellt folgende Fragen:

Was ziehen Sie in Betracht, wenn sie das Risiko dieses Produktes bewerten?

An was denken Sie, wenn Sie das Risiko dieses Produktes bewerten? (oder an was haben Sie dabei gedacht?)

Warum bewerten Sie das Risiko dieses Produktes mit „ "?

Interviewerin notiert Nennungen auf **Blatt I Gewürz A _Risiko"**

Was ziehen Sie in Betracht, wenn Sie den Nutzen dieses Produktes bewerten?

An was denken Sie dabei? (oder an was haben Sie dabei gedacht)

Warum bewerten Sie den Nutzen dieses Produktes mit „ "?

Interviewerin notiert Nennungen auf Blatt I **„Gewürz A _Nutzen"**

Gewürz B & C

Gleiches Verfahren mit Gewürz B&C! **Nicht Gewürz D!**

! Wirklich versuchen alle Attribute zu elizitieren! *(„Ist sonst noch was wichtig?")*

! Den Teilnehmer/innen wird der Fragebogen zu den Soziodemographika ausgehändigt (Fragebogen II)

E) Attributsortierung & Ranking nach Wichtigkeit

Attributsortierung

Interviewerin schreibt Attribute auf Blatt „". Es ist sehr wahrscheinlich, dass sich die Nennungen auf die LM-Risiken beziehen (Schimmelpilzgifte, Bestrahlung, Pestizide).

Interviewerin sortiert Nennungen nun zu den LM-Risiken (am besten daneben auch schreiben, ob Nennungen sich auf „Keine xy" bezieht oder auf „enthält xy" bezieht. Das geht zwar aus den einzelnen Produktbewertungen und deren Begründung hervor, erleichtert aber das Interview nachher.

Interviewerin bezieht auch die Nennungen, die unter der Frage nach Assoziationen/Gedanken/Gefühle geschrieben wurden mit ein. (ev. nachfragen, was genau diese Assoziation ausgelöst hat)

Ranking nach Wichtigkeit

Interviewerin bittet die Teilnehmer/in die Nennungen nach Wichtigkeit für die Nutzen und Risikobewertung zu sortieren.--> Interviewerin schreibt Ziffern zum Ranking daneben.

Wenn sie an Ihre Bewertung der Risiken und Nutzen der Produkte denken, was ist Ihnen davon persönlich am wichtigsten? Ordnen Sie diese bitte der Wichtigkeit nach in absteigender Reihenfolge.

Bei der Sortierung der Attribute nach LM-Risiko und Wichtigkeit kann man gut nochmal nachfragen, was mit manchen Aussagen gemeint ist.....

Ranking für jedes LM-Risiko einzeln machen!!!

(Interviewerin kann die drei wichtigsten Attribute je LM-Risiko farbig markieren→ diese werden im Anschluss „geleitert")

Die Elizitierung der Eigenschaften ist ein sehr sensibler Punkt im Leiterinterview! Also bereits an dieser Stelle bei Unklarheiten nachfragen. Z.B.: Der Teilnehmer sagt so was wie „Was soll das?" Dann kann man nachfragen: „ Was meinen Sie damit?"

Teilnehmer/in antwortet dann vielleicht: „ *Was soll das mit der Bestrahlung*? *Für was ist die Bestrahlung gut"?*

F) Laddering

Je LM-Risiko werden die 3 wichtigsten **Attribute** geleitert. → DIN A 3 Bögen

Fragemöglichkeiten:

1) *Warum ist das wichtig/ für Sie?*
2) *Warum haben Sie (gerade) das erwähnt?*
3) *Warum wollen Sie Produkte mit einer solchen Eigenschaft vermeiden?*
4) *Warum beunruhigt/besorgt Sie das?*
5) *Was glauben Sie, warum haben Sie daran gedacht?*

6) *Warum glauben Sie müssen/sollen sich andere Leute Sorgen/Gedanken darüber machen?*
7) *Was bedeutet das für Sie?*
8) *Was für Gefühle weckt das bei Ihnen?*
9) *Was wäre, wenn diese Eigenschaft (oder Konsequenz) fehlen würde?*

Erklärungen zu den Frageweisen und Interviewereffekte: Siehe Dokument „Intervieweffekte“

G) Ausgangsfragebogen

H) Geldauszahlung & Quittung unterschreiben lassen

Appendix C 2: Entry Questionnaire

Sehr geehrte Studienteilnehmer/innen!

Vielen Dank dafür, dass Sie an unserer Studie teilnehmen!

Diese Studie wird vom Lehrstuhl für BWL der Technischen Universität München durchgeführt. Bitte lesen Sie die jeweilige Frage genau durch, bevor Sie diese beantworten. Es gibt keine „falschen“ oder „richtigen“ Antworten. Bitte äußern Sie Ihre ehrliche Meinung!

1. Zu Beginn möchten wir gerne wissen, wer in Ihrem Haushalt für den Lebensmitteleinkauf zuständig ist.

☐ Überwiegend kaufe ich die Lebensmittel

☐ Überwiegend kauft eine andere Person im Haushalt die Lebensmittel

☐ Eine andere Person und ich sind gleichermaßen für den Lebensmitteleinkauf zuständig.

2. Produktranking

	Produkt___

	Produkt___

	Produkt___

	Produkt___

Wir möchten nun gerne wissen, was Sie über die Ihnen vorgestellten Lebensmittelprodukte denken und wie Sie diese Produkte bewerten.

Bitte beantworten Sie die unter den jeweiligen Produkten stehenden Fragen.

Bitte beachten Sie weiterhin, dass sich die verschiedenen Gewürzkräuter in Geschmack, Preis und Gewicht **nicht unterscheiden**. Sie unterscheiden sich lediglich in den neben den Produkten stehenden Kriterien.

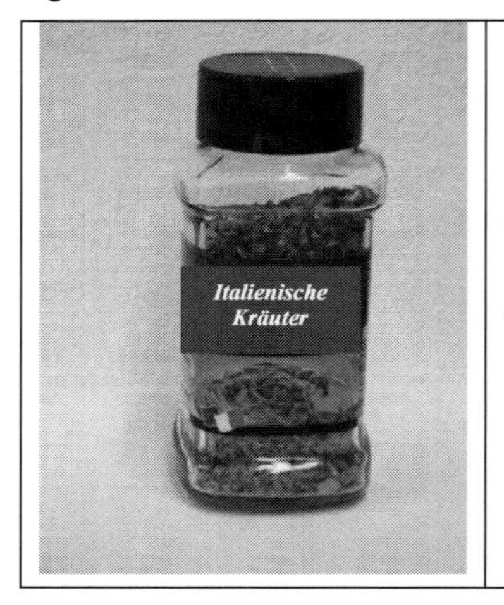

A

- Herkömmliche Herstellung
- **Kann** Schimmelpilzgifte enthalten
- **Frei von** Pestiziden

3a. Welche spontanen **Assoziationen/Gedanken/Gefühle** weckt dieses Produkt bei Ihnen? Bitte schreiben Sie diese auf:

____

____

3b. Dieses Produkt löst ein ______ Gefühl bei mir aus:

1 sehr schlechtes Gefühl	2	3	4	5 sehr gutes Gefühl

3c. Bitte beantworten sie inwiefern folgende Aussagen auf Sie zutreffen:

1 bedeutet, dass die Aussage **überhaupt nicht zutrifft** &

5 bedeutet, dass die Aussage **sehr zutreffend** ist.

Dieses Produkt löst ein zufriedenes Gefühl in mir aus	1	2	3	4	5
Dieses Produkt irritiert mich.	1	2	3	4	5
Dieses Produkt macht mich besorgt.	1	2	3	4	5
Dieses Produkt macht mich ärgerlich.	1	2	3	4	5
Dieses Produkt macht mich nervös	1	2	3	4	5
Dieses Produkt löst ein erfülltes Gefühl in mir aus.	1	2	3	4	5
Dieses Produkt frustriert mich.	1	2	3	4	5
Dieses Produkt löst Anspannung in mir aus.	1	2	3	4	5

3d.Wie würden Sie bei regelmäßigem Konsum dieser Gewürzkräuter das Risiko dieses Produktes bewerten? Bitte kreuzen Sie betreffendes an:

Überhaupt nicht risikoreich 1	2	3	4	**sehr risikoreich** 5

3e.Wie würden Sie bei regelmäßigem Konsum dieser Gewürzkräuter den Nutzen dieses Produktes bewerten? Bitte kreuzen Sie betreffendes an:

Überhaupt nicht nützlich 1	2	3	4	**sehr nützlich** 5

<table>
<tr>
<td>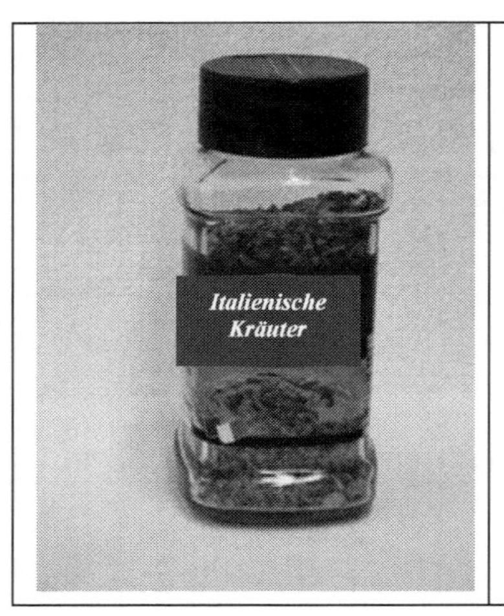
</td>
<td>B

• Herkömmliche Herstellung
• **Frei von** Schimmelpilzgiften
• **Kann** Pestizide **enthalten**</td>
</tr>
</table>

4a. Welche spontanen **Assoziationen/Gedanken/Gefühle** weckt dieses Produkt bei Ihnen? Bitte schreiben Sie diese auf:

____

____

4b. Dieses Produkt löst ein ______ Gefühl bei mir aus:

1 sehr schlechtes Gefühl	2	3	4	5 sehr gutes Gefühl

4c. Bitte beantworten sie inwiefern folgende Aussagen auf Sie zutreffen:

1 bedeutet, dass die Aussage **überhaupt nicht zutrifft** &

5 bedeutet, dass die Aussage **sehr zutreffend** ist.

Dieses Produkt löst ein zufriedenes Gefühl in mir aus	1	2	3	4	5

Dieses Produkt irritiert mich.	1	2	3	4	5
Dieses Produkt macht mich besorgt.	1	2	3	4	5
Dieses Produkt macht mich ärgerlich.	1	2	3	4	5
Dieses Produkt macht mich nervös	1	2	3	4	5
Dieses Produkt löst ein erfülltes Gefühl in mir aus.	1	2	3	4	5
Dieses Produkt frustriert mich.	1	2	3	4	5
Dieses Produkt löst Anspannung in mir aus.	1	2	3	4	5

4d. Wie würden Sie bei regelmäßigem Konsum dieser Gewürzkräuter das **Risiko** dieses Produktes bewerten? Bitte kreuzen Sie betreffendes an:

Überhaupt nicht risikoreich 1	2	3	4	**sehr risikoreich** 5

4e. Wie würden Sie bei regelmäßigem Konsum dieser Gewürzkräuter den **Nutzen** dieses Produktes bewerten? Bitte kreuzen Sie betreffendes an:

Überhaupt nicht nützlich 1	2	3	4	**sehr nützlich** 5

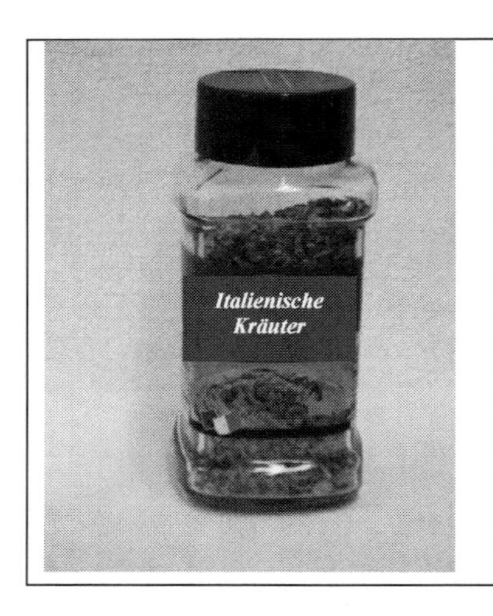	 • Bestrahlung • **Frei von** Schimmelpilzgiften • **Frei von** Pestiziden

5a. Welche spontanen **Assoziationen/Gedanken/Gefühle** weckt dieses Produkt bei Ihnen? Bitte schreiben Sie diese auf:

____

____

5b. Dieses Produkt löst ein ______ Gefühl bei mir aus:

1 sehr schlechtes Gefühl	2	3	4	5 sehr gutes Gefühl

5c. Bitte beantworten sie inwiefern folgende Aussagen auf Sie zutreffen:

1 bedeutet, dass die Aussage **überhaupt nicht zutrifft**

& **5** bedeutet, dass die Aussage **sehr zutreffend** ist.

Dieses Produkt löst ein zufriedenes Gefühl in mir aus	1	2	3	4	5
Dieses Produkt irritiert mich.	1	2	3	4	5

Dieses Produkt macht mich besorgt.	1	2	3	4	5
Dieses Produkt macht mich ärgerlich.	1	2	3	4	5
Dieses Produkt macht mich nervös	1	2	3	4	5
Dieses Produkt löst ein erfülltes Gefühl in mir aus.	1	2	3	4	5
Dieses Produkt frustriert mich.	1	2	3	4	5
Dieses Produkt löst Anspannung in mir aus.	1	2	3	4	5

5d. Wie würden Sie bei regelmäßigem Konsum dieser Gewürzkräuter das **Risiko** dieses Produktes bewerten? Bitte kreuzen Sie betreffendes an:

Überhaupt nicht risikoreich 1	2	3	4	**sehr risikoreich** 5

5e. Wie würden Sie bei regelmäßigem Konsum dieser Gewürzkräuter den **Nutzen** dieses Produktes bewerten? Bitte kreuzen Sie betreffendes an:

Überhaupt nicht nützlich 1	2	3	4	**sehr nützlich** 5

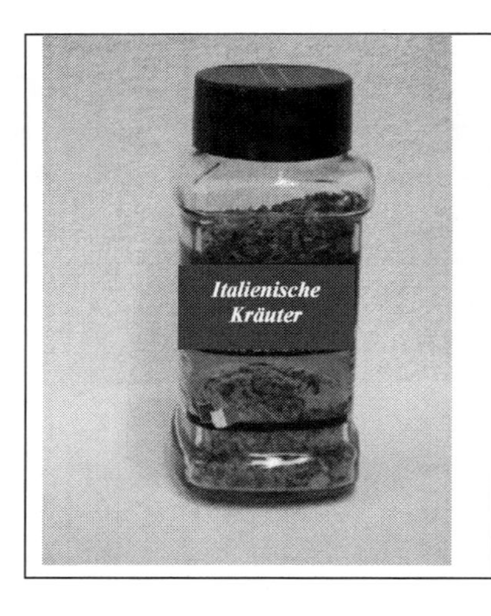 	 • Herkömmliche Herstellung • **Frei von** Schimmelpilzgiften • **Frei von** Pestiziden

6a. Welche spontanen **Assoziationen/Gedanken/Gefühle** weckt dieses Produkt bei Ihnen? Bitte schreiben Sie diese auf:

____

____

6b. Dieses Produkt löst ein ______ Gefühl bei mir aus:

1 sehr schlechtes Gefühl	2	3	4	5 sehr gutes Gefühl

6c. Bitte beantworten sie inwiefern folgende Aussagen auf Sie zutreffen:

1 bedeutet, dass die Aussage **überhaupt nicht zutrifft** &

5 bedeutet, dass die Aussage **sehr zutreffend** ist.

Dieses Produkt löst ein zufriedenes Gefühl in mir aus	1	2	3	4	5
Dieses Produkt irritiert mich.	1	2	3	4	5
Dieses Produkt macht mich besorgt.	1	2	3	4	5
Dieses Produkt macht mich ärgerlich.	1	2	3	4	5
Dieses Produkt macht mich nervös	1	2	3	4	5
Dieses Produkt löst ein erfülltes Gefühl in mir aus.	1	2	3	4	5
Dieses Produkt frustriert mich.	1	2	3	4	5
Dieses Produkt löst Anspannung in mir aus.	1	2	3	4	5

6d. Wie würden Sie bei regelmäßigem Konsum dieser Gewürzkräuter das **Risiko** dieses Produktes bewerten? Bitte kreuzen Sie betreffendes an:

Überhaupt nicht risikoreich 1	2	3	4	**sehr risikoreich** 5

6e. Wie würden Sie bei regelmäßigem Konsum dieser Gewürzkräuter den **Nutzen** dieses Produktes bewerten? Bitte kreuzen Sie betreffendes an:

Überhaupt nicht nützlich 1	2	3	4	**sehr nützlich** 5

Appendix C 3: Exit Questionniare

Um Ihre Angaben besser einordnen zu können, beantworten Sie bitte noch folgende Fragen.

7. Bitte tragen Sie Ihr Geschlecht ein

□ männlich

□ weiblich

08. Bitte geben Sie Ihr Geburtsjahr an

19___

9. Wie viele Personen leben ständig in Ihrem Haushalt, Sie selbst eingeschlossen?

____

10. Leben Kinder in Ihrem Haushalt?

□ Ja

□ Nein →weiter mit Frage 12

11. Wenn ja, wie viele Kinder leben in Ihrem Haushalt und wie alt sind sie?

Bitte kreuzen Sie die zutreffende(n) Antwort(en) an und tragen die entsprechende Anzahl ein.

Anzahl:

□ 0 - 2 Jahre _________

□ 2 - 6 Jahre ________

□ 7 - 12 Jahre ________

□ älter als 12 Jahre ________

12. Was ist Ihr höchster Bildungsabschluss?

☐ kein Abschluss

☐ Hauptschulabschluss (Volksschulabschluss)

☐ Realschulabschluss (Mittlere Reife)

☐ Allgemeine oder fachgebundene Hochschulreife (Abitur)

☐ Hochschulabschluss / Fachhochschulabschluss

☐ keine Angabe

13. Zu welcher Gruppe gehören Sie momentan?

☐ in der Ausbildung:

☐ Schüler/in, Lehrling

☐ Student/in

☐ Hausfrau/-mann

☐ Rentner/in, Pensionär/in, im Vorruhestand

☐ arbeitslos

☐ berufstätig:

  ☐ Vollzeit

  ☐ Teilzeit

☐ sonstiges und zwar:________________________________

☐ keine Angabe

14. Im Folgenden sind verschiedene Einkommensklassen angegeben. Bitte geben Sie an, welche der Einkommensklassen dem monatlichen Nettoeinkommen Ihres Haushaltes entspricht (einschließlich Verdienst, Kindergeld, andere Einkommensquellen).

1	Unter 600 Euros
2	600 bis 900 Euros
3	901 bis 1200 Euros
4	1201 bis 1500 Euros
5	1501 bis 2300 Euros
6	2301 bis 3000 Euros
7	3001 bis 6000 Euros
8	Über 6000 Euros
9	Ich weiß es nicht

15. Würden Sie sagen, dass es der Welt durch Entwicklungen in Wissenschaft und Technik schlechter oder besser geht?

1 bedeutet, dass es der Welt viel schlechter dadurch geht und 10 bedeutet, dass es der Welt dadurch viel besser geht.

Die Welt ist viel schle chter dran									**Die Welt ist viel besser dran**
1	2	3	4	5	6	7	8	9	10

16. Sind Sie oder jemand in Ihrem Bekanntenkreis in der Landwirtschaft oder anderweitig im Lebensmittel produzierenden Gewerbe tätig?

☐ Ja

☐ Nein

Wenn ja, als was?:__________________________________

17. Wie informiert fühlen Sie sich bezüglich Lebensmittelrisiken?
1 bedeutet, dass Sie sich sehr schlecht informiert fühlen und 10 bedeutet, dass Sie sich sehr gut informiert fühlen.

Sehr schlecht Infor-miert									**Sehr gut infor-miert**
1	2	3	4	5	6	7	8	9	10

18. **Woher erhalten** Sie Informationen bezüglich Lebensmittelrisiken?
*Bitte kreuzen Sie **eine oder mehrere** zutreffende Antworten an.*

☐ Direkt/mündlich (über einen Freund/Freundin, Verwandte/n; Bekannte/n; Kollegen/in)

☐ Über das Fernsehen

☐ Internet

☐ Zeitungen

☐ Sonstige:____________________

19. Zu welchem Anteil wählen Sie für Ihre tägliche Ernährung Lebensmittel aus, die Sie als gesund einstufen?

- ☐ Zu einem sehr großen Anteil
- ☐ Zu einem großen Anteil
- ☐ Zu einem durchschnittlichen Anteil
- ☐ Zu einem geringen Anteil
- ☐ Zu einem sehr geringen Anteil
- ☐ Ich weiß es nicht

20. Wie sicher sind Sie, dass die Lebensmittel, die Sie kaufen unbedenklich für Sie und Ihre Familie sind?

- ☐ Ich bin vollkommen sicher
- ☐ Ich bin sehr sicher
- ☐ Teils/teils sicher
- ☐ Eher nicht sicher
- ☐ Überhaupt nicht sicher
- ☐ Ich weiß es nicht

21. Wir möchten jetzt mehr über Ihren Konsum von Biolebensmittel wissen. Haben Sie während der letzten drei Monate Lebensmittel aus biologischem Anbau gegessen?

☐ Ja

☐ Nein → *weiter mit Frage 23*

22. Wenn ja, gemessen an Ihrem Gesamtverbrauch von Lebensmitteln, wie groß war Ihr Anteil an Biolebensmittel während der letzten drei Monate?

- ☐ Äußerst gering
- ☐ Gering
- ☐ Ungefähr die Hälfte
- ☐ Der Großteil
- ☐ 100% bzw. fast 100%
- ☐ Ich weiß es nicht

Bitte betrachten Sie nochmals die Ihnen bereits vorgestellten Produkte und beantworten Sie die darunter stehenden Fragen:

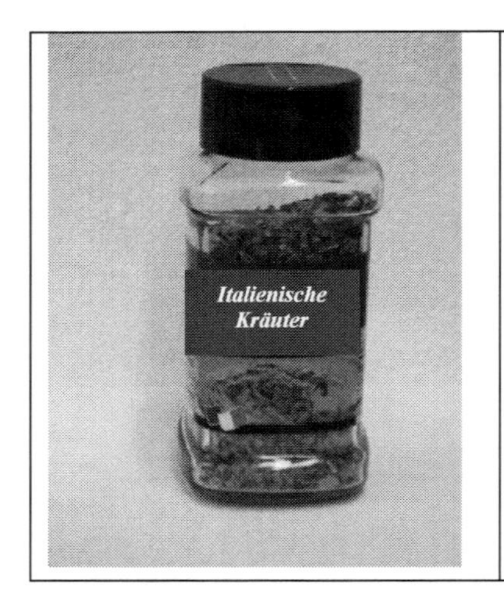

A

- Herkömmliche Herstellung
- **Kann** Schimmelpilzgifte enthalten
- **Frei von** Pestiziden

23a. Wie würden Sie bei regelmäßigem Konsum dieser Gewürzkräuter das **Risiko** dieses Produktes bewerten? Bitte kreuzen Sie betreffendes an:

Überhaupt nicht risikoreich 1	2	3	4	**sehr risikoreich** 5

23b. Wie würden Sie bei regelmäßigem Konsum dieser Gewürzkräuter den **Nutzen** dieses Produktes bewerten? Bitte kreuzen Sie betreffendes an:

Überhaupt nicht nützlich 1	2	3	4	**sehr nützlich** 5

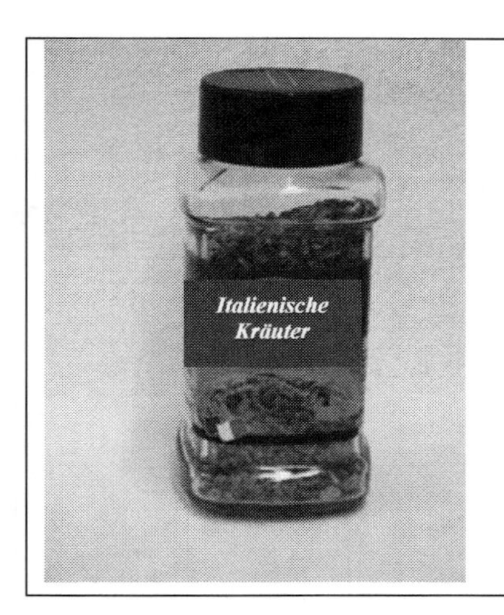 	**B** • Herkömmliche Herstellung • **Frei von** Schimmelpilzgiften • **Kann** Pestizide **enthalten**

24a. Wie würden Sie bei regelmäßigem Konsum dieser Gewürzkräuter das **Risiko** dieses Produktes bewerten? Bitte kreuzen Sie betreffendes an:

Überhaupt nicht risikoreich 1	2	3	4	**sehr risikoreich** 5

24b. Wie würden Sie bei regelmäßigem Konsum dieser Gewürzkräuter den **Nutzen** dieses Produktes bewerten? Bitte kreuzen Sie betreffendes an:

Überhaupt nicht nützlich 1	2	3	4	**sehr nützlich** 5

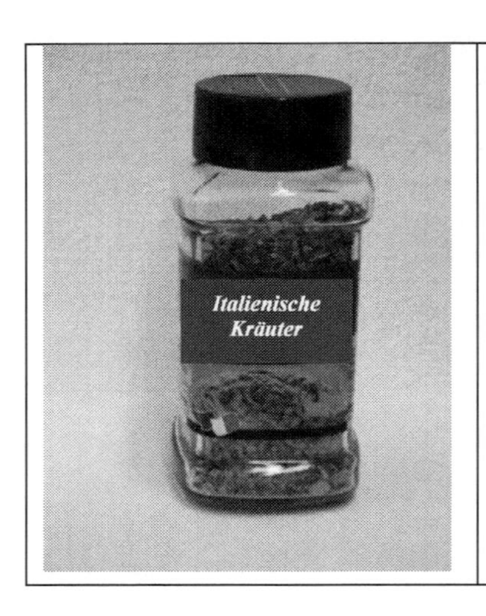	 • Bestrahlung • **Frei von** Schimmelpilzgiften • **Frei von** Pestiziden

25a. Wie würden Sie bei regelmäßigem Konsum dieser Gewürzkräuter das **Risiko** dieses Produktes bewerten? Bitte kreuzen Sie betreffendes an:

Überhaupt nicht risiko-reich 1	2	3	4	**sehr risiko-reich** 5

25b. Wie würden Sie bei regelmäßigem Konsum dieser Gewürzkräuter den **Nutzen** dieses Produktes bewerten? Bitte kreuzen Sie betreffendes an:

Überhaupt nicht nütz-lich 1	2	3	4	**sehr nütz-lich** 5

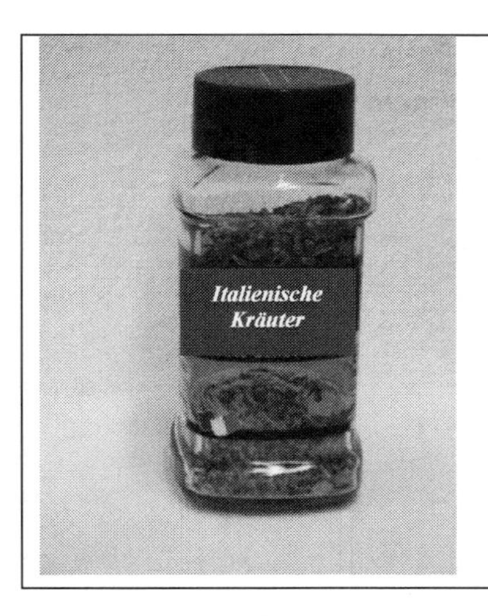 	**D** • Herkömmliche Herstellung • **Frei von** Schimmelpilzgiften • **Frei von** Pestiziden

26a. Wie würden Sie bei regelmäßigem Konsum dieser Gewürzkräuter das **Risiko** dieses Produktes bewerten? Bitte kreuzen Sie betreffendes an:

Überhaupt nicht risikoreich 1	2	3	4	**sehr risikoreich** 5

26b. Wie würden Sie bei regelmäßigem Konsum dieser Gewürzkräuter den **Nutzen** dieses Produktes bewerten? Bitte kreuzen Sie betreffendes an:

Überhaupt nicht nützlich 1	2	3	4	**sehr nützlich** 5

Vielen Dank für Ihre Zeit und Unterstützung

Appendix C4: Consent

Studie zum Thema „Lebensmittelwahl"

Allgemeine Informationen

Sie sind eingeladen, an einer Studie zum Thema „Lebensmittelwahl" teilzunehmen. Diese Studie wird vom Lehrstuhl für BWL – Marketing und Konsumforschung der Technischen Universität München durchgeführt. Der folgende Text beschreibt diese Studie kurz. Lesen Sie diesen bitte aufmerksam durch und zögern Sie nicht, uns Fragen zu stellen.

Während dieser Studie, werden wir Sie bitten, einige Fragen zu beantworten (per Fragebogen) und in einem Gespräch (Interview) werden Sie zu Ihrer Meinung bzgl. einiger Lebensmittel befragt. Dieses Gespräch wird auf Tonband aufgezeichnet.

Diese Befragung wird anonym ausgewertet und dient ausschließlich der wissenschaftlichen Analyse im Rahmen eines Projektes, das von der Deutschen Forschungsgemeinschaft gefördert wird.

Die Befragung dauert circa eine Stunde. Wenn Sie Fragen haben, können Sie diese jetzt gerne stellen.

Wenn alle Punkte geklärt sind, können Sie sich entscheiden, ob Sie an der Studie teilnehmen wollen. Wenn Sie sich dazu entscheiden teilzunehmen, lesen und unterschreiben Sie bitte die Einwilligungserklärung auf der nächsten Seite. Mit Ihrer Unterschrift geben Sie an, dass Sie verstanden haben, worum es in der Studie geht und bereit sind den Anweisungen, die Ihnen im Laufe der Studie gegeben werden zu folgen.

Einwilligungserklärung

Ich habe die allgemeinen Informationen auf der ersten Seite gelesen.

Hiermit nehme ich freiwillig an der Studie zum Thema „Lebensmittelwahl" teil. Im Rahmen dieser Studie werde ich einige Fragen beantworten und Informationen lesen.

Für meine Teilnahme an der Studie erhalte ich eine Aufwandsentschädigung von 15 €.

Ich wurde darüber informiert, dass alle Angaben anonym ausgewertet werden und alle Informationen bezüglich meiner Person vertraulich behandelt werden und unter keinen Umständen an Dritte weitergegeben werden.

Ich kann meine Teilnahme an dieser Studie zu jedem Zeitpunkt und ohne Angabe von Gründen abbrechen.

Name, Vorname:

____

Adresse:

____

Datum, Unterschrift:

____

Appendix D1: Frequency of the Order in which each Hazard was laddered

Order of hazards	Women N=32	Men N=35
Mycotoxins first	46.9%	45.7%
Mycotoxins second	28.1%	12.8%
Mycotoxins third	15.7%	22.8%
Pesticides first	25.1%	37.1%
Pesticides second	34.4%	45.7%
Pesticides third	37.5%	17.1%
Irradiation first	28.1%	17.1%
Irradiation second	28.2%	22.8%
Irradiation third	37.5%	51.4%

Appendix D2: Example of a Transcribed Interview with Keyword in Context and MS-Word Track Changes Function

First the original transcribed interview with respondent 22 is presented, followed by the same interview with keyword in context and MS-word track changes function. The arrows (→) indicate, that the interviewer asked the typical 'why is this important to you?' question or a similar question. Otherwise, the arrow (→) marks a further step in the cognition elicitation, that the respondent mentioned without the typicial 'why is this important to you?' probe.

'Meaning' in parentheses (*Meaning*) specifies the meaning of the statement, when interviewee's words might be arbitrary.

Numbers indicate the beginning of a ladder and letters (a, b) indicate that a ladder is split.

ID_22 (weiblich)

Reihenfolge: Pestizide, Schimmelpilzgifte, Bestrahlung

Pestizide

P. müssten erklärt werden→müsste wissen, was man sich darunter vorstellen soll→ wäre für Kaufentscheidung wichtig→wenn nix Schlechtes→ könnte ich es kaufen→ könnte dann entscheiden→ (*so*)reicht die Info nicht→so würde ich es nicht kaufen→ klingt ungesund

Klingt ungesund→gibt genug Umweltgifte

(1) → brauche ich nicht→ (möchte) so natürlich wie möglich →(Planze meine Tomaten auf Balkon)

(1a)→ nix drin, nix Gespritztes→da weiß ich genau was drin ist→ ich weiß ja nicht was die Bauern da draußen machen

(1b)→schmeckt nach nix→(*meaning*: Gemüse) gibt es das ganze Jahr aus Gewächshaus→ die spritzen, das es länger hält

→Geschmack ist wichtig→ viele LM schmecken nicht mehr→traurig→ (*meaning: man zahlt)* viel Geld und es schmeckt nicht

(2)krebs auslösend→auf Dauer andere Krankheiten→ich muss keine Krankheit vom Essen bekommen→möchte möglichst alt, aber gesund werden→ es ist schön auf der Welt

(3) (es ist) unnötig→zu viel Konsum→Verfügbarkeit jeden Tag→man freut sich nicht mehr richtig, weil man immer alles essen kann→ anderes Lebensgefühl

Klingt gesünder (frei von Pestiziden)→achte beim Essen auf Gesundheit→ für meine Gesundheit→habe eine leicht Herzkrankheit→ man kann Einiges ändern (*meaning: über Essen*)→ körperliches befinden kann man beeinflussen→Elan für den Tag→fühlt sich besser→ wenn man voll vom Essen ist, fühlt man sich nicht mehr wohl→ keine Trägheit

(*meaning: wenn man liest*) kann Pestizide enthalten→ negatives Gefühl, das ist auch eine Kopfsache: schlechtes Wohlbefinden im Kopf

Aufklärung ist sehr wichtig→ dann weiß ich was und wie, was das überhaupt ist→ Hersteller sollten das draufschreiben

Schimmelpilzgifte

Giftig→ nehme nicht freiwillig Gifte zu mir

(1) →Gesundheitsschäden auf Dauer→muss nicht noch zusätzlich sein→ muss auf Gesundheit achten→ weil ich eine angeschlagene Gesundheit habe→ das ist wie Dauergifteinnahme

(2)SPG in der Wohnung: geht auf die Lunge→ Nein, im Essen brauche ich die nicht auch noch

Ekel→ möchte ich nicht essen→ vergeht mir der Appetit→Ekel

Steht nicht drauf, ob auf Dauer gesundheitsschädlich ist→ brauche Gewürze regelmäßig→denke, dass auf Dauer Auswirkungen→ länger gesund belieben

(1)→ jeder sollte auf Gesundheit achten

(2) muss sowieso man Medikamente nehmen, haben Nebenwirkungen

Wenn es drauf steht→kann jeder selbst entscheiden→ möchte mich nicht einfach anschließen an alle anderen (*meaning: was alle anderen machen*)→muss schon drauf stehen-möchte keine Bedenken haben→ Sicherheit brauche ich→ möchte jeden Tag essen→ besser ganz ohne

Bestrahlung

Müsste drauf stehen→möchte wissen, wie bestrahlt

(1) Gute Bestrahlung

(1a)→ Keim tötend/Pilz tötend

(1a_1)→ wäre gut, dann(vielleicht) frei von Giftstoffen/Pestiziden→ eher natürlich→ frei von Giftstoffen

(1a_1a)→schmeckt wie's schmecken soll

(1a_1b)→ natürlich gewachsen, ohne Geschmacksverstärker

(1a_2)→ bin im Widerspruch: muss man erst spritzen und dann (deswegen) bestrahlen→ warum erst rein und dann wieder raus

(1b) schöne rote Tomaten→ wäre (aber) nicht toll→ lieber naturgewachsen→ haben dann keinen Geschmack mit Bestrahlung→ sollten nachdem schmecken, was ich esse→ sonst könnte ich ja irgendwas essen→ möchte kein künstliches Aussehen/Geschmack

(2) Schlechte Bestrahlung→ Röntgenstrahlen→ unnatürlich→ das Ding muss bestrahlt werden, dass es gut aussieht, oder gut schmeckt-Aufzucht mit künstlichem Licht

Bestrahlung macht Angst→(möchte) einkaufen ohne schlechte Gedanken→steht alles drauf→ muss nicht lange suche→ nicht überlegen was die da rein machen→ kann regelmäßig kaufen, ohne nachzulesen

(1) Wenn ich keine Brille mein Einkaufen dabei habe

(2) Gutes Gefühl→ kaufe nix Schlechtes→ kann Kochen in Ruhe, ohne gesundheitliche Bedenken→ Zufriedenheit

[Notiz: Teilnehmerin hatte Herzinfarkt→ seitdem achtet sie beim Essen ganz besonders auf ihre Gesundheit]

Gekürztes Interview_ID 22 mit Nachvollziehbarkeit der Änderungen Reihenfolge: Pestizide, Schimmelpilzgifte, Bestrahlung

Weiblich

Pestizide

1: Pestizide müssten erklärt werden; 2: klingt ungesund; 3: klingt gesünder (Frei von Pestiziden)

Leiter 1: **P. müssten erklärt werden**, müsste wissen, was man sich darunter vorstellen soll (~~aA~~fC: ~~unbekannt~~keine Information)→ wäre für Kaufentscheidung wichtig (→wenn nix Schlechtes→ könnte ich es kaufen→ könnte dann entscheiden pC: Entscheidungsfreiheit)~~(pC: wichtig für Kaufentscheidung)~~ (~~*so*)reicht die Info nicht→so würde ich es nicht kaufen (fC: Nicht Kauf)→ klingt ungesund~~**Ende Leiter 1**

Leiter 2: Klingt ungesund (**aA: schädlich**~~**aA: ungesund)**→gibt genug Umweltgifte~~

(1) ~~→~~brauche ich nicht (aA: ~~unnötig~~kein Nutzen)→(1) (2)

(1) (möchte) so natürlich wie möglich (~~fV~~pC: Natürlichkeit) ~~→(Planze meine Tomaten auf Balkon)~~

(1a)→ nix drin, nix Gespritztes→da weiß ich genau was drin ist (fC: ~~Wissen über Qualität)~~ausreichend Information? Gewissheit??)→ ich weiß ja nicht was die Bauern da draußen machen

(1b)→schmeckt nach nix→(fC: kein Geschmack)(*meaning*: Gemüse) gibt es das ganze Jahr aus Gewächshaus→ die spritzen, das es länger hält

→~~Geschmack ist wichtig(fV: Geschmack)→ viele LM schmecken nicht mehr→traurig→ (*meaning: man zahlt*) viel Geld und es schmeckt nicht~~

(2) zu viel Konsum, Verfügbarkeit jeden Tag (fC: Konsum)→man freut sich nicht mehr richtig, weil man immer alles essen kann (pC: keine Freude)→ anderes Lebensgefühl (tV: Lebensqualität)**Ende Leiter 2**

Leiter 3: ~~(2)~~**K~~k~~rebs auslösend**, auf Dauer andere Krankheiten, ungesund (fC:

negative gesundheitliche Folgen für Körper)→ich muss keine Krankheit vom Essen bekommen (ifV: Krank werden durch ErnährungGesundheit erhalten)→möchte möglichst alt, aber gesund werden (tfV: langes, gesundes Leben)→ es ist schön auf der Welt (tV: Lebensfreude ist schön)

(3) (es ist) unnötig→zu viel Konsum→Verfügbarkeit jeden Tag→man freut sich nicht mehr richtig, weil man immer alles essen kann→ anderes Lebensgefühl**Ende Leiter 3**

frei von Pestiziden

Leiter 4: **Klingt gesünder** (frei von Pestiziden)→achte beim Essen auf Gesundheit, körperliches Befinden kann man beeinflussen (ifV: achte auf Gesundheit erhalten)→

(1) für meine Gesundheit (tV. Gesundheit/Wohlbefinden)→habe eine leicht Herzkrankheit→ man kann Einiges ändern (*meaning: über Essen*)→ körperliches befinden kann man beeinflussen

→(2)Elan für den Tag, keine Trägheit (pC: Leistungsfähigkeit)→fühlt sich besser (fV: Wohlbefinden)→ wenn man voll vom Essen ist, fühlt man sich nicht mehr wohl→ keine **Trägheit****Ende Leiter 4**

Leiter 5: (*meaning: wenn man"... „liest*) kann Pestizide enthalten→ negatives Gefühl, das ist auch eine Kopfsache: schlechtes Wohlbefinden im Kopf (pC: Sorgen) **Ende Leiter 5**

Aufklärung ist sehr wichtig→ dann weiß ich was und wie, was das überhaupt ist→ Hersteller sollten das draufschreiben

Schimmelpilzgifte

Leiter 1:Gifte→ negativ; 2: würde ich nicht nehmen→ Ekel; 3: steht nicht drauf, ob auf Dauer gesundheitsschädlich

Leiter 1: Giftig (aA:giftigschädlich)→ nehme nicht freiwillig Gifte zu mir (fV: Gesundheit erhalten)

(1)→Gesundheitsschäden auf Dauer (fC: negative gesundheitliche Folgen ~~für Körper~~)→muss nicht noch zusätzlich sein→ muss auf Gesundheit achten(i~~f~~V: Gesundheit erhalten)~~→ weil ich eine angeschlagene Gesundheit habe→ das ist wie Dauergifteinnahme~~

~~(2)SPG in der Wohnung: geht auf die Lunge (fC: negative Folgen für Körper) Nein, im Essen brauche ich die nicht auch noch~~**Ende Leiter 1**

Leiter 2: ~~möchte ich nicht essen→~~ vergeht mir der Appetit ~~(fC: kein Appetit mehr→~~ Ekel (pC:Appetit/Ekel)**Ende Leiter 2**

Leiter 3: Steht nicht drauf, ob auf Dauer gesundheitsschädlich ist (fC: keine Information)→

(1) brauche Gewürze regelmäßig→denke, dass auf Dauer Auswirkungen (fC: negative gesundheitliche Folgen ~~für Körper~~von Dauer/Dosis abhängig) → länger gesund ~~belieben~~ bleiben, jeder sollte auf Gesundheit (i~~t~~V: Gesundheit erhalten)

→~~jeder sollte auf Gesundheit~~ achten (fV: Gesundheit erhalten)

(2) muss sowieso man Medikamente nehmen, haben Nebenwirkungen

(2) Wenn es drauf steht→kann jeder selbst entscheiden (pC: freie Entscheidung)→ möchte mich nicht einfach anschließen an alle anderen (*meaning: was alle anderen machen*)→muss schon drauf stehen-möchte keine Bedenken haben(~~fV~~pC:~~ möchte keine~~ Sorgen)→ Sicherheit brauche ich (tV: Sicherheit)~~)→ möchte jeden Tag essen→ besser ganz ohne~~**Ende Leiter 3**

Bestrahlung

1: müsste draufstehen, welche Bestrahlung, sonst würde ich es nicht nutzen

2: wenn gute Bestrahlung→ macht es frei von Pestiziden und SPG?

3:weiß nicht wie bestrahlt→ Angst, erste Gedanken sind Röntgenstrahlen=negativ

Leiter 1: Müsste drauf stehen→möchte wissen, wie bestrahlt (aA: ~~zu wenig~~keine Information)

(1)Gute Bestrahlung

(1a)→ keim tötend/Pilz tötend (fC: ~~Schädlinge bekämpfend~~Pflanzenschutz)

→wäre gut, dann(vielleicht) frei von Giftstoffen/Pestiziden(~~fC: frei von Giften~~aA:unschädlich)→ eher natürlich ~~natürlich gewachsen, ohne Geschmacksverstärker~~ (fC: Natürlichkeit)~~→ frei von Giftstoffen~~

→schmeckt wie's schmecken soll (fC: ~~richtiger~~ guter Geschmack)

(1a_1b)~~→~~

(1b)→ bin im Widerspruch: muss man erst spritzen und dann (deswegen) bestrahlen--> warum erst rein und dann wieder raus? (fC: kein Nutzen)

(~~1c~~b)schöne rote Tomaten (kA: ~~schönes~~ Aussehen ~~der Produkte~~)→ wäre (aber) nicht toll→ lieber naturgewachsen(~~fV~~pC: keine Natürlichkeit)→ haben dann keinen Geschmack mit Bestrahlung (~~aA~~fC: ~~keinen~~ Beeinträchtigung des Geschmacks)~~→ sollten nachdem schmecken, was ich esse (→ sonst könnte ich ja irgendwas essen→ möchte kein künstliches Aussehen/Geschmack (tV: natürlicher Geschmack(Aussehen) Natürlichkeit)~~Ende Leiter 1

~~(1a_2)→ bin im Widerspruch: muss man erst spritzen und dann (deswegen) bestrahlen--> warum erst rein und dann wieder raus? (pC: unnötig)~~

(2) Schlechte Bestrahlung→ Röntgenstrahlen→ unnatürlich, künstlich (aA: ~~nicht~~ unnatürlich)~~→ das Ding muss bestrahlt werden, dass es gut aussieht, oder gut schmeckt Aufzucht mit künstlichem Licht~~

Bestrahlung macht Angst (pC: Angst)→(möchte) einkaufen ohne schlechte Gedanken ~~(pC: Angst, Sorge)~~→steht alles drauf→ muss nicht lange suche→ nicht überlegen was die da rein machen→ kann regelmäßig kaufen, ohne nachzulesen(pC: ~~Einkaufen ohne~~keine Sorgen) →kaufe nix Schlechtes/ kann Kochen in Ruhe, ohne gesundheitliche Bedenken (pC: gesunde Ernährung)

~~(1) Wenn ich keine Brille mein Einkaufen dabei habe~~

Gutes Gefühl~~→ kaufe nix Schlechtes~~→ ~~kann Kochen in Ruhe, ohne gesundheitliche Bedenken~~→ Zufriedenheit (tV: Zufriedenheit)

[Notiz: Teilnehmerin hatte Herzinfarkt→ seitdem achtet sie beim Essen ganz besonders auf ihre Gesundheit]

Appendix D3 to D10 can be found on OnlinePlus at www.springer.com

Appendix D3: Implication Matrix Mycotoxins (Women)

Appendix D4: Implication Matrix Mycotoxins (Men)

Appendix D5: Implication Matrix Pesticides (Women)

Appendix D6: Implication Matrix Pesticidess (Men)

Appendix D7: Implication Matrix Irradiation (Women)

Appendix D8: Implication Matrix Irradiation (Men)

Appendix D9: Implication Matrix Irradiation Positive (Women)

Appendix D10: Implication Matrix Irradiation Positive (Men)

Appendix E: Results

Appendix E 1: Frequencies of Associations Related to Mycotoxins Spilt by Gender (Product A: Mycotoxins)

The following table presents the number of times a concept is mentioned and the related percentage of women and men who mention that concept in parentheses (Columns with the headings 'general associations', 'associations related to risk' and 'associations related to benefit). As the analysis of the first concepts mentioned ('top of mind' concepts) also focus on the role that emotions play, emotions are classified here under a separate category next to attributes, consequences and values.

Concepts are split according to elicitation task: the column 'general associations' presents the results of the content analysis of the mentioned concepts, when respondents were asked about their general associations, thoughts and feelings with regard to product *A (mycotoxins).* The columns 'associations related to risk' and 'associations related to benefits' present the results of the content analysis of the mentioned concepts, when respondents were asked what they considered when ratings the risks and rating the benefits of the product. The last column 'sum of all' outlines the results of the content analysis across the three elicitation tasks. Here, the results take into account that the same concept might be mentioned several times by an individual. In the last column, the percentages in parentheses outline the relative share of each concept against the total number of concepts that were mentioned.
As an example, four women and thus 14.3% of the women mention the concept 'bad feeling' when being asked about their general associations. Two women and thus 6.9% of the women mentiond that concept ('bad feeling'), when being asked what they considered during risk rating and one women and thus 3.7% of the women mentioned that concept ('bad feeling'), when being asked what they considered during benefit rating. In total the concept 'bad feeling' was mentioned seven times by women and constitutes 4.3% of the total number of mentioned concepts.

Mycoto-xins		General associa-tions		Associations related to risk		Associations related to benefit		Sum of all[3]	
		Women (N=28)	Men (N=32)	Women (N=29)	Men (N=33)	Women (N=27)	Men (N=32)	Women (N*=164)	Men (N*=184)
		N (%)	N (%)	N (%)	N (%)	N (%)	N (%)		
Emotions	Anger			1 (3.4)	1 (3.0)			1 (0.6)	1 (0.5)
	Anxiety				1 (3.0)				1 (0.5)
	Bad feeling	4 (14.3)	12 (37.5)	2 (6.9)	1 (3.0)	1 (3.7)		7 (4.3)	13 (7.1)
	Feeling of uncertainty[1]	1 (3.6)	4 (12.5)	1 (3.4)	2 (6.1)	1 (3.7)		3 (1.8)	6 (3.3)
	Worry	3 (10.7)		2 (6.9)				5 (3.0)	
Attribu-tes/Associ ations	Beneficial type of mycotoxins	1 (3.6)		2 (6.9)	3 (9.1)		1 (3.1)	3 (1.8)	4 (2.2)
	Conventio-nal produc-tion	1 (3.6)	3 (9.4)			1 (3.7)	1 (3.1)	2 (1.2)	4 (2.2)
	Comparison with other hazards			3 (10.3)	1 (3.0)			3 (1.8)	1 (0.5)

Mycoto-xins		General associa-tions		Associations related to risk		Associations related to benefit		Sum of all[3]	
		Women (N=28)	**Men (N=32)**	**Women (N=29)**	**Men (N=33)**	**Women (N=27)**	**Men (N=32)**	**Women (N*=164)**	**Men (N*=184)**
		N (%)	**N (%)**	**N (%)**	**N (%)**	**N (%)**	**N (%)**		
Attribu-tes/Associ ations	Disasters			1 (3.4)				1 (0.6)	
	Free of pesticides	3 (10.7)	4 (12.5)	1 (3.4)	2 (6.1)	2 (7.4)	1 (3.1)	6 (3.7)	7 (3.8)
	Harmful not (always)	1 (3.6)		1 (3.4)	4 (12.1)	1 (3.7)		3 (1.8)	4 (2.2)
	Harmful	11 (39.3)	10 (31.3)	11 (37.9)	11 (33.3)	1 (3.7)	1 (3.1)	23 (14.0)	22 (12.0)
	Labelling (no)		1 (3.1)						1 (0.5)
	Artificial (not)	2 (7.1)	1 (3.1)		1 (3.0)			2 (1.2)	2 (1.1)
	Artificial		1 (3.1)		1 (3.0)				2 (1.1)
	Visible			1 (3.4)					1 (0.5)
	Visible (not)			1 (3.4)				1 (0.6)	

Mycoto-xins		General associa-tions		Associations related to risk		Associations related to benefit		Sum of all[3]	
		Women (N=28)	Men (N=32)	Women (N=29)	Men (N=33)	Women (N=27)	Men (N=32)	Women (N*=164)	Men (N*=184)
		N (%)	N (%)	N (%)	N (%)	N (%)	N (%)		
Attribu-tes/Associ ations (cont.)	Producer's profit								
	Widespread	1 (3.6)						1 (0.6)	
Conse-quences	Benefit reduction due to mycotoxins					4 (14.8)	7 (21.9)	4 (2.4)	7 (3.8)
	Beneficial (not) when harmful					13 (48.1)	7 (21.9)	13 (7.9)	7 (3.8)
	Buy/Use[2]	1 (3.6)				1 (3.7)		2 (2.4)	
	Buy/Use (not)	6 (21.4)	6 (18.8)	6 (20.7)	7 (21.2)	4 (14.8)	5 (15.6)	16 (9.8)	18 (9.8)
	Contamina-tion of nature (no)		1 (3.1)						1 (0.5)

Mycotoxins		General associations		Associations related to risk		Associations related to benefit		Sum of all[3]	
		Women (N=28)	Men (N=32)	Women (N=29)	Men (N=33)	Women (N=27)	Men (N=32)	Women (N*=164)	Men (N*=184)
		N (%)	N (%)	N (%)	N (%)	N (%)	N (%)		
Consequences (cont.)	Consumer control				1 (3.0)				1 (0.5)
	Don't know					1 (3.7)	1 (3.1)	1 (0.6)	1 (0.5)
	Disgust	3 (10.7)	2 (6.3)		1 (3.0)	1 (3.7)		4 (2.4)	3 (1.6)
	Flavor					2 (7.4)	1 (3.1)	2 (1.2)	1 (0.5)
	Food control			2 (6.9)	2 (6.1)		1 (3.1)	2(1.2)	3 (1.6)
	Food quality	1 (3.6)	1 (3.1)	1 (3.4)		5 (18.5)	3 (9.4)	7 (4.3)	4 (2.2)
	Food quality (no)	3 (10.7)	4 (12.5)	3 (10.3)	5 (15.2)	2 (7.4)	3 (9.4)	8 (4.9)	12 (6.5)
	Freedom of choice					1 (3.7)		1 (0.6)	

Mycoto-xins		General associa-tions		Associations related to risk		Associations related to benefit		Sum of all[3]	
		Women (N=28)	Men (N=32)	Women (N=29)	Men (N=33)	Women (N=27)	Men (N=32)	Women (N*=164)	Men (N*=184)
		N (%)	N (%)	N (%)	N (%)	N (%)	N (%)		
Conse-quences	Freedom of choice (no)			1 (3.4)				1 (0.6)	
	Frequency /amount of use			1 (3.4)				1 (0.6)	
	Health risk	8 (28.6)	9 (28.1)	15 (51.7)	17 (51.5)	1 (3.7)	3 (9.4)	24 (14.6)	29 (15.8)
	Health risk (no)			1 (3.4)	2 (6.1)			1 (0.6)	2 (1.1)
	Health risk (family/ others)	1 (3.6)		3 (10.3)	3 (9.1)		1 (3.1)	4 (2.4)	4 (2.2)
	Healthy diet				1 (3.0)				1 (0.5)
	Information (no)	1 (3.6)		1 (3.4)	2 (6.1)	2 (7.4)	3 (9.4)	4 (2.4)	5 (2.7)
	Intake in human body	1 (3.6)	2 (6.3)	2 (6.9)	1 (3.0)			3 (1.8)	3 (1.6)
	Pleasure (no)				1 (3.0)		1 (3.1)		2 (1.1)

Mycotoxins		General associations		Associations related to risk		Associations related to benefit		Sum of all[3]	
		Women (N=28)	Men (N=32)	Women (N=29)	Men (N=33)	Women (N=27)	Men (N=32)	Women (N*=164)	Men (N*=184)
		N (%)	N (%)	N (%)	N (%)	N (%)	N (%)		
Consequences	Producer's profit				1 (3.0)				1 (0.5)
	Uncertainty			1 (3.4)	2 (6.1)		1 (3.1)	1 (0.6)	3 (1.6)
Values	Benevolence			1 (3.4)	1 (3.0)			1 (0.6)	1 (0.5)
	Long, healthy life (no)		1 (3.1)		1 (3.0)				2 (1.1)
	Preservation humanity			1 (3.4)				1 (0.6)	
	Responsibility producer (no)			1 (3.4)			1 (3.1)	1 (0.6)	1 (0.5)
	Social trust			1 (3.4)	2 (6.1)		1 (3.1)	1 (0.6)	3 (1.6)

N= Number of respondents that mentioned that concept; N*=Total number of mentioned concepts; [1]including feelings of irritation, unease, discomfort; [2]Often framed as 'buy when (really) necessary'; [3]Number of times each concept has been mentioned for all association tasks (general, risk and benefit together), taking into account that multiple mentions of one association per individal were counted.

Appendix E 2: Frequencies of Associations Related to Pesticides Spilt by Gender (Product B: Pesticides)

The following table presents the number of times a concept is mentioned and the related percentage of women and men who mention that concept in parentheses (Columns with the headings 'general associations', 'associations related to risk' and 'associations related to benefit). As the analysis of the first concepts mentioned ('top of mind' concepts) also focus on the role that emotions play, emotions are classified here under a separate category next to attributes, consequences and values.
Concepts are split according to elicitation task: the column 'general associations' presents the results of the content analysis of the mentioned concepts, when respondents were asked about their general associations, thoughts and feelings with regard to product **B (pesticides).** The columns 'associations related to risk' and 'associations related to benefits' present the results of the content analysis of the mentioned concepts, when respondents were asked what they considered when ratings the risks and rating the benefits of the product. The last column 'sum of all' outlines the results of the content analysis across the three elicitation tasks. Here, the results take into account that the same concept might be mentioned several times by an individual. In the last column, the percentages in parentheses outline the relative share of each concept against the total number of concepts that are mentioned.
As an example, four women and thus 14.3% of the women mention the concept 'bad feeling' when being asked about their general associations. Three women and 10.7% of the women mention that concept ('bad feeling'), when being asked what they considered during risk rating and one women and thus 3.6% of the women mention that concept ('bad feeling'), when being asked what they considered during benefit rating. In total the concept 'bad feeling' is mentioned eight times by women and constitutes 5.3% of the total number of mentioned concepts.

Pestici-des		General associations		Associations related to risk		Associations rela-ted to benefit		Sum of all[3]	
		Women (N=28)	Men (N=31)	Women (N=28)	Men (N=34)	Women (N=28)	Men (N=29)	Women (N*=152)	Men (N*=144)
		N (%)	N (%)	N (%)	N (%)	N (%)	N (%)		
Emoti-ons	Anger	2 (7.1)						2 (1.3)	
	Bad fee-ling	4 (14.3)	1 (3.2)	3 (10.7)	1 (2.9)	1 (3.6)		8 (5.3)	2 (1.4)
	Feeling of uncertain-ty[1]	1 (3.6)	1 (3.2)					1 (0.7)	1 (0.7)
	Worry	4 (14.3)	1 (3.2)					4 (2.6)	1 (0.7)
Attribu-tes/ Associa-tions	Compari-son with other hazards	3 (10.7)	3 (9.7)	2 (7.1)	7 (20.6)			5 (3.3)	10 (6.9)
	Conventi-onal pro-duction	1 (3.6)	2 (6.5)	2 (7.1)	1 (2.9)			3 (2.0)	3 (2.1)
	Disasters			1 (3.6)	2 (5.9)			1 (0.7)	2 (1.4)

Pestici-des		**General associations**		**Associations related to risk**		**Associations rela-ted to benefit**		**Summ of all[3]**	
		Women (N=28)	**Men (N=31)**	**Women (N=28)**	**Men (N=34)**	**Women (N=28)**	**Men (N=29)**	**Women (N*=152)**	**Men (N*=144)**
		N (%)	**N (%)**	**N (%)**	**N (%)**	**N (%)**	**N (%)**		
Attribu-tes/Asso ciations (cont.)	Free of mycoto-xins	3 (10.7)	1 (3.2)	1 (3.6)	2 (5.9)		2 (6.9)	4 (2.6)	5 (3.5)
	Harmful not (al-ways)					1 (3.6)		1 (0.7)	
	Harmful	5 (17.9)	7 (22.6)	14 (50.0)	11 (32.4)	1 (3.6)	1 (3.4)	20 (13.2)	19 (13.2)
	Labelling (no)			1 (3.6)				1 (0.7)	
	Natural types of pesticides						1 (3.4)		1 (0.7)
	Natural (not)	1 (3.6)	2 (6.5)	1 (3.6)	3 (8.8)	1 (3.6)	1 (3.4)	3 (2.0)	6 (4.2)
	Producer's profit			1 (3.6)	1 (2.9)	1 (3.6)		2 (1.3)	1 (0.7)

Pestici-des		General associations		Associations related to risk		Associations rela-ted to benefit		Summ of all[3]	
		Women (N=28)	Men (N=31)	Women (N=28)	Men (N=34)	Women (N=28)	Men (N=29)	Women (N*=152)	Men (N*=144)
		N (%)	N (%)	N (%)	N (%)	N (%)	N (%)		
Attribu-tes/Asso ciations	Wides-pread	3 (10.7)	1 (3.2)	2 (7.1)	1 (2.9)	1 (3.6)		6 (3.9)	2 (1.4)
Conse-quences	Benefit reduction due to pesticides					3 (10.7)	2 (6.9)	3 (2.0)	2 (1.4)
	Beneficial (not) when harmful					5 (17.9)	7 (24.1)	5 (3.3)	7 (4.9)
	Buy/Use[2]	2 (7.1)		1 (3.6)			3 (10.3)	3 (2.0)	3 (2.1)
	Buy/Use (not)	5 (17.9)	2 (6.5)	2 (7.1)	2 (5.9)	3 (10.7)	5 (17.2)	10 (6.6)	9 (6.3)
	Certainty (no)	1 (3.6)			2 (5.9)	1 (3.6)	1 (3.4)	2 (1.3)	3 (2.1)

Pestici-des		**General associa-tions**	**Associ-ations related to risk**	**Associa-tions related to benefit**	**Sum of all[3]**	**Pestici-des**		**General associa-tions**	**Associa-tions related to risk**
		Women (N=28)	**Men (N=31)**	**Women (N=28)**	**Men (N=34)**	**Women (N=28)**	**Men (N=29)**	**Women (N*=152)**	**Men (N*=144)**
		N (%)	**N (%)**	**N (%)**	**N (%)**	**N (%)**	**N (%)**		
Conse-quences (cont.)	Contami-nation of nature	2 (7.1)	1 (3.2)		1 (2.9)			2 (1.3)	2 (1.4)
	Deception		1 (3.2)		1 (2.9)				2 (1.4)
	'Don't know'						1 (3.4)		1 (0.7)
	Disgust		1 (3.2)		1 (2.9)				2 (1.4)
	Flavor					3 (10.7)		3 (2.0)	
	Food cont.	1 (3.6)		2 (7.1)			1 (3.4)	3 (2.0)	1 (0.7)
	Food quality	1 (3.6)	2 (6.5)	1 (3.6)	1 (2.9)	3 (10.7)	1 (3.4)	5 (3.3)	5 (3.5)
	Food quality (no)	1 (3.6)	1 (3.2)	2 (7.1)	2 (5.9)	3 (10.7)	1 (3.4)	6 (3.9)	4 (2.8)
	Freedom of choice			1 (3.6)				1 (0.7)	

Pestici-des		General associations		Associations related to risk		Associations related to benefit		Sum of all[3]	
		Women (N=28)	Men (N=31)	Women (N=28)	Men (N=34)	Women (N=28)	Men (N=29)	Women (N*=152)	Men (N*=144)
		N (%)	N (%)	N (%)	N (%)	N (%)	N (%)		
	Frequency of use				3 (8.8)				3 (2.1)
Conse-quences	Health risk (family)			1 (3.6)	2 (5.9)		1 (3.4)	1 (0.7)	3 (2.1)
	Information	1 (3.6)	1 (3.2)	2 (7.1)		1 (3.6)		4 (2.6)	1 (0.7)
	Information (no)			1 (3.6)		1 (3.6)	1 (3.4)	2 (1.3)	1 (0.7)
	Intake in human bod.	1 (3.6)	3 (9.7)	3 (10.7)	5 (14.7)			4 (2.6)	8 (5.6)
	Plant protec-tion	1 (3.6)	2 (6.5)	2 (7.1)	1 (2.9)	1 (3.6)	2 (6.9)	4 (2.6)	5 (3.5)
Values	Social trust	1 (3.6)		2 (7.1)	1 (2.9)			3 (2.0)	1 (0.7)
	Responsibi-lity prod.			1 (3.6)				1 (0.7)	

N= Number of respondents that mentioned that concept; N*=Total number of mentioned concepts ; [1]including feelings of irritation, unease, discomfort; [2]Often framed as 'buy when (really) necessary'; [3]Number of times each concept has been mentioned for all association tasks (general, risk and benefit together), taking into account that multiple mentions of one association per individual were counted.

Appendix E 3: Frequencies of Associations Spilt by Gender (Product C: Irradiation)

The following table presents the number of times a concept is mentioned and the related percentage of women and men who mention that concept in parentheses (Columns with the headings 'general associations', 'associations related to risk' and 'associations related to benefit). As the analysis of the first concepts mentioned ('top of mind' concepts) also focus on the role that emotions play, emotions are classified here under a separate category next to attributes, consequences and values.

Concepts are split according to elicitation task: the column 'general associations' presents the results of the content analysis of the mentioned concepts, when respondents were asked about their general associations, thoughts and feelings with regard to product **C (irradiation).** The columns 'associations related to risk' and 'associations related to benefits' present the results of the content analysis of the mentioned concepts, when respondents were asked what they considered when ratings the risks and rating the benefits of the product. The last column 'sum of all' outlines the results of the content analysis across the three elicitation tasks. Here, the results take into account that the same concept might be mentioned several times by an individual. In the last column, the percentages in parentheses outline the relative share of each concept against the total number of concepts that are mentioned.

As an example, five women and thus 16.7% of the women mention the concept 'bad feeling' when being asked about their general associations. Three women and 10.3% of the women mention that concept ('bad feeling'), when being asked what they considered during risk rating and no women mention that concept ('bad feeling'), when being asked what they considered during benefit rating. In total the concept 'bad feeling' is mentioned eight times by women and constitutes 4.4% of the total number of mentioned concepts.

Irradiation		**General associations**		**Associations related to risk**		**Associations related to benefit**		**Sum of all[4]**	
		Women (N=30)	**Men (N=34)**	**Women (N=29)**	**Men (N=33)**	**Women (N=23)**	**Men (N=30)**	**Women (N*=181**	**Men (N*=163)**
		N (%)	**N (%)**	**N (%)**	**N (%)**	**N (%)**	**N (%)**		
Emotions	Anger	1 (3.3)		1 (3.4)	1 (3.0)			2 (1.1)	1 (0.6)
	Anxiety	2 (6.7)					1 (3.3)	2 (1.1)	1 (0.6)
	Bad feeling	5 (16.7)	7 (20.6)	3 (10.3)				8 (4.4)	7 (4.3)
	Beneficial					1 (4.3)		1 (0.6)	
	Beneficial (not)	1 (3.3)						1 (0.6)	
	Controllable (not)								
	Good feeling		1 (2.9)					1 (0.6)	
	Feeling of uncertainty[1]	4 (13.3)	5 (14.7)	2 (6.9)		1 (4.3)		7 (3.9)	5 (3.1)
	Worry	4 (13.3)	4 (11.8)	1 (3.4)				5 (2.8)	4 (2.5)
	Worry (no)		1 (2.9)		1 (3.0)				2 (1.2)
Attributes/Associations	Comparison with other hazards	1 (3.3)	4 (11.8)	2 (6.9)			1 (3.3)	3 (1.7)	5 (3.1)

Irradiation		**General associations**		**Associations related to risk**		**Associations related to benefit**		**Sum of all[4]**	
		Women (N=30)	**Men (N=34)**	**Women (N=29)**	**Men (N=33)**	**Women (N=23)**	**Men (N=30)**	**Women (N*=181)**	**Men (N*=163)**
		N (%)	**N (%)**	**N (%)**	**N (%)**	**N (%)**	**N (%)**		
Attributes/Assoications (cont.)	Disasters	3 (10.0)	6 (17.6)	4 (13.8)	1 (3.0)			7 (3.9)	7 (4.3)
	Free of mycotoxins	3 (10.0)	3 (8.8)	1 (3.4)	3 (9.1)	3 (13.0)	4 (13.3)	7 (3.9)	10 (6.1)
	Free of pesticides	3 (10.0)	3 (8.8)	1 (3.4)		3 (13.0)	3 (10.0)	7 (3.9)	6 (3.7)
	Harmful	4 (13.3)	5 (14.7)	11 (37.9)	2 (6.1)	3 (13.0)		18 (9.9)	6 (3.7)
	Harmful not (always)	1 (3.3)	3 (8.8)	2 (6.9)	1 (3.0)		2 (6.7)	3 (1.7)	4 (2.5)
	Artificial	2 (6.7)	1 (2.9)	3 (10.3)			1 (3.3)	5 (2.8)	2 (1.2)
	Natural type of radiation	1 (3.3)		3 (10.3)		1 (4.3)		5 (2.8)	
	Organic				1 (3.0)				1 (0.6)
	Radioactive	6 (20.0)	5 (14.7)	3 (10.3)		1 (4.3)	1 (3.3)	10 (5.5)	6 (3.7)

Irradiation		General associations		Associations related to risk		Associations related to benefit		Sum of all[4]	
		Women (N=30)	Men (N=34)	Women (N=29)	Men (N=33)	Women (N=23)	Men (N=30)	Women (N*=181	Men (N*=163)
		N (%)	N (%)	N (%)	N (%)	N (%)	N (%)		
Attributes/Associations (cont.)	Roentgen	1 (3.3)		1 (3.4)				2 (1.1)	
	Ultraviolet		1 (2.9)						1 (0.6)
	Visible		1 (2.9)						1 (0.6)
	Visible (not)			1 (3.4)	2 (6.1)			1 (0.6)	2 (1.2)
	Widespread	1 (3.3)	3 (8.8)	2 (6.9)	2 (6.1)		2 (6.7)	3 (1.7)	7 (4.3)
Consequences	Benefit reduction due to irradiation				10 (30.3)	1 (4.3)	2 (6.7)	1 (0.6)	12 (7.4)
	Beneficial (not) when harmful				1 (3.0)	7 (30.4)	10 (33.3)	7 (3.9)	11 (6.7)
	Buy/Use[3]		1 (2.9)	1 (3.4)	1 (3.0)		1 (3.3)	1 (0.6)	3 (1.8)
	Buy/Use (not)	6 (20.0)	2 (5.9)	7 (24.1)	1 (3.0)	5 (21.7)	1 (3.3)	18 (9.9)	4 (2.5)
	Certainty (no)						1 (3.3)		1 (0.6)

Irradia-tion		**General associa-tions**		**Associations related to risk**		**Associations related to benefit**		**Sum of all[4]**	
		Women (N=30)	**Men (N=34)**	**Women (N=29)**	**Men (N=33)**	**Women (N=23)**	**Men (N=30)**	**Women (N*=181)**	**Men (N*=163)**
		N (%)	**N (%)**	**N (%)**	**N (%)**	**N (%)**	**N (%)**		
Conse-quences	Contaminati-on of nature	1 (3.3)						1 (0.6)	
	Consumer control (no)		1 (2.9)		1 (3.0)				2 (1.2)
	Deception				2 (6.1)		1 (3.3)		3 (1.8)
	'Don't know'			1 (3.4)		2 (8.7)	2 (6.7)	3 (1.7)	2 (1.2)
	Flavor					1 (4.3)	1 (3.3)	1 (0.6)	1 (0.6)
	Food control		1 (2.9)	1 (3.4)	2 (6.1)			1 (0.6)	3 (1.8)
	Food quality		5 (14.7)	2 (6.9)	2 (6.1)		2 (6.7)	2 (1.1)	9 (5.5)
	Food quality (no)		2 (5.9)	2 (6.9)	4 (12.1)	2 (8.7)	2 (6.7)	4 (2.2)	6 (3.7)
	Frequency & amount of use		1 (2.9)	1 (3.4)	1 (3.0)			1 (0.6)	2 (1.2)
	Health risk	7 (23.3)	5 (14.7)	7 (24.1)	1 (3.0)	3 (13.0)	1 (3.3)	17 (9.4)	7 (4.3)
	Health risk (no)			1 (3.4)			1 (3.3)	1 (0.6)	
	Health risk (family)				1 (3.0)				1 (0.6)

Irradiation		**General associations**		**Associations related to risk**		**Associations related to benefit**		**Sum of all[4]**	
		Women (N=30)	**Men (N=34)**	**Women (N=29)**	**Men (N=33)**	**Women (N=23)**	**Men (N=30)**	**Women (N*=181)**	**Men (N*=163)**
		N (%)	**N (%)**	**N (%)**	**N (%)**	**N (%)**	**N (%)**		
Consequences	Plant protect.	2 (6.7)			1 (3.0)			2 (1.1)	1 (0.6)
	Pleasure				1 (3.0)		1 (3.3)		2 (1.2)
	Pleasure (no)						1 (3.3)		1 (0.6)
	Producer's profit	1 (3.3)						1 (0.6)	
Values	Long, healthy life (no)	1 (3.3)		1 (3.4)				2 (1.1)	
	Preservation nature	1 (3.3)						1 (0.6)	
	Responsibility producer			1 (3.4)				1 (0.6)	
	Social trust		1 (2.9)						1 (0.6)

N= Number of respondents that mentioned that concept
N*=Total number of mentioned concepts
[1] including feelings of irritation, unease, discomfort; [2]microwave, mobile phone;; [3]Often framed as 'buy when (really) necessary'
[4]Number of times each concept has been mentioned for all association tasks (general, risk and benefit together), taking into account that multiple mentions of one association per individual were counted.

Appendix E 4: Ranking of the Most Important General Associations by Gender

The following table depicts the four most important concepts in descending order for each of the products and split according to gender, that are mentioned by the respondents when they were asked about their general associations, thoughts and feelings. This table is based on the results presented in the columns 'general associations' in Appendix E1, Appendix E2 and Appendix E3. Numbers in parentheses are percentages of women/men that mention a concept. For instance, 31.3% of men mention the concept 'harmful' as a general association with regard to mycotoxins, and the concept constitutes the second most important concept for men.

General 'top of mind' associations					
Mycotoxins		**Pesticides**		**Irradiation**	
Women	**Men**	**Women**	**Men**	**Women**	**Men**
1. Harmful (39.3)	1. Bad feeling (37.5)	1. Health risk (25)	1. Harmful (22.6)	1. No information (30)	1. No information (35.3)
2. Health risk (28.6)	2. Harmful (31.3)	2. Harmful (17.9)	2. Health risk (19.4)	2. Health risk (23.3)	2. Bad feeling (20.6)
3. Buy (not) (21.4)	3. Health risk (28.1)	2. Buy (not) (17.9)	3. Comparison with other hazards (9.7)	3. Radioactive (20)	3. Disasters (17.6)
4. Bad feeling (14.3)	4. Buy (not) (18.8)	3. Bad feeling (14.3)	3. Intake human body (9.7)	3. Buy (not) (20)	4. Feeling of uncertainty (14.7)
		3. Worry (14.3)	4.Conventional production (6.5)	4. Feeling of uncertainty (13.3)	4. Harmful (14.7)
		4. Comparison with other hazards (10.7)	4. Natural (not) (6.5)	4. Worry (13.3)	4. Radioactive (14.7)
		4. Widespread (10.7)	4. Buy (not) (6.5)		4. Food quality (14.7)
		4. Free of mycoto-xins (10.7)	4.Food quality (6.5)		4. Health risk (14.7)
			4.Plant prot. (6.5)		

Appendix E 5: Ranking of the Most Important Associations Related to Risk by Gender

The following table depicts the four most important concepts in descending order for each of the products and split according to gender, that are mentioned by the respondents when they were asked about what they considered when rating the risks. This table is based on the results presented in the columns 'associations related to risks' in Appendix E1, Appendix E2 and Appendix E3.

Numbers in parentheses are percentages of women/men that mention a concept. For instance, 51.5% of men mention the concept 'health risk' with regard to mycotoxins, and the concept constitutes the most important concept for men.

'Top of mind' associations related to risk					
Mycotoxins		**Pesticides**		**Irradiation**	
Women	**Men**	**Women**	**Men**	**Women**	**Men**
1. Health risk (51.7)	1. Health risk (51.5)	1. Harmful (50)	1. Health risk (41.2)	1. Harmful (37.9)	1. Benefit reduction due to irr. (30.3)
2.Harmful (37.9)	2. Harmful (33.3)	2. Health risk (32.1)	2. Harmful (32.4)	2. Buy (not) (24.1)	2. Food quality (no) (12.1)
3. Buy (not) (20.7)	3. Health risk (28.1)	3. Health risk (no) (17.9)	3. Comparison other hazards (20.6)	2. Health risk (24.1)	3. Free of mycoto-xins (9.1)
4. Comparison with hazards (10.3)	4. Buy (not) (21.2)	4. Consumer control (no) (14.3)	4. Intake human body (14.7)	2. No information (24.1)	3. Health risk (9.1)
4.Food quali-ty(no)(10.3)				3.Disasters (13.8)	4. Harmful (6.1)
4. Health risk (family) (10.3)				4. Bad feeling (10.3)	4. Visible (not) (6.1)
				4. Artificial (10.3)	4. Widespr. (6.1)
				4. Natural type of irradiation (10.3)	4. Deception (6.1)
				4. Radioactive (10.3)	4. Food control (6.1)
					4. Food quality (6.1)

Appendix E 6: Ranking of the Most Important Associations Related to Benefit by Gender

The following table depicts the three (due to a large amount of equally important concepts at rank 4, only the three most important concepts are depicted for irradiation) most important concepts in descending order for each of the products and split according to gender, that are mentioned by the respondents when they were asked about what they considered when rating the benefits. This table is based on the results presented in the columns 'associations related to benefits' in Appendix E1, Appendix E2 and Appendix E3.

Numbers in parentheses are percentages of women/men that mention a concept. For instance, 18.5% of women mention the concept 'food quality' with regard to mycotoxins, and the concept constitutes the second most important concept for women.

'Top of mind' associations related to benefit					
Mycotoxins		Pesticides		Irradiation	
Women	Men	Women	Men	Women	Men
1. Beneficial (not) when harmful (48.1)	1. Benefit reduction due to mycotoxins (21.9)	1. Beneficial (not) when harmful (17.9)	1. Beneficial (not) when harmful (24.1)	1. Beneficial (not) when harmful (30.4)	1. Beneficial (not) when harmful (33.3)
2. Food quality (18.5)	1. Beneficial (not) when harmful (21.9)	2. Benefit reduction due to pesticides (10.7)	2. Buy (not) (17.2)	2. Buy (not) (21.7)	2. Free of mycotoxins (13.3)
3. Benefit reduction due to mycotoxins (14.8)	2. Buy (not) (15.6)	3. Buy (not) (10.7)	3. Buy (10.3)	3. Free of mycotoxins (13.0)	3. Free of pesticides (10.0)
3. Buy (not) (14.8)	3. Food quality (no) (9.4)	3. Flavor (10.7)		3. Free of pesticides (13.0)	
	3. Free of pesticides (9.4)	3. Food quality (10.7)		3. Harmful (13.0)	
	3. Health risk (9.4)	3. Food quality (no) (10.7)		3. Health risk (13.0)	
	3. No information (9.4)				

Appendix E 7: Results of the Content Analysis for Mycotoxins (Negative Concepts)

The following table presents the results of the content analysis of the laddering interviews with regard to the **negative** ladders that are mentioned for mycotoxins and split by gender. The columns headed with N* present the number of times a concept is mentioned and the numbers in parentheses present the related share against the total number of mentioned concepts. Thus, results consider that some concepts were mentioned several times by the respondents.

The columns headed with N** present the number of women or men that mention a concept and the numbers in parentheses present the related percentage of women or men that mention that concept.

As an example, women mentioned the concept 'harmful' 52 times and this constitutes 7.4% of the total number of mentioned concepts (703). Moreover, 15 women and thus 51.7% of the women mentioned the concept 'harmful'.

Mycotoxins	**Women (N=29)**		**Men (N=26)**	
	N* **703**	**N** (%)**	**N*** **499**	**N** (%)**
Abstract attributes				
Artificial	3 (0.4)	1 (3.4)	1 (0.2)	2 (7.7)
Beneficial (not)			1 (0.2)	1 (3.8)
Harmful	52 (7.4)	15 (51.7)	42 (8.4)	13 (50.0)
Unlikely	2 (0.3)	2 (6.9)		
Visible	6 (0.9)	2 (6.9)	1 (0.2)	1 (3.8)
Visible (not)	12 (1.7)	2 (6.9)	1 (0.2)	1 (3.8)
Functional consequences				
Economic consequences	3 (0.4)	1 (3.4)		
Environmental contamination	3 (0.4)	1 (3.4)		
Food quality	29 (4.1)	14 (48.3)	20 (4.0)	11 (42.3)
Health risk	89 (12.7)	27 (93.1)	80 (16.0)	25 (96.2)
Health risk (family/others)	8 (1.1)	5 (17.2)	5 (1.0)	3 (11.5)

Intake in human body	8 (1.1)	5 (17.2)	16 (3.2)	6 (23.1)
No information	10 (1.4)	7 (24.1)	7 (1.4)	3 (11.5)
Plant protection			1 (0.2)	1 (3.8)
Psychosocial consequences				
Anger	4 (0.6)	3 (10.3)	2 (0.4)	2 (7.7)
Anxiety	8 (1.1)	6 (20.7)	5 (1.0)	3 (11.5)
Bad look	6 (0.9)	5 (17.2)	1 (0.2)	1 (3.8)
Burden to others	5 (0.7)	3 (10.3)	3 (0.6)	3 (11.5)
Certainty	1 (0.1)	1 (3.4)		
Certainty (no)	13 (1.8)	8 (27.6)	6 (1.2)	2 (7.7)
Change in mood	4 (0.6)	3 (10.3)	1 (0.2)	1 (3.8)
Consumer consciousness			1 (0.2)	1 (3.8)
Control by consumers	6 (0.9)	2 (6.9)	3 (0.6)	3 (11.5)
Control by consumers (no)			6 (1.2)	2 (7.7)
Deception	3 (0.4)	2 (6.9)	4 (0.8)	4 (15.4)
Disgust	9 (1.3)	6 (20.7)	7 (1.4)	7 (26.9)
Feeling of guilt	1 (0.1)	1 (3.4)		
Financial/time burden	18 (2.6)	10 (34.5)	3 (0.6)	3 (11.5)
Food control	2 (0.3)	2 (6.9)	6 (1.2)	3 (11.5)
Freedom of choice	12 (1.7)	8 (27.6)	7 (1.4)	5 (19.2)
Health (own)	61 (8.7)	17 (58.6)	42 (8.4)	24 (92.3)
Health (family/others)	8 (1.1)	4 (13.8)	10 (2.0)	6 (23.1)
Healthy diet	9 (1.3)	4 (13.8)	10 (2.0)	5 (19.2)
Human beauty	1 (0.1)	1 (3.4)		
Inspiration	3 (0.4)	3 (10.3)	1 (0.2)	1 (3.8)
Leisure/ education	10 (1.4)	7 (24.1)	8 (1.6)	4 (15.4)
Naturalness	1 (0.1)	1 (3.4)		
Performance	23 (3.3)	10 (34.5)	8 (1.6)	5 (19.2)
Pleasure	13 (1.8)	9 (31.0)	17 (3.4)	9 (34.6)
Producer’s profit	3 (0.4)	2 (6.9)	3 (0.6)	2 (7.7)

Product expectations	2 (0.3)	2 (6.9)	2 (0.4)	2 (7.7)
Regeneration	8 (1.1)	5 (17.2)		
Restriction disease	28 (4.0)	13 (44.8)	13 (2.6)	6 (23.1)
Shame	1 (0.1)	1 (3.4)		
Social contact	11 (1.6)	9 (31.0)	5 (1.0)	4 (15.4)
Social relationships	7 (1.0)	5 (17.2)		
Stigmatization	1 (0.1)	1 (3.4)	2 (0.4)	2 (7.7)
Subsistence	10 (1.4)	6 (20.7)	3 (0.6)	3 (11.5)
Success			1 (0.2)	1 (3.8)
Well-being (own)	34 (4.8)	18 (62.1)	9 (1.8)	11 (42.3)
Worry	6 (0.9)	4 (13.8)	3 (0.6)	1 (3.8)
Worry (no)	5 (0.7)	4 (13.8)	3 (0.6)	3 (11.5)
Instrumental values				
Benevolence	25 (3.6)	14 (48.3)	12 (2.4)	6 (23.1)
Honesty	2 (0.3)	2 (6.9)		
Justice	1 (0.1)	1 (3.4)	4 (0.8)	4 (15.4)
Social trust	1 (0.1)	1 (3.4)		
Responsibility (own)	1 (0.1)	1 (3.4)	2 (0.4)	2 (7.7)
Responsibility producer	3 (0.3)	3 (10.3)	3 (0.6)	2 (7.7)
Terminal values				
Hedonism	47 (6.7)	19 (65.5)	29 (5.8)	15 (57.7)
Long, healthy life	13 (1.8)	10 (34.5)	23 (4.6)	13 (50.0)
Preservation nature	1 (0.1)	1 (3.4)		
Preservation humanity	1 (0.1)	1 (3.4)	4 (0.8)	3 (11.5)
Security	4 (0.6)	4 (13.8)	6 (1.2)	6 (23.1)
Self-direction	15 (2.1)	11 (37.9)	8 (1.6)	6 (23.1)
Self-esteem	11 (1.6)	5 (17.2)	10 (2.0)	4 (15.4)
Self-fulfillment	6 (0.9)	6 (20.7)	15 (3.0)	8 (30.8)
Sense of belonging	2 (0.3)	2 (6.9)	3 (0.6)	2 (7.7)

Social recognition	4 (0.6)	4 (13.8)	2 (0.4)	2 (7.7)
Universalism	4 (0.6)	3 (10.3)	8 (1.6)	5 (19.2)
	703 (100)	**29 (100)**	**499 (100)**	**26 (100)**

N*= Number of times a concept has been mentioned at least once per respondent

N**= Number of respondents that mentioned that concept

Appendix E 8: Results of the Content Analysis for Mycotoxins (Positive Concepts)

The following table presents the results of the content analysis of the laddering interviews with regard to the **positive** ladders that are mentioned for mycotoxins and split by gender. The columns headed with N* present the number of times a concept is mentioned and the numbers in parentheses present the related share against the total number of mentioned concepts. Thus, results consider that some concepts are mentioned several times by the respondents.

The columns headed with N** present the number of women or men that mention a concept and the numbers in parentheses present the related percentage of women or men that mention that concept.

As an example, women mention the concept 'artificial (not)' 4 times and this constitutes 14.3% of the total number of positive concepts mentioned (28). Moreover, 2 women mention the concept 'artificial (not)' and this constitutes 50% of the women who mention positive concepts with regard to mycotoxins.

Mycotoxins	**Women (N=4)**		**Men (N=1)**	
Positive concepts	**N* 28**	**N** (%)**	**N* 3**	**N** (%)**
Attributes				
Artificial (not)	4 (14.3)	2 (50.0)		
Functional consequences				
Food quality	5 (17.9)	3 (75.0)		
Health risk (no)			1 (33.3)	1 (100)
Information	1 (3.6)	1 (25.0)		
Psychosocial consequences				
Control by consumers	1 (3.6)	1 (25.0)		
Health	2 (7.1)	1 (25.0)		
Naturalness	2 (7.1)	1 (25.0)	1 (33.3)	1 (100)
Pleasure			1 (33.3)	1 (100)
Well-being (own)	1 (3.6)	1 (25.0)		
Instrumental values				
Hedonism	2 (7.1)	2 (50.0)		

Responsibility (own)	1 (3.6)	1 (25.0)		
Responsibility producer	1 (3.6)	1 (25.0)		
Social trust	1 (3.6)	1 (25.0)		
Terminal values				
Preservation nature	2 (7.1)	1 (25.0)		
Preservation humanity	1 (3.6)	1 (25.0)		
Self-direction	2 (7.1)	2 (50.0)		
Self-esteem	2 (7.1)	1 (25.0)		
	28 **(100)**	**4** **(100)**	**3** **(100)**	**1** **(100)**

N*= Number of times a concept has been mentioned at least once per respondent

N**= Number of respondents that mentioned that concept

4 of 4 women also elicited negative ladders, but one men only elicited positive ladders.

Appendix E 9: Results of the Content Analysis for Pesticides (Negative Concepts)

The following table presents the results of the content analysis of the laddering interviews with regard to the **negative** ladders mentioned for pesticides and split by gender. The columns headed with N* present the number of times a concept is mentioned and the numbers in parentheses present the related share against the total number of mentioned concepts. Thus, results consider that some concepts are mentioned several times by the respondents. The columns headed with N** present the number of women or men that mention a concept and the numbers in parentheses present the related percentage of women and men that mention that concept.

As an example, the concept 'artificial' is mentioned 29 times and this constitutes 4.5% of the total number of negative concepts mentioned (640).

Moreover, 8 women and thus 28.6% of the women mention the concept 'artificial'.

Pesticides	**Women (N=28)**		**Men (N=33)**	
	N* **640**	**N** (%)**	**N*** **855**	**N** (%)**
Attributes				
Artificial	29 (4.5)	8 (28.6)	20 (2.3)	7 (21.2)
Beneficial	3 (0.5)	2 (7.1)		
Beneficial (not)	14 (2.2)	8 (28.6)	8 (0.9)	5 (15.2)
Harmful	43 (6.7)	12 (42.9)	65 (7.6)	18 (54.5)
No labeling	3(0.5)	3 (10.7)		
Functional consequences				
Economic consequences	1 (0.2)	1 (3.6)	4 (0.5)	3 (9.1)
Environmental contamination	7 (1.1)	5 (17.9)	11 (1.3)	4 (12.1)
Food quality	14 (2.2)	8 (28.6)	21 (2.5)	11 (33.3)
Food control	1 (0.2)	1 (3.6)	4 (0.5)	3 (9.1)
Health risk	78 (12.2)	27 (96.4)	100 (11.7)	33 (100.0)
Health risk (family/others)	2 (0.3)	2 (7.1)	13 (1.5)	4 (12.1)

Intake in human body	21 (3.3)	5 (17.9)	19 (2.2)	10 (30.3)
Plant protection	18 (2.8)	6 (21.4)	8 (0.9)	5 (15.2)
Spreading in nature	11 (1.7)	6 (21.4)	14 (1.6)	7 (21.2)
Psychosocial consequences				
Anger	4 (0.6)	4 (14.3)	5 (0.6)	3 (9.1)
Anxiety	10 (1.6)	4 (14.3)	10 (1.2)	3 (9.1)
Bad look	2 (0.3)	2 (7.1)	6 (0.7)	2 (6.1)
Burden to others	2 (0.3)	2 (7.1)	7 (0.8)	5 (15.2)
Certainty	4 (0.6)	4 (14.3)	2 (0.2)	1 (3.0)
Certainty (no)	14 (2.2)	10 (35.7)	16 (1.9)	12 (36.4)
Change in mood	4 (0.6)	3 (10.7)	3 (0.4)	2 (6.1)
Consumer consciousness	3 (0.5)	1 (3.6)	1 (0.1)	1 (3.0)
Control by consumers	5 (0.8)	3 (10.7)	2 (0.2)	2 (6.1)
Control by consumers (no)	9 (1.4)	5 (17.9)	5 (0.6)	4 (12.1)
Deception	3 (0.5)	3 (10.7)	10 (1.2)	6 (18.2)
Disgust			1 (0.1)	1 (3.0)
Feeling of guilt			3 (0.4)	2 (6.1)
Financial/time burden	2 (0.3)	2 (7.1)	23 (2.7)	13 (39.4)
Freedom of choice	23 (3.6)	14 (50.0)	11 (1.3)	8 (24.2)
Health (own)	33 (5.2)	20 (71.4)	67 (7.8)	22 (66.7)
Health (family/others)	10 (1.6)	6 (21.4)	10 (1.2)	5 (15.2)
Healthy diet	9 (1.4)	6(21.4)	9 (1.1)	6 (18.2)
Human beauty	4 (0.6)	1 (3.6)	1 (0.1)	1 (3.0)
Inspiration			3 (0.4)	3 (9.1)
Leisure/ education	6 (0.9)	5 (17.9)	16 (1.9)	10 (30.3)
Naturalness	13 (2.0)	6 (21.4)	15 (1.8)	6 (18.2)
Performance	10 (1.6)	5 (17.9)	16 (1.9)	11 (33.3)
Pleasure	13 (2.0)	10 (35.7)	24 (2.8)	12 (36.4)
Producer's profit	7 (1.1)	4 (14.3)	10 (1.2)	6 (18.2)
Product expectations	2 (0.3)	2 (7.1)		
Regeneration	1 (0.2)	1 (3.6)	7 (0.8)	3 (9.1)
Restriction disease	16 (2.5)	8 (28.6)	14 (1.6)	10 (30.3)

Shame	1 (0.1)	1 (3.6)	1 (0.1)	1 (3.0)
Social contact	3 (0.5)	3 (10.7)	10 (1.2)	7 (21.2)
Social relationships	3 (0.5)	3 (10.7)	1 (0.1)	1 (3.0)
Subsistence	5 (0.8)	4 (14.3)	2 (0.2)	3 (9.1)
Well-being (own)	19 (2.8)	12 (42.9)	23 (2.7)	16 (48.5)
Worry	6 (0.9)	4 (14.3)	7 (0.8)	4 (12.1)
Worry (no)	5 (0.7)	3 (10.7)	8 (0.9)	5 (15.2)
Instrumental values				
Benevolence	11 (1.7)	7 (25.0)	29 (3.4)	7 (21.2)
Honesty	3 (0.5)	2 (7.1)	1 (0.1)	1 (3.0)
Justice	4 (0.6)	5 (10.7)	12 (1.4)	8 (24.2)
Social trust	3 (0.5)	2 (7.1)	5 (0.6)	5 (15.2)
Responsibility (own)	6 (0.9)	5 (17.9)		
Responsibility producer	4 (0.6)	3 (10.7)	5 (0.6)	4 (12.1)
Terminal values				
Hedonism	40 (6.3)	21 (75.0)	45 (5.3)	20 (60.6)
Long, healthy life	13 (2.0)	9 (32.1)	23 (2.7)	17 (51.5)
Preservation nature	13 (2.0)	8 (28.6)	8 (0.9)	5 (15.2)
Preservation humanity	5 (0.8)	4 (14.3)	4 (0.5)	3 (9.1)
Security	3 (0.5)	3 (10.7)	9 (1.1)	6 (18.2)
Self-direction	12 (1.9)	8 (28.6)	19 (2.2)	13 (39.4)
Self-esteem	4 (0.6)	4 (14.3)	15 (1.8)	7 (21.2)
Self-fulfillment	3 (0.5)	3 (10.7)	11 (1.3)	6 (18.2)
Social recognition	2 (0.3)	1 (3.6)	6 (0.7)	3 (9.1)
Universalism	4 (0.6)	3 (10.7)	6 (0.7)	4 (12.1)
	640 (100)	**28 (100)**	**855 (100)**	**33 (100)**

N*= Number of times (and percent of the total number of concepts) a concept has been mentioned at least once per respondent

N**= Number of respondents that mentioned that concept

Appendix E 10: Results of the Content Analysis for Pesticides (Positive Codes)

The following table presents the results of the content analysis of the laddering interviews with regard to the **positive** ladders that are mentioned for pesticides and split by gender. The columns headed with N* present the number of times a concept is mentioned and the numbers in parentheses present the related share against the total number of mentioned concepts. Thus, results consider that some concepts are mentioned several times by the respondents.

The columns headed with N** present the number of women or men that mention a concept and the numbers in parentheses present the related percentage of women or men that mention that concept.

As an example, women mention the concept 'food quality' 13 times and this constitutes 28.9% of the total number of positive concepts mentioned (45). Moreover, 2 women mention the concept 'food quality' and this constitutes 33.3% of the women who mention positive concepts with regard to pesticides.

Pesticides	**Women (N=6)**		**Men (N=4)**	
Positive concepts	**N* 45**	**N** (%)**	**N* 13**	**N** (%)**
Attributes				
Beneficial	1 (2.2)	1 (16.7)	1 (7.7)	1 (25.0)
Harmful (not)	2 (4.4)	1 (16.7)		
Functional consequences				
Economic consequences	1 (2.2)	1 (16.7)		
Food quality	13 (28.9)	2 (33.3)	1 (7.7)	1 (25.0)
Health risk (no)	2 (4.4)	2 (33.3)	1 (7.7)	1 (25.0)
Plant protection			2 (15.4)	2 (50.0)
Spreading in nature			1 (7.7)	1 (25.0)
Psychosocial consequences				
Change in mood	1 (2.2)	1 (16.7)		
Disgust			1 (7.7)	1 (25.0)
Health (own)	4 (8.9)	2 (33.3)		
Leisure/education	3 (6.7)	1 (16.7)	1 (7.7)	1 (25.0)

Performance	2 (4.4)	1 (16.7)	1 (7.7)	1 (25.0)
Well-being (own)	6 (13.3)	1 (16.7)		
Instrumental values				
Benevolence	1 (2.2)	1 (16.7)		
Hedonism	6 (13.3)	2 (33.3)	2 (15.4)	2 (50.0)
Social trust	1 (2.2)	1 (16.7)		
Terminal values				
Long, healthy life	1 (2.2)	1 (16.7)		
Self-direction	1 (2.2)	1 (16.7)		
Self-esteem	1 (2.2)	1 (16.7)		
Self-fulfillment	1 (2.2)	1 (16.7)		
	45 (100)	**6 (100)**	**13 (100)**	**4 (100)**

N*= Number of times a concept has been mentioned at least once per respondent

N**= Number of respondents that mentioned that concept

6 of 6 women and 4 of 4 men also elicited negative ladders.

Appendix E 11: Results of the Content Analysis for Irradiation (Negative Concepts)

The following table presents the results of the content analysis of the laddering interviews with regard to the **negative** ladders mentioned for irradiation and split by gender. The columns headed with N* present the number of times a concept is mentioned and the numbers in parentheses present the related share against the total number of mentioned concepts. Thus, results consider that some concepts are mentioned several times by the respondents.

The columns headed with N** present the number of women or men that mention a concept and the numbers in parentheses present the related percentage of women or men that mention that concept.

As an example, women mention the concept 'artificial' 14 times and this constitutes 2.5% of the total number of negative concepts mentioned (568). Moreover, 6 women mention the concept 'artificial' and this constitutes 20% of the women.

Irradiation	**Women (N=30)**		**Men (N=29)**	
	N*	**N** (%)**	**N***	**N** (%)**
Attributes				
Artificial	14 (2.5)	6 (20.0)	4 (0.8)	4 (13.8)
Beneficial (not)	7 (1.2)	6 (20.0)	8 (1.7)	6 (20.7)
Harmful	21 (3.7)	8 (26.7)	8 (1.7)	5 (17.2)
Irreversible	1 (0.2)	1 (3.3)	2 (0.4)	2 (6.9)
Radioactive	8 (1.4)	4 (13.3)	17 (3.6)	6 (20.7)
Roentgen	4 (0.7)	3 (10.0)	4 (0.8)	2 (6.9)
Visible (not)	8 (1.4)	4 (13.3)	7 (1.5)	4 (13.8)
Functional consequences				
Environmental contamination	5 (0.9)	4 (13.3)	4 (0.8)	2 (6.9)
Food control			12 (2.5)	4 (13.8)
Food quality	21 (3.7)	12 (40.0)	21 (4.4)	12 (41.4)
Food security (no)	2 (0.4)	1 (3.3)		
Health risk	66 (11.6)	24 (80.0)	60 (12.7)	21 (72.4)
Health risk (family/others)	6 (1.1)	5 (16.7)	8 (1.7)	5 (17.2)
Intake in human body	9 (1.6)	5 (16.7)	9 (1.9)	6 (20.7)

No information	27 (4.8)	13 (43.3)	32 (6.8)	14 (48.3)
Plant protection	2 (0.4)	2 (6.7)	3 (0.6)	2 (6.9)
Spreading in nature	2 (0.4)	2 (6.7)	12 (2.5)	5 (17.2)
Psychosocial consequences				
Anger	2 (0.4)	1 (3.3)		
Anxiety	11 (1.9)	7 (23.3)	5 (1.1)	4 (13.8)
Bad look	6 (1.1)	2 (6.7)	1 (0.2)	1 (3.4)
Burden to others	4 (0.7)	3 (10.0)	1 (0.2)	1 (3.4)
Certainty	3 (0.5)	2 (6.7)	4 (0.8)	2 (6.9)
Certainty (no)	23 (4.0)	10 (33.3)	24 (4.7)	13 (44.8)
Change in mood	4 (0.7)	3 (10.0)	2 (0.4)	2 (6.9)
Control by consumers	8 (1.4)	4 (13.3)	7 (1.4)	4 (13.8)
Control by consumers (no)	1 (0.2)	1 (3.3)	3 (0.6)	3 (10.3)
Deception			6 (1.2)	5 (17.2)
Feeling of guilt	1 (0.2)	1 (3.3)	1 (0.2)	1 (3.4)
Financial/time burden	5 (0.9)	5 (16.7)	2 (0.4)	2 (6.9)
Freedom of choice	18 (3.2)	9 (30.0)	23 (4.5)	13 (44.8)
Health (own)	35 (6.2)	17 (56.7)	37 (7.3)	13 (44.8)
Health (family/others)	8 (1.4)	3 (10.0)	4 (0.8)	4 (13.8)
Healthy diet	7 (1.2)	4 (13.3)	5 (1.0)	3 (10.3)
Inspiration	1 (0.2)	1 (3.3)		
Leisure/ education	9 (1.6)	8 (26.7)	4 (0.8)	2 (6.9)
Naturalness	4 (0.7)	4 (13.3)	7 (1.4)	4 (13.8)
Performance	7 (1.2)	4 (13.3)	6 (1.2)	6 (20.7)
Pleasure	5 (0.9)	5 (16.7)	12 (2.4)	8 (27.6)
Producer's profit	4 (0.7)	2 (6.7)	3 (0.6)	3 (10.3)
Product expectations			2 (0.4)	2 (6.9)
Regeneration	4 (0.7)	1 (3.3)	1 (0.2)	1 (3.4)
Restriction disease	17 (3.0)	10 (33.3)	11 (2.2)	10 (34.5)
Social contact	4 (0.7)	2 (6.7)	2 (0.4)	2 (6.9)
Social relationships			1 (0.2)	1 (3.4)

Stigmatization	5 (0.9)	2 (6.7)		
Subsistence	4 (0.7)	4 (13.3)	5 (1.0)	4 (13.8)
Success	2 (0.4)	1 (3.3)	1 (0.2)	1 (3.4)
Well-being (own)	17 (3.0)	7 (23.3)	11 (2.2)	9 (31.0)
Worry	11 (1.9)	9 (30.0)	4 (0.8)	4 (13.8)
Worry (no)	10 (1.8)	4 (13.3)	3 (0.6)	3 (10.3)
Instrumental values				
Benevolence	18 (3.2)	12 (40.0)	11 (2.2)	8 (27.6)
Justice	2 (0.4)	2 (6.7)	3 (0.6)	3 (10.3)
Social trust			2 (0.4)	2 (6.9)
Responsibility (own)	3 (0.5)	3 (10.0)	3 (0.6)	3 (10.3)
Responsibility producer	3 (0.5)	3 (10.0)	1 (0.2)	1 (3.4)
Terminal values				
Hedonism	32 (5.6)	16 (53.3)	28 (5.5)	13 (44.8)
Long, healthy life	14 (2.5)	10 (33.3)	14 (2.7)	12 (41.4)
Preservation nature	6 (1.1)	3 (10.0)	3 (0.6)	1 (3.4)
Preservation humanity	1 (0.2)	1 (3.3)	6 (1.2)	6 (20.7)
Security	5 (0.9)	4 (13.3)	6 (1.2)	5 (17.2)
Self-direction	19 (3.3)	13 (43.4)	11 (2.2)	8 (27.6)
Self-esteem	8 (1.4)	6 (20.0)	2 (0.4)	2 (6.9)
Self-fulfillment	5 (0.9)	5 (16.7)	7 (1.4)	5 (17.2)
Sense of belonging	1 (0.2)	1 (3.3)	1 (0.2)	1 (3.4)
Social recognition	2 (0.4)	2 (6.7)	1 (0.2)	1 (3.4)
Universalism	6 (1.1)	2 (6.7)	2 (0.4)	1 (3.4)
	568 (100)		**510 (100)**	

N*= Number of times a concept has been mentioned at least once per respondent

N**= Number of respondents that mentioned that concept

Appendix E 12: Results of the Content Analysis for Irradiation (Positive Concepts)

The following table presents the results of the content analysis of the laddering interviews with regard to the **positive** ladders mentioned for irradiation and split by gender. The columns headed with N* present the number of times a concept is mentioned and the numbers in parentheses present the related share against the total number of mentioned concepts. Thus, results consider that some concepts are mentioned several times by the respondents.

The columns headed with N** present the number of women or men that mention a concept and the numbers in parentheses present the related percentage of women or men that mention that concept.

As an example, women mention the concept 'artificial (not)' 6 times and this constitutes 11.3% of the total number of positive concepts mentioned (53). Moreover, 5 women mention the concept 'artificial (not)' and this constitutes 45.5% of the women who mention positive concepts with regard to irradiation.

Irradiation	**Women (N=11)**		**Men (N=11)**	
Positive concepts	**N* 53**	**N** (%)**	**N* 123**	**N** (%)**
Attributes				
Artificial (not)	6 (11.3)	5 (45.5)	3 (2.4)	3 (27.3)
Beneficial	2 (3.8)	2 (18.2)	7 (5.7)	3 (27.3)
Harmful (not)	7 (13.2)	3 (27.3)	5 (4.1)	4 (36.4)
Functional consequences				
Economic consequences			2 (1.6)	1 (9.1)
Environmental contamination			1 (0.8)	1 (9.1)
Food quality	5 (9.4)	3 (27.3)	15 (12.2)	5 (45.5)
Food security	3 (5.7)	1 (9.1)		
Health risk	5 (9.4)	4 (36.4)	14 (11.4)	6 (54.5)
Health risk (family/others) (no)			1 (0.8)	1 (9.1)
Intake in human body			4 (3.3)	2 (18.2)
No information			3 (2.4)	

Plant protection	6 (11.3)	4 (36.4)	7 (5.7)	3 (27.3)
Spreading in nature	1 (1.9)	1 (9.1)	1 (0.8)	1 (9.1)
Psychosocial consequences				
Anger (no)			1 (0.8)	1 (9.1)
Bad look			1 (0.8)	1 (9.1)
Burden to others	1 (1.9)	1 (9.1)	1 (0.8)	1 (9.1)
Change in mood			1 (0.8)	1 (9.1)
Deception			1 (0.8)	1 (9.1)
Disgust			2 (1.6)	2 (18.2)
Financial/time burden			2 (1.6)	2 (18.2)
Freedom of choice	1 (1.9)	1 (9.1)	1 (0.8)	1 (9.1)
Health (own)	1 (1.9)	1 (9.1)	2 (1.6)	2 (18.2)
Healthy diet	2 (3.8)	1 (9.1)	1 (0.8)	1 (9.1)
Human beauty			1 (0.8)	1 (9.1)
Leisure/ education			2 (1.6)	2 (18.2)
Naturalness	1 (1.9)	1 (9.1)	1 (0.8)	1 (9.1)
Performance			2 (1.6)	1 (9.1)
Pleasure	1 (1.9)	1 (9.1)	2 (1.6)	2 (18.2)
Product expectations			1 (0.8)	1 (9.1)
Restriction disease			3 (2.4)	2 (18.2)
Social contact			2 (1.6)	1 (9.1)
Subsistence			1 (0.8)	1 (9.1)
Success			1 (0.8)	1 (9.1)
Well-being (own)			9 (7.3)	5 (45.5)
Worry (no)	1 (1.9)	1 (9.1)	2 (1.6)	2 (18.2)
Instrumental values				
Benevolence			2 (1.6)	2 (18.2)
Hedonism	1 (1.9)	1 (9.1)	6 (4.9)	5 (45.5)
Justice	2 (3.8)	1 (9.1)	2 (1.6)	2 (18.2)

Terminal values				
Long, healthy life	2 (3.8)	1 (9.1)	1 (0.8)	1 (9.1)
Preservation nature			1 (0.8)	1 (9.1)
Preservation humanity	1 (1.9)	1 (9.1)	3 (2.4)	2 (18.2)
Security			2 (1.6)	2 (18.2)
Self-direction	2 (3.8)	2 (18.2)		
Self-esteem			2 (1.6)	1 (9.1)
Social recognition			1 (0.8)	1 (9.1)
Universalism	2 (3.8)	1 (9.1)		
	53 (100)		**123 (100)**	

N*= Number of times a concept has been mentioned at least once per respondent

N**= Number of respondents that mentioned that concept

10 of 11 women and 9 of 11 men also elicited negative ladders.

Appendix F: Strength of Relations between Concepts in the HVMs with the Percentage of Repondents That Mentioned a Relation and the Related Number of Times a Relation is Mentioned.

A relation between two concepts that was mentioned by less than 15% of women and men is presented as a thin arrow in the HVMs. Taking the example of mycotoxins, this means that a thin arrow is a relation that was mentioned by three or four women and by three men, but not less than three women and men due to selected cut-off levels. Moreover, a relation between two concepts that was mentioned by greater equal 15% and less than 35% of women and men is represented as a medium arrow in the HVMs.

Appendix F1: Strength of Relations in HVMs and the Number of Times a Relation is Mentioned (Mycotoxins)

Mycotoxins	**Women (N=29)**	**Men (N=26)**
% of respondents mentioning a relation	**Number of times a relation is mentioned**	**Number of times a relation is mentioned**
<15% (thin arrow)	3, 4	3
≥15% and<35% (medium arrow)	5-9	4-8
≥35% (thick arrow)	10-19	9-15

Appendix F2: Strength of Relations in HVM and Number of Times a Relation is Mentioned (Pesticides)

Pesticides	**Women (N=28)**	**Men (N=33)**
% of respondents mentioning a relation	**Number of times a relation is mentioned**	**Number of times a relation is mentioned**
<15% (thin arrow)	3, 4	3, 4
≥15% and <35% (medium arrow)	5-9	5-11
≥35% (thick arrow)	10-16	12-18

Appendix F3: Strength of Relations in HVM and Number of Times a Relation is Mentioned (Irradiation)

Irradiation	**Women (N=28)**	**Men (N=33)**
% of respondents mentioning a relation	**Number of times a relation is mentioned**	**Number of times a relation is mentioned**
<15% (thin arrow)	2-4	2-4
≥15% and <35% (medium arrow)	5-10	5-9
≥35% (thick arrow)	11, 12	10, 11